The Actions and Uses of Ophthalmic Drugs

Third Edition

by
P. H. O'Connor Davies, FBCO, FBOA HD, DCLP, DOrth, MPS
Formerly Associate Lecturer, Department of Optometry, and
Visiting Lecturer, Welsh School of Pharmacy,
University of Wales Institute of Science and Technology

Third edition revised by
G. A. Hopkins, BPharm, PhD, MRPharm, S
Ophthalmic Manager, Smith & Nephew Pharmaceuticals Ltd, Romford

Optometric Adviser
R. M. Pearson, MPhil, FBOA HD, FBCO, DCLP, DOrth
Senior Lecturer, Department of Optometry and Visual Science,
The City University, London

Butterworths

London   Boston   Singapore   Sydney   Toronto   Wellington

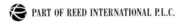
PART OF REED INTERNATIONAL P.L.C.

First published 1989

© Butterworth & Co. (Publishers) Ltd, 1989

British Library Cataloguing in Publication Data
Davies, P. H. O'Connor (Patrick Henry O'Connor), 1922–
    The actions and uses of ophthalmic drugs. – 3rd ed.
    1. Man. Eyes. Effects of drugs
    I. Title II. Hopkins, G. A. III. Pearson, R. M.
    (Richard M.)
    615′.7

    ISBN 0–407–00799–7

Library of Congress Cataloging in Publication Data
Davies, P. H. O'Connor (Patrick Henry O'Connor), 1922–
    The actions and uses of ophthalmic drugs / P. H. O'Connor Davies,
    G. A. Hopkins, R. M. Pearson, — 3rd ed.
        p.   cm
        Includes bibliographies and index.
        ISBN 0–407–00799–7:
        1. Ophthalmic drugs.   I. Hopkins, G. A.   II. Pearson, R. M.
    (Richard M.) III. Title.
        [DNLM: 1. Eye Diseases—drug therapy. 2. Ophthalmic Solutions–
    –pharmacology. WW 166 D257a]
    RE994.D38   1989
    617.7′061—dc20
    DNLM/DLC
    for Library of Congress   89–15840
                                                                   CIP

Photoset by Tec-Set Ltd, Wallington, Surrey
Printed and bound in Great Britain by Butler and Tanner, Frome, Somerset
This book is printed on acid-free paper

Foreword

It was with great sadness that, during the closing stages of the preparation of this book, we learnt of the death of Paddy O'Connor-Davies, who was for many years associate lecturer at the Department of Optometry, University of Wales Institute of Science and Technology.

In 1972 Paddy wrote the first edition of **The Actions and Uses of Opthalmic Drugs**, and although he decided to involve other people in the production of the third edition of this book, he has been constantly involved with its progress and his help, encouragement and enthusiasm made an initially daunting task very much easier. Only someone of Paddy's stature would have considered writing such an important and well-needed text book and the profession of optometry will miss his input in the various discussions about the use of drugs by optometrists. We are lucky that he has put some of his wealth of knowledge on paper for us and I hope that this book, along with the previous two editions, will serve as an appropriate memorial to the name of P. H. O'Connor-Davies, FBCO, FBOA, HD, DCLP, DOrth, MPS

G A Hopkins, BPharm, PhD, MRPharm, S

Since it was first published in 1972 *The Action and Uses of Ophthalmic Drugs* has become established as the standard textbook in ophthalmic drugs for all who practise optometry. The Third Edition will further enhance this status: the new and revised material is extensive and has been very effectively incorporated into the main body of the text by two experienced and skilful writers. The collaboration between pharmacologist and optometrist has produced a work which gives a sound theoretical basis for the application of drugs, and emphasis on care and discrimination in the use of drugs and, particularly welcome, guidance on many key practical issues such as, for example, the use of mydriatic and miotic agents.

The new Edition thus takes account of the significant and inexorable developments which have taken place in pharmaceutical science and optometric practice over the last decade: a comprehensive survey is given of recent contact lens preparations; there is a concise outline of developments in drugs used by ophthalmologists that are relevant to optometry; a splendid review of ocular adverse reactions to systemic and topical medications will greatly assist the optometrist in the detection, management and reporting of these conditions; readers will be introduced to the principles of the use of therapeutic drugs, now already a feature of optometric practice in many parts of the USA. The above are just a few examples of the topics which have undergone signicant revision: I could cite many more.

The initiative and enthusiasm for the subject demonstrated by the late Paddy O'Connor Davies in earlier editions remains evident in this revised text. The Third Edition consolidates the book's reputation as a standard reference text and represents essential reading for optometry students, pre-registration students and registered practitioners.

Bernard Gilmartin BSc, PhD, FBCO
Lecturer in Ophthalmic Drugs, Aston University
Chief Examiner in Ophthalmic Drugs for the British College of Optometrists

Preface to the third edition

The optometrist has always had a responsibility to himself and his patients to keep his knowledge up to date. This is particularly true today in the light of his changing role in eye care. He is called upon to have an increasing depth of knowledge in the areas of his expertise. This is particularly true in the area of drugs, where pharmaceutical products used by ophthalmologists and general practitioners influence his finding during examination.

It is with this situation in mind that I was particularly pleased to be invited to contribute to the third edition of Paddy O'Connor Davies' textbook. I have re-organized the information, not to provide a better order, but to make it easier to introduce some new material. At this stage, the author must balance existing material with new, always mindful of the need to restrict the size of the book to readable proportions.

I have included a chapter on microbiology because the advent of new infections such as AIDS and acanthamoeba keratitis has highlighted a requirement for some knowledge in this area.

I have separated the drugs to which optometrists do not have access into a chapter of drugs used in ophthalmology. I realize that the separation is somewhat arbitrary, as the ophthalmologist will probably use all the drugs mentioned in the book, but this is an attempt to separate the therapeutic drugs from the diagnostic.

It has been a far more difficult task than I envisaged and it is thanks mainly to my co-writer, Richard Pearson, that the book is complete. His helpful suggestions and encouragement have been a great support. Paddy O'Connor Davies has also been most helpful in the planning stages and in agreeing to find text.

My thanks are also due to Dr Bernard Gilmartin for this help during the planning stage and to various colleagues at Smith & Nephew who gave help and advice.

G. A. Hopkins
St Albans

Preface to the first edition

The contents of this book are based mainly on the lectures and practical teaching given to third year students in the Department of Ophthalmic Optics at the University of Wales Institute of Science and Technology.

The introductory chapters discuss general pharmacological principles, mechanism of drug action and neurohumoral transmissions. The comments of Dr. W. M. Lyle, Associate Professor, The School of Optometry, University of Waterloo, Canada, on the pharmacological content have proved very helpful in this initial section, as also have those of Dr. G. L. Ruskell, Reader in Ocular Anatomy, The City University, on the relevant anatomy and physiology. It is hoped that an adequate theoretical pharmacological basis has thus been laid for what is essentially intended as a clinical approach to the use of ophthalmic drugs in routine ophthalmic optical practice.

The author is very conscious of how much he has been taught and influenced by the writings of others and, in this respect, he feels particularly indebted to Sir Stewart Duke-Elder and D. W. A. Mitchell. I would like also to express my appreciation to the publishers of these authorities and to those of Goodman and Gilman's classic treatise *The Pharmacological Basis of Therapeutics* for permission to use information and quote from their publications.

Following the opening chapters, special reference is made to therapeutic drugs mainly employed in ophthalmology, a knowledge of which, particularly the sulphonamides, antibiotics and corticosteroids, is of considerable interest and value to the ophthalmic optician, even though the prescribing of drugs in the latter two groups is restricted to, or their use only permitted under the supervision of, the medically qualified practitioner.

The classification of the standard diagnostic ophthalmic drugs includes a more detailed discussion of the main examples of these, followed by some references to those less frequently employed by ophthalmic opticians, or mainly used by ophthalmologists. Local anaesthetics, staining agents, conjunctival decongestants and anti-infective preparations are next considered. The toxicology of ophthalmic drugs then precedes chapters on those important aspects—the sterility of ocular preparations and solutions used in contact lens practice.

I am grateful to Professor R. J. Fletcher, J. H. Stewart-Jones and G. A Hopkins of the Department of Ophthalmic Optics, The City University, and to W. J. Porter, for their very useful suggestions on a review of the main principles involved in carrying out ocular first aid and the action to be taken in emergencies.

A résumé of 'official' ophthalmic preparations and a chapter on the legal aspects concerning drugs and prescription writing is then undertaken. The final chapter serves as an introduction to a subject which is rapidly assuming an increasingly important role in daily ophthalmic practice—possible adverse ocular effects of systemically and topically prescribed drugs. Only those adverse effects caused by some of the most commonly prescribed medications are reviewed, as an index is required, and one has been written by H. Green and J. Spencer, to endeavour to cover the large number of preparations that are involved.

I should like to express my sincere thanks to Dr. P. J. Nicholls, Senior Lecturer in pharmacology at the Welsh School of Pharmacy, University of Wales Institute of Science and Technology, Emeritus Professor A. D. W. Macdonald and Dr. Barry Cox of the Department of Pharmacology, University of Manchester Medical School, Dr. D. F. J. Mason, Senior Lecturer in pharmacology, St. Bartholomew's Hospital Medical School, R. M. Pearson, Lecturer, The City University, and colleagues in my own and other Departments of the Institute for their invaluable assistance, advice and co-operation throughout the preparation of the clinical material.

The publishers and Mr. G. M. Dunn, Secretary of the British Optical Association, have, at all times, given me every encouragement and guidance in dealing with the manuscript, and I am also grateful to the General Medical Council, The British Medical Association and the Council of the Pharmaceutical Society for permission to incorporate information and formulae from their publications.

Finally, my thanks are due to Mrs. B. J. Andrews for her great patience and thoroughness in interpreting and typing the manuscript from my original longhand.

P. H. O'Connor Davies
Cardiff

Contents

Chapter 1

General pharmacological principles

Introduction

In order to use drugs safely and efficiently, it is necessary to have an understanding of how drugs produce their effects. Drugs are chemicals and produce their action by reacting chemically with biological structures. Pharmacy is the study of drugs and is divided into several disciplines.

Pharmacognosy deals with the natural sources of drugs, plants and animals.

Pharmaceutics is the science of compounding and formulating drugs into suitable dosage forms for human and veterinary administration.

Pharmacology covers the absorption, metabolism, mechanism of action, detoxification and excretion of drugs.

Therapeutics is the application of drugs to produce the desired effect, whether this is therapeutic or prophylactic.

Sources of drugs

Although there are a few inorganic drugs, for example lithium salts, the majority of drugs are organic compounds and can be derived from several sources.

(1) Naturally occurring compounds which are extracted from plants or animals are probably the oldest type of drugs. Such drugs tend to be expensive and, because some of the source plants are grown in exotic locations, the supply can be erratic. In the past, crude extracts such as tinctures or decoctions were used but now discrete compounds are isolated for formulating into medicinal products.

(2) Drugs produced purely by synthetic means have many advantages over natural drugs and have become one of the principal sources of drugs. Not only are synthetic drugs usually cheaper and more certain in supply but it is possible to 'tailor-make' drugs by using structure-activity relationships. This, in theory, makes it possible to enhance the desirable effects and reduce the adverse ones.

(3) Some natural drugs can be modified in order to produce better and more efficacious drugs. Porcine insulin can be modified so that it is closer to the human hormone and semi-synthetic penicillins are an important group of compounds in the treatment of infections.

(4) Genetic engineering is the newest and most modern method by which drugs can be made. Human insulin can be made by incorporating the necessary gene into *Escherichia coli*, a Gram negative rod.

Drug nomenclature

A drug can have a variety of names:

(1) *Chemical name*. This is the full name according to conventions for naming chemical compounds. Such names are usually too lengthy and complicated to use.

(2) *Approved or official name*. Also known as the generic name, it allows different products with the same ingredient to be identified as such. Unfortunately, some compounds have different approved names in different countries, for example the catecholamine extracted from the adrenal medulla is known as adrenaline in the United Kingdom but epinephrine in America. This sometimes makes it difficult to compare products from different countries.

(3) *Proprietary names*. These are also known as trade marks and are unique to particular manufacturers.

Pharmacological classification

As most drugs have a variety of actions, often not easily interrelated, a rigid system for drug classification is not really possible. A complication increasingly encountered is that many drugs possess actions that would permit their categorization in several groups, using any one classification system, for example, lignocaine may be used as a local anaesthetic (in the eye and elsewhere), but it also used intravenously for its cardiac effects as an anti-arrhythmic agent.

One or two major systems of drug classification are commonly employed either grouping drugs according to (1) their actions or effects, or (2) on the basis of their chemistry; or a combination of these systems in an endeavour to include all drugs.

The principal classes of drugs (slightly modified) are enumerated according to the system which they affect, as follows.

Notes on the Use of Drugs are introduced under the following main headings.

Drugs Acting on the Alimentary System
Drugs Acting on the Cardiovascular System
Drugs Acting on the Respiratory System
Drugs Affecting Allergic Reactions
Drugs Acting on the Nervous System
Obstetric and Gynaecological Preparations
Drugs Acting on Infections
Endocrinological Preparations
Drugs for the Suppression of Malignant Disease
Drugs Affecting Nutrition and the Blood
Drugs Used in Rheumatic Diseases
Drugs Acting on the Ear, Nose and Nasopharynx
Drugs Acting on the Eye
Drugs Acting on the Skin
Vaccines and Related Products

In the last few decades with the advent of a vastly increased range of systemic drugs, it is becoming ever more apparent that not infrequently a drug's effectiveness is linked to its potential toxicity.

As part of this milieu, adverse effects from therapeutic drug therapy are now seen more often, and the eye is not infrequently one of the locations of these unwanted reactions. This aspect of adverse ocular reactions to systemic drug therapy is dealt with in some detail in Chapter 18.

Optometry students, as future primary health care practitioners, need to possess an increasingly wider knowledge of general pharmacology and its specific application to the ocular problems presented by their patients. Happily, greater emphasis on general pharmacology is currently occurring in the teaching institutions, thereby also enhancing the understanding of ocular pharmacology.

General pharmacological principles

A revision of the general principles underlying basic pharmacological concepts applying to all drugs greatly facilitates the subsequent study of ophthalmic drugs. Briefly, these factors may be considered, according to Fingl and Woodbury (1975), under the following main headings.

Pharmacokinetics, which deals with the absorption, distribution, biotransformation and excretion of drugs.

Pharmacodynamics, which is the study of the biochemical and physiological effects of drugs and their mechanisms of action: it includes the dose-effect relationship; mechanisms (modes) of drug action; factors modifying drug effects and dosage; and drug toxicity.

Development and use of drugs.

Pharmacokinetics

Absorption, distribution, biotransformation and excretion
To achieve its characteristic effects a drug must reach adequate concentration at its sites of action. The amount of drug administered will obviously affect its concentration at its active site (or locus of action), but this latter will also vary with the rate of absorption, distribution, binding or location in tissues, inactivation and excretion. Factors affecting the absorption of a drug are its routes of administration and its pharmaceutical presentation or formulation.

Latent period: the time interval between administration and onset of effects. This factor is influenced by the following.

(1) Route of administration: via the skin (ointments, etc.); mucous membranes (mouth, rectum, bladder, conjunctiva, etc.); gastrointestinal (oral); respiratory tracts (inhalation), or by injection (parenteral).

(2) Form of administration. The formulation of the drug can have a great influence on the rate of absorption. Eye preparations can be given in the form of eye drops or eye ointments.

Duration: the rate of inactivation and excretion determines this to a large extent, but redistribution to other tissues and accumulation in storage depots (for example, fat) may be important.

Physico-chemical factors in transfer of drugs across membranes. Whatever the route of administration, the drug usually must cross one or several semi-permeable membranes before reaching the site of action.

Passive transport processes. Cell membranes consist of a bimolecular layer of lipoid material interspersed with minute water-filled pores and bound on both sides by protein. The size of these pores varies in different membranes (4–40 Å). Lipid-soluble substances readily penetrate the lipoid sheet. Small water-soluble polar materials pass through the pores, some of which are charged, and some are not. The passage of a drug across the cell membrane is, therefore, strongly influenced by its lipid solubility, molecular size, degree of ionization and solubility of its ionized and non-ionized forms.

Lipid-soluble substances and both non-polar and polar substances, as long as the last named two possess sufficient lipid solubility, move across the membrane by a process of passive diffusion. Hydrostatic and osmotic differences are involved in passage through the pores by the further passive process of filtration. Water-soluble molecules in solution must be small enough to pass through the pores, and this is a common route for many small, water-soluble, polar and non-polar substances: most inorganic ions are also sufficiently small. This filtration proceeds until the concentration of the drug is the same on both sides of the membrane.

Many drugs are the salts of weak bases and strong acids, e.g. atropine sulphate, cyclopentolate hydrochloride. Salts are highly ionized and hydrophilic but are poorly soluble in lipids. The free base is, on the other hand, non-ionized and therefore lipophilic. Cell membranes contain lipids and thus lipophilic drugs tend to pass through them more easily than hydrophilic ones.

In any solution of drugs, there will be a mixture of the salt and the free base, the ratio of which will depend on the pH and a property of the compound known as its pKa. From the equation below it will be seen that the pKa is the pH at which there are equal concentrations of base and salt.

$$pH = pKa + \log_{10} \frac{[base]}{[salt]}$$

The lower the pKa, the higher will be the proportion of base at a given pH. Because the corneal epithelium favours absorption of lipophilic substances, compounds with a low pKa are better absorbed than those with a high one.

Although the pKa of a drug cannot be altered, the pH of an eyedrops solution may be changed within certain limits without causing ocular tissue irritation. As the pH of eyedrops is raised, the degree of ionization of a weak base will be reduced, thus improving corneal epithelial absorption. The effects of pH variation on the solubility and stability of the drugs—as well as the primary consideration of avoidance of tissue irritation—must, however, also be allowed for in reaching a balanced formulation. The pH of the solution is of particular importance in eyedrops, an acceptable range being pH 5–pH 9.

Active transport processes. Specialized active transport processes appear to be responsible for the transfer of certain water-soluble drugs, as well as naturally occurring sugars, amino acids and pyrimidines. Carriers (membrane components) form complexes with the selected substance and, with the aid of energy, transport it through the membrane by a diffusion process, releasing it from the complex on the other side, against an electro-chemical gradient. These processes rely in part on the Na^+ gradient across the membrane and are affected by drugs that modify Na–K transport. Active transport differs from passive processes by requiring metabolic energy, and also exhibiting selectivity and saturability.

Absorption

Absorption is directly related to solubility, being far more rapid from solution than solid form. High concentration of the drug and good circulation of blood at the site are helpful, as also is a greater rather than smaller area of absorbing surface; for example, this is one reason for the oral (which involves the gastro-intestinal tract with its large surface area) route of administration for suitably soluble drugs, not inactivated by the secretions encountered. Absorption may take place at the following sites.

(1) The alimentary tract.

(2) By subcutaneous or intramuscular injection; (intravenous injection circumvents the factors involved in absorption).

(3) Via mucous membranes (for example, the conjunctiva* and corneal epithelium, or pulmonary epithelium).

(4) Via the skin.

Bio-availability. The active principle of any given dose form of a drug may be only a very small proportion of the whole, for example, in many potent tablets and capsules, in eyedrops and eye ointments. It has been conclusively proved that the biological availability (*bio-availability*—the facility with which the drug is absorbed) can be greatly influenced by the formulation (the active ingredient plus the other constituents), for example, the active principle in an eyedrops formulation is absorbed much more rapidly than if it were in an eye ointment. Adequate absorption of such drugs as carbachol and bethanechol chloride in eyedrops requires a wetting agent in the formula.

Distribution

After absorption into the blood stream by one of these routes the drug enters or passes through various body fluid compartments: plasma, interstitial fluid and cellular fluids. Those drugs that pass through all cell membranes redistribute throughout all fluid compartments, whereas other drugs which cannot pass through all cell membranes are restricted in their distribution and potential effects.

Many drugs are bound to plasma proteins, especially the albumin fraction, the extent of this varying with the particular drugs. Although this binding is usually reversible, it limits the drug's distribution and therapeutically effective blood concentration, as only the unbound (free) drug is pharmacologically active. Accumulation in tissues at higher concentrations than in plasma may be the result of pH gradients, binding, active transport or dissolving in fat.

The site of accumulation may serve as a drug reservoir that prolongs the effects of the drug. This occurs if the stored drug is in equilibrium with that in the plasma and is released as the plasma concentration declines. Drug bound to plasma protein may act as an important drug reservoir. However, the effect of drug reservoirs on the distribution of the drug is such that larger doses of the drug are required initially in order to provide an effective therapeutic concentration.

The ability of drugs to pass across capillary walls varies greatly according to the tissue in which the latter are situated. Capillaries in the brain are very impermeable and the term 'blood/brain barrier' is used to describe this. Ionized and water-

---

* Absorption through mucous membranes, such as the conjunctiva, occurs readily. Local anaesthetics applied topically may sometimes be absorbed so rapidly that they produce systemic toxicity.

soluble compounds are retained in the blood and even some lipophilic compounds pass into the brain very slowly.

In the eye, there is a marked variation between different tissues. The retinal capillaries have similar properties to those in the brain and the blood/retina barrier is as difficult to pass as the blood/brain barrier. The blood/aqueous barrier is somewhat more permeable. Drugs pass from the blood into the aqueous humour by two main routes.

(1) Through the epithelium of the ciliary body; this involves secretion (from those secretory cells into which the drug diffuses from the blood capillaries), and direct diffusion from non-secretory ciliary cells.

(2) Some diffusion from iris capillaries.

Cornea. Most drugs cross the cornea at rates related to their degree of ionization and to their lipid solubility. The proportion of non-ionized molecules is dependent on the dissociation constant of the drug and the pH of the medium, and is related in many drugs to the rate of passage from the corneal surface into the aqueous humour. The lipoidal barrier of the cornea has been shown by experiment to be located within the anterior epithelial layer.

Although the penetration of various substances into the cornea is assumed to be in inverse relationship to the size of their individual molecules, this factor, as Swann and White (1942) have shown, is not now believed to be as important as their phase solubilities. The lipid-soluble, non-polar, non-ionized moiety of a drug solution penetrates the corneal epithelium (and endothelium) most readily, whereas the water-soluble, polar, ionized moiety crosses the stroma more easily. For any substance to pass through the intact cornea it must be soluble in both water and fat. The cornea has been aptly compared to a fat–water–fat sandwich (Havener, 1978).

Penetration of an alkaloid through the cornea (Figure 1.1). Adler's (1975) illustration shown here conveys V. E. Kinsey's concept of how a weak base, such as the alkaloid homatropine, penetrates the intact cornea according to this differential solubility theory. R_3N represents the non-ionized, fat-soluble, water-insoluble form of the alkaloid. This exists, as a small amount of free base, in equilibrium with the ionized, water-soluble, fat-insoluble form, R_3N^+, the pH of the solution determining the relative proportion of ionized to non-ionized substance. Bromide ions bear a negative charge Br^-, and hydrogen ions a positive charge, H^+.

When a drop of the clinically used solution (which has a pH of approximately 6.0) is placed on the cornea, the amount of dissociation will not be the same as that of this solution in the bottle (where the ratio of homatropine ions to free base is about 1000:1), as the pH of the tears is about 7.4, but the homatropine will still exist in both charged and free base (uncharged) forms. Only the non-ionized form (fat-soluble free base) penetrates the epithelium; the homatropine ion penetrates the epithelium poorly since it is relatively insoluble in lipid. The stroma resists entry by the non-ionized moiety until it again ionizes, but having done so, this form of the alkaloid (water-soluble) now passes freely through the stroma, dissolving in the stroma water, until it is again blocked, this time by the endothelium. Here the alkaloid changes back to the non-ionized form to pass through the endothelial barrier. Charged homatropine finally leaves the endothelium for the aqueous humour.

The homatropine is able, therefore, to penetrate the cornea because of the difference in solubility of the two forms in which it exists. Exhaustion of the

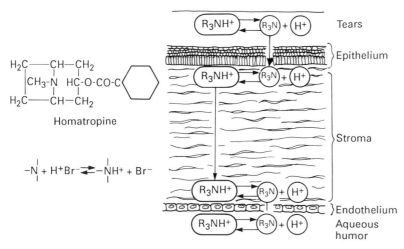

Figure 1.1 Penetration of an alkaloid through the cornea illustrating differential solubility character-istics (reproduced from *Adler's Physiology of the Eye*, 1975, by courtesy of Mosby, St Louis)

alkaloid in one form does not limit the process, since equilibrium between the forms is re-established as soon as one particle of either form (charged or uncharged) leaves the layer. Drugs leave the aqueous via the drainage route through the canal of Schlemm into the blood stream, and lipid-soluble drugs can also leave by diffusing across lipoidal membranes separating the aqueous from the blood.

Biotransformation

Although *redistribution* from its locus of action into other tissues or sites may be a factor in terminating drug effect (primarily with highly lipid-soluble drugs admi-nistered rapidly by intravenous route or by inhalation), biotransformation and secretion are usually the principal factors.

Biotransformation of drugs involves non-synthetic reactions—oxidation, reduc-tion or hydrolysis—which may result in activation, change in activity, or inactiva-tion of the parent drug. If the metabolite is active further biotransformation, or excretion in the urine, terminates its activity.

Synthetic reactions (*conjugate reactions*) also occur; the drug or its metabolite is coupled (conjugated) enzymatically with an endogenous substrate, usually a carbohydrate or an amino acid or a derivation of these, resulting almost invariably in inactivation of this parent drug.

Some compounds may be enzymatically inactivated during intermediate meta-bolism, and again tissues, including plasma, kidney and gastro-intestinal tract, contribute to drug biotransformation, but for the majority of drugs this process is mediated through the hepatic microsomal systems.

Fragments of the hepatic endoplasmic reticulum, in which are located the enzyme systems frequently involved with metabolism of many drugs, are usually called microsomes, following their isolation by centrifugation of liver homogenates.

Some drugs are excreted largely unchanged but the majority are metabolized via extremely complex routes, the number of different metabolites sometimes exceeding a hundred (Penn, 1980).

Genetic, physiological (for example, age), pharmacodynamic (for example, chronic administration; drug interaction), and environmental (for example, smoking, food additives) factors all influence the metabolism of a drug.

Microsomal enzymes catalyse a few conjugations (coupling of drugs or their metabolites with an endogenous substrate) and most of the oxidation, reduction and hydrolysis of the majority of drugs. All the remainder of conjugations and some oxidation, reduction and hydrolysis reactions of a small number of drugs are catalysed by non-microsomal enzymes, primarily in the liver but also in plasma and other tissues.

Not all biotransformation reactions involve inactivation of the drug. Prodrugs are compounds which have no *in vitro* activity but are activated by enzymes to produce new compounds which are active *in vivo*. Dipivalylepinephrine is a prodrug of adrenaline which is better absorbed than the parent compound. It passes across the corneal epithelium unmodified and when it gains access to the aqueous humour, adrenaline is released to produce its effects (Figure 1.2).

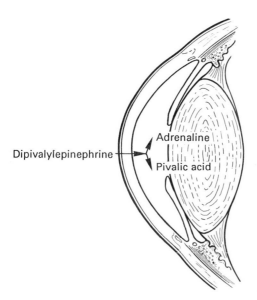

Figure 1.2 Mode of action of a prodrug

Excretion

Drugs or their metabolites are eliminated from the body mainly by excretion via the kidneys. In general the more polar, ionized, less lipid-soluble compounds, or drugs metabolized to this form, are poorly reabsorbed and so excreted. Excretion in urine involves three processes: (1) glomerular filtration; (2) active tubular secretion (in the proximal renal tubules); and (3) passive tubular reabsorption (in the proximal and distal tubules). It is the non-ionized form of weak acids and bases that undergoes reabsorption, which depends primarily on the permeability of the tubular epithelium for this non-ionic moiety.

Alteration in the excretion rate of a compound from the kidneys may be assisted if necessary (for example, in poisoning or use of urinary antiseptics) by increasing the formation of urine (with diuretics) and by decreasing its reabsorption by appropriate changes of urinary pH.

Weak acids are secreted more readily if the tubular urine is made more alkaline, mainly because they are more ionized and less readily reabsorbed. The reverse occurs if the urine is made more acid. Alkalinization and acidification of the urine in the case of weak bases have the opposite effects—decreasing and increasing excretion, respectively.

Those drugs which remain unabsorbed after oral administration, and metabolites which enter the gut in the bile, are excreted in the faeces. Excretion of drugs via the milk is not appreciable *per se*, but is of considerable importance as a potential source of unwanted effects in the nursing infant. The lungs are involved in the elimination of gaseous general anaesthetics.

The metabolites of some drugs are not excreted but deposited in certain tissues. For example, when adrenaline is oxidized to adrenochrome, it can be deposited in the conjunctiva and corneal epithelium. Some phenothiazines, used in the treatment of psychoses, form a pigment which can be deposited in the skin, the cornea and the lens.

Pharmacodynamics

The dose-response relationship
The relationship between the dose of a drug and the response it produces is not a linear one. It is normal to plot the logarithm of the dose on the x-axis and the response on the y-axis. The resultant curve usually has a characteristic S or sigmoid shape (Figure 1.3). At the lower end of the dose range there is no response, as the concentration is below the threshold. Above the threshold, the response increases in proportion to the logarithm of the dose until a maximum is reached. After this point, no increase in response is achieved with an increased dose. If more than one drug is plotted on a curve the distance between the lines is a measure of their relative potencies. Agents which cause a shift to the left of the dose-response curve represent potentiation, while a move to the right is inhibition.

The slope of the dose-response curve indicates how sharply the response will vary with dose. A steep curve will show that there is little margin for error and an overdose situation can be quickly reached.

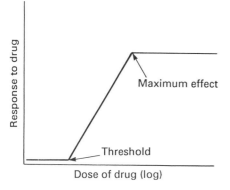

Figure 1.3 Dose-response curve

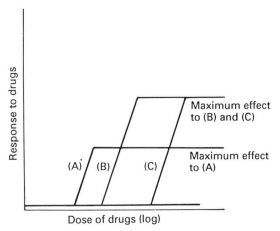

Figure 1.4 Potency and efficacy. (B) is more potent than (C) but both have the same efficacy. (B) and (C) have a greater efficacy than (A)

The height of the curve, in other words the maximum response, is a measure of the drug's efficacy. Potency and efficacy are different terms (Figure 1.4).

Biological variations
Even when allowing for the control of all known sources of variation, drug effects are never identical in all individuals, or even in the same individual on a different occasion. A drug-response curve applies only to a particular individual or the average individual of a group, and another individual may not respond to the same dose in exactly the same manner, although the variation will probably be quantitative rather than qualitative.

The median effective dose (ED_{50}) is that dose which is required to produce a standard effect on 50 per cent of a population.

Terminology
An individual is *hyper-reactive* if a drug produces its usual effect at an unexpectedly low dosage, and *hypo-reactive* if the reverse is true.

The term *hypersensitivity* (not to be confused with hyper-reactivity) should be confined to effects associated with *drug allergy*, that is, an altered reactivity to a drug which acts as an antigen and causes antigen-antibody reactions. *Idiosyncracy* is an apparently abnormal response to a drug. *Tolerance* is hypo-reactivity acquired as a result of previous exposure to a drug, and if this occurs after only a few doses it is termed *tachyphylaxis*.

Mechanisms of drug action
The most essential aspect of pharmacodynamics is that which concerns the mechanisms of drug action. Analysis of drug action aims to identify the primary action, the details of the chemical reaction between the drug and the cell, and the characterization of the complete action-effects sequence. Only such a complete analysis provides a truly adequate basis for the therapeutic use of a drug, but at present much remains to be learned of the basic mechanisms of action of most drugs.

Most drugs are thought to produce their effects by combining with enzymes, cell membranes, or other specialized cell components. The function of the cell component, it is presumed, is thereby altered by this drug-cell interaction, and biochemical and physiological changes are initiated. Only the initial consequences of the drug-cell combination should be called the action of the drug, the subsequent events being more correctly termed drug effects.

Structure-activity relationship
There is an intimate relationship between the chemical structure of a drug and its actions. Minor changes of molecular configuration to give a *congener* of the parent compound may, or may not, alter some or all of a drug's actions. This has on occasion resulted in the synthesis of a greatly improved drug, with a more favourable therapeutic index or more acceptable secondary characteristics than its parent drug.

Drug receptors
The specific functional unit or cell component which becomes directly involved in the action of a drug is called its receptor. Receptors exist in certain tissues and cells, and structurally specific drugs undergo chemical and/or physical reaction with them to form a drug receptor complex. Claude Bernard, in his classical experiments in 1857, showed that skeletal muscle poisoned with the South American arrow poison, curare, no longer exhibited a contractual response to electrical stimulation of its nerve, although the nerve still conducted the stimulation and the muscle still contracted to direct electrical stimulation.

Langley (1878) and a number of other scientists, including Lewandowsky (1898), Elliot (1905) and Dixon (1907) developed the concept of drug-cell combinations, where the receptors were envisaged as chemically defined areas of large molecules to which foreign molecules, such as drugs, supplied complementary areas. The first named scientist suggested the term receptive substance, for what is now called a receptor, around 1905. Clark (1933) developed his occupation theory, assuming that a drug's action commenced when, and lasted only as long as its molecules occupied the receptors. He also considered that the maximal biological response only occurred when all the receptors were occupied. This occupation theory was supplemented in the 1960s by Paton's rate theory (Paton, 1961). This proposes it is not necessary for all the receptors to be occupied to obtain a maximal response, but that this response may depend on the rate of formation of drug-receptor complex and rapidity of dissociation, freeing the receptors for further combination with another drug molecule. The view that drugs interact with receptors still remains the cornerstone for theories on drug action, and it bears a close relationship to theories of enzyme action. Another modification of the receptor theory is the concept of spare receptors—this proposes that maximal effect may be obtained providing a critical proportion of receptors are occupied. The various drug-receptor theories are not initially exclusive as one or other of them may be applicable for individual circumstances. Drugs capable of forming a drug-receptor complex which initiates physiological activity have both affinity and efficacy and are called agonists. A drug can bind with receptors without initiating a physiological response and may hinder an agonist from doing so. It is then said to possess affinity but not efficacy (or intrinsic activity), and is called an antagonist. This reaction against the natural agonist is, in time, reversible. If the inhibition can be reversed by increasing the concentration of the agonist, the latter ultimately achieving maximal effect, the antagonist is described as competitive or surmountable.

The cell is eloquently described by Penn (1980) as 'essentially a pool of enzymes bounded by a membrane and has energy-using and energy-producing reactions', and it is not unexpected that interference by a drug at only one site could initiate marked biochemical and physiological changes in such a structure.

The receptor sites (the receptor and adjacent areas, the latter helping or hindering access of the drug) for most drugs have not yet been identified. The motor end-plate (investigated originally in Bernard's experiments), however, is such a specialized site that can be demonstrated anatomically. Nevertheless, despite the difficulty of precise location there remains little doubt that the drug-cell complexes obey mass-law kinetics and are involved in drug action. The binding of drugs to plasma, to cell proteins and to enzymes concerned with biotransformation and transport of drugs, that does not initiate drug action is said to involve secondary or silent receptors, or storage sites.

Irreversible inactivation of a receptor site is said to be unsurmountable antagonism. An antagonist may be classified as acting in a reversible (competitive) or irreversible (non-competitive) manner if it binds at the active site for the agonist, but if binding elsewhere the description would not be applicable.

Classification of receptors and drug effects. Receptors are now classified according to the effects or lack of effects initiated by representative agonists and antagonists. The effects of the alkaloids muscarine and nicotine are used to categorize the receptors for acetylcholine (ACh), which is released on stimulation of all pre-ganglionic autonomic fibres, parasympathetic and sympathetic, all post-ganglionic parasympathetic and all somatic motor nerve fibres (Figures 1.5 and 1.6). It is the combination of this transmitter with the post-junctional receptors that initiates the subsequent biochemical and physiological activity of the next membrane in the chain, be it post-ganglionic neurone (in the case of all autonomic ganglion synapses), smooth muscle fibre, cardiac muscle fibre or gland cell (in the case of post-ganglionic parasympathetic), or skeletal muscle fibre (in the case of somatic motor nerve). Muscarine mimics the action of acetylcholine released at the parasympathetic neuro-effector sites only, whereas nicotine mimics its action at autonomic ganglia and skeletal neuromuscular junctions. Both muscarine and nicotine stimulate in low doses and paralyse in high dosage (that is, they cause a cholinomimetic effect or a cholinergic blockade, respectively). The receptor types of the post-ganglionic parasympathetic system are therefore called muscarinic, and those of the autonomic ganglia and skeletal muscle are termed nicotinic.

Drugs can, therefore, be described as having muscarinic (or antimuscarinic) and nicotinic (or antinicotinic) effects, such designation immediately conveying where and what type of effect is initiated by them.

The adrenergic fibres, comprising the majority of post-ganglionic sympathetic fibres, release on stimulation the transmitter noradrenaline (usually referred to as norepinephrine in America). Exceptions are the post-ganglionic sympathetic fibres to the sweat glands, and those that cause vasodilatation in blood vessels to skeletal muscle; these release acetylcholine and, therefore, their receptor types are muscarinic like those of post-ganglionic parasympathetic fibres. The closely related amine adrenaline is secreted along with noradrenaline, in a ratio of about 4:1, by the adrenal medulla. The receptors for noradrenaline and adrenaline have been designated alpha- or beta-adrenergic receptors on the basis of the effects of several representative sympathomimetic amines, and adrenergic blocking agents. Again,

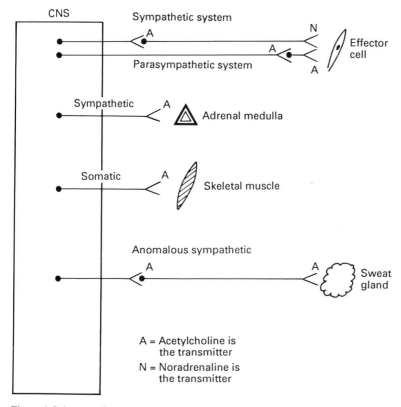

Figure 1.5 Autonomic nervous system

a statement that a drug activates or blocks a specified type of adrenergic receptor gives considerable information on the effects to be expected from its use (Chapter 2).

Sites of action

The receptor for a drug may be considered to be any functional macro-molecular component present in the organism. The drug is capable of altering (increasing or decreasing) the rate of any bodily function, but by interaction with such receptors it cannot initiate any function not already characteristic of a tissue acted upon.

If the drug interacts with receptors involved in functions common to most cells then its effects will be extensive throughout the body. This will not be so if the interaction of the drug is with more specialized receptors concerned with tissues involved solely with specific bodily functions. Not all drug activity involves receptors. Some agents may act by virtue of their physical or chemical properties; for example, antacids have a direct chemical interaction.

Therefore, these sites of action may be localized (for example, affecting a restricted area or particular organ), or generalized, affecting most of the cells throughout the body. Even though the concentration of a drug is the same in all body fluids its effects may still be localized; some drugs act only on certain cells, tissues or organs, and this explains their localized effect. A drug may have a direct

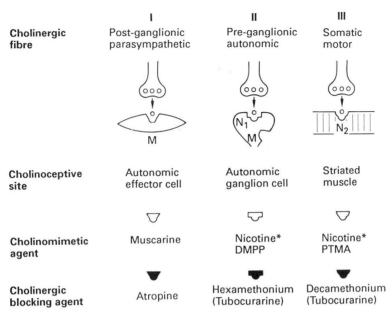

	I	II	III
Cholinergic fibre	Post-ganglionic parasympathetic	Pre-ganglionic autonomic	Somatic motor
Cholinoceptive site	Autonomic effector cell	Autonomic ganglion cell	Striated muscle
Cholinomimetic agent	Muscarine	Nicotine* DMPP	Nicotine* PTMA
Cholinergic blocking agent	Atropine	Hexamethonium (Tubocurarine)	Decamethonium (Tubocurarine)

Figure 1.6 Acetylcholine is represented above by open circles. On release following the nerve AP it combines with the corresponding cholinergic post-junctional cell receptors. Individual chemical configurations immediately adjacent to these receptors are assumed to give relative specificity by restricting the approach of various ACh-like drugs according to their 'shape' or 'fit' of the total receptor complex. Nicotine at cholinergic sites (II and III) causes stimulation in small doses and blockade (causing paralysis) in large doses. The receptors of autonomic effector cells (I) are classified as muscarinic (M) and those of autonomic ganglion cells (II) and striated muscle (III) are classified as nicotinic (N). Although certain drugs act at nicotinic receptors on both autonomic ganglion cells and striated muscle, for example, *d*-tubocurarine, others are relatively selective for II (for example, hexamethonium) or III (for example, decamethonium); hence their designation here as N_1 and N_2, respectively. It is now known that autonomic ganglion cells (II) also contain a proportion of muscarinic receptors (M), although these may not participate in normal ganglion transmission. Examples of drugs that act selectively to produce cholinomimetic effects at cholinoceptive sites are muscarine (I); dimethylphenylpiperazine (DMPP) (II); and phenyltrimethyl-ammonium (PTMA) (III) (adapted from Figure 21.8 in *Goodman and Gilman's Pharmacological Basis of Therapeutics*, 5th edn, after Koelle, Macmillan; New York, 1975)

action on certain cells (that is, it is an agonist), or it may exert this action indirectly, by promoting or preventing the activity of another substance, by stimulating release of a natural mediator, or blockading the effect of this (competitive antagonism), respectively.

Factors modifying drug effects and dosage
These relate to the following:

(1) Medication error and patient compliance: the former may be due to errors in prescription writing or dispensing; the latter involves the factor of whether or not the patient consistently takes his medication as the physician intended.

(2) Placebo effects: these are present with the taking of any drug, active or inert, and depend largely on the physician–patient relationship. They are, however, most commonly associated with dummy medication used in controlled clinical trials.

(3) Age: smaller dosages for children and the aged are usually necessary as both categories are often hyperreactive.

(4) Bodyweight: dosages for adults should be adjusted in direct ratio to weight.

(5) Sex: women are more susceptible to effects of certain drugs, especially during pregnancy.

(6) Route of administration: absorption differs; for example, drug effects are normally achieved faster and are more intense after intravenous than after oral or subcutaneous administration. Absorption after topical administration to the eye may be as rapid as if the drug was given by slow intravenous injection.

(7) Time of administration: for example, with oral therapy absorption is quicker when the drug is taken on an empty stomach (that is, before meals).

(8) Rate of inactivation and excretion: maintenance dose must be adjusted to balance the rate of inactivation and excretion, and any impaired excretory organ (for example, kidney) must be allowed for to prevent cumulative effects causing toxicity with maintenance doses of continued therapy.

(9) Tolerance: acquired especially for opiates, barbiturates and other central nervous system drugs (for example, depressants and stimulants). This necessitates increased dosage to obtain the same degree of effect, or change to another drug giving the same type and degree of effect.

(10) Physiological variables: changes in water and electrolyte balance, acid base states, and body temperature may modify drug effects.

(11) Pathological states: diseased states modify effects of certain drugs.

(12) Milieu: environmental factors are important with some drugs, especially mood and behaviour agents.

(13) Genetic factors: inherited susceptibilities may occur with certain drugs.

(14) Drug interaction: combined medication may be beneficial or cause serious adverse reactions. Combined effects of drugs equal to individual effects are said to exhibit summation and if the drugs act by the same mechanism they are termed additive. When only one of a pair of drugs initiates an effect, but the combined effects are greater than those of the active agent alone it is called synergism, for example, the cycloplegia caused by homatropine, with cocaine or ephedrine being instilled at the same time.

This definition of synergism or potentiation assumes the two drugs to be heterergic for a particular effect, that is, this effect is exhibited by one of the drugs but is not included in the spectrum of the other. If the combined effect in such a combination of heterergic drugs is less than that of the active component alone, the interaction may be termed antagonism.

Two drugs producing the same effect are termed homergic, and their combined effects may be equal to (additive), or greater, or less than, those expected by simple addition.

There is equivocation over the meaning of some of the terms describing the combined effects of drugs, which can lead to some ambiguity in their use. For example, some interpretations assume synergism to occur when two drugs act together in the same manner and if the total effect is the simple sum of the individual effects; this is described as addition. On the other hand, potentiation occurs if the magnitude of the effects of a mixture of drugs is greater than the individual effects of the component drugs (Penn, 1974). These interpretations of synergism and potentiation as different qualities, includes homergic rather than (as with Loewe) heterergic drugs in their meaning.

Many drug interactions are desired but the prevention of unwanted drug interactions is assuming a role of ever-increasing clinical significance. Some references to undesirable ophthalmic/systemic drug interactions, of significance to the ophthalmic practitioner, are discussed in Chapter 17.

Drug toxicity
Briefly, it might be mentioned that some adverse reactions to drugs are trivial but others may be serious and even fatal. All drugs have some toxic effects. Hypersensitive (or allergic) reactions to most drugs are infrequent, but they may include mild to severe skin rashes, drug fever, asthma, blood dyscrasias, liver and kidney toxaemias, psychotic states, and in some instances repeated administration may lead to drug dependence, which may be of the psychic or physical type (often referred to as habituation and addiction respectively).

Direct toxic effects of drugs, including blood dyscrasias, hepatotoxicity and nephrotoxicity, teratogenic effects, and behavioural toxicity, are not uncommon, especially when prolonged administration is employed for therapeutic purposes.

Development and use of drugs

New drugs are discovered by three main processes.

(1) *Screening* during which a large number of substances are investigated with reference to specific pharmacological activity, for example, the considerable range of antibiotics now available resulted from the testing of thousands of soil samples seeking micro-organisms capable of producing antibiotic activity.

(2) *Structural modification* of established therapeutic agents or endogenous substances in the hope of producing useful congeners with pharmacological properties different or superior to the parent, for example, the development of a whole family of more effective sulphonamides from the parent sulphonilamide.

(3) *By accident* or fortuitous discovery of a new use for a known substance, for example, the original antibiotic penicillin; the use of α-chymotrypsin for cataract extraction illustrates a fortuitous example in ophthalmology.

Evaluation is by means of controlled clinical trials on volunteer humans, after first extensive research on animals has evaluated the full pharmacological spectrum and toxicity and indicated a potentially useful new therapeutic agent.

In Great Britain, under the Medicines Act, 1968, only a licensing authority, under the direct control of the Health Minister and Parliament, may issue a certificate permitting clinical trials on any new drug. One of the several committees advising the licensing authority is the Committee on Safety of Medicines, which is responsible for drugs used in humans, and the latter committee has an Adverse Reactions Sub-committee which continually maintains a surveillance on the safety of drugs already on the market. The Medicines Commission (*see* Chapter 16) also acts in an advisory role to the licensing authority.

It is true to say that only a relatively small fraction of the new drugs released each year represent a significant advance on their precursors, particularly as it may be some time before the efficacy and safety of the newer agents, relative to the older ones, may be finally assessed by continuing usage. Application of basic pharmacological knowledge and a critical attitude towards the necessity of the need or otherwise of the use of any drug, whether for therapeutic, prophylactic or diagnostic purposes, is a necessary attribute of the student or practitioner at all times.

References

Clark, A. J. (1933) *The Mode of Action of Drugs on Cells*, Edward Arnold, London

Cotlier, E. (1975) *Adler's Physiology of the Eye—Clinical Application*, 6th ed, Mosby, St Louis, p. 52

Dixon, W. D. (1907) On the mode of action of drugs. *Med. Mag.*, **16**, 454–457

Elliot, T. R. (1905) The action of adrenaline. *J. Physiol*, **32**, 401–467

Fingl, E. and Woodbury, D. M. (1975) In Goodman and Gilman's *The Pharmacological Basis of Therapeutics*, 5th ed, pp. 1–46, Macmillan, New York

Havener, W. H. (1978) *Ocular Pharmacology*, 4th ed, Mosby, St Louis, p. 18

Langley, J. N. (1905) On the reactions of cells and nerve-endings to certain poisons, chiefly as regards the reactions of striated muscles to nicotine and curare. *J. Physiol.*, **33**, 374–413

Lewandowsky, M. (1898) Ueber eine Wirkung des Nebennierenextractes auf das Auge. *Zent Bl. Physiol.*, **12**, 599–600

Moses, R. A. (1975) *Adler's Physiology of the Eye—Clinical Application*, 6th ed, Mosby, St Louis, p. 52

Paton, W. D. M. (1961) A theory of drug action based on the rate of drug-receptor combination. *Proc. R. Soc. B.*, **154**, 21–69

Penn, R. G. (1980) *Pharmacology*, 3rd ed, Baillière Tindall, London, pp. 1–41

Swann, K. and White, N. (1942) Corneal permeability. Factors affecting penetration of drugs into the cornea. *Am. J. Ophthal.*, **25**, 1043

Chapter 2

Ocular autonomic innervation and neurohumoral transmission

Many of the diagnostic drugs used in ophthalmic practice, in particular cycloplegics, mydriatics, and miotics, directly or indirectly produce their effects by stimulating or inhibiting a part of the autonomic nervous system supplying the intra-ocular muscles. They may, in addition, also have an effect on other smooth muscles or glands in the orbit. Therefore, it is essential before proceeding to a more detailed discussion on the actions and uses of ophthalmic autonomic drugs to have a basic understanding of the structure and function of this involuntary nervous system in the orbital region.

Intra-ocular musculature

Ciliary muscle

This muscle consists of flat bundles of unstriped fibres which may be classified as follows.
  (1) Meridional fibres (Brücke's muscle)
  (2) Radial fibres
  (3) Circular fibres (Müller's muscle) (Figure 2.1)

Parasympathetic innervation of the eye (Colour Plate I)

The ciliary muscle is innervated by cholinergic fibres of the parasympathetic running in the third cranial nerve (the oculomotor), and their origin is in the Edinger–Westphal nucleus near the third nucleus in the floor of the aqueduct of Sylvius. From there they pass out of the midbrain in the main trunk of the third nerve, which, just before entering the orbit, divides into superior and inferior divisions. The parasympathetic fibres continue in the inferior division and pass into its inferior oblique branch, which they leave to form the motor root of the ciliary ganglion. In this ganglion the parasympathetic fibres synapse, their post-ganglionic components, which are atypical in being medullated, entering the globe via the short ciliary nerves (6–10), which pierce the sclera around the optic nerve. The parasympathetic fibres then pass forward in the perichoroidal space to supply the ciliary and sphincter pupillae muscles.

The Edinger–Westphal nucleus, according to Miller (1978), receives excitatory connections from the frontal and occipital (psycho-optical) cortex.

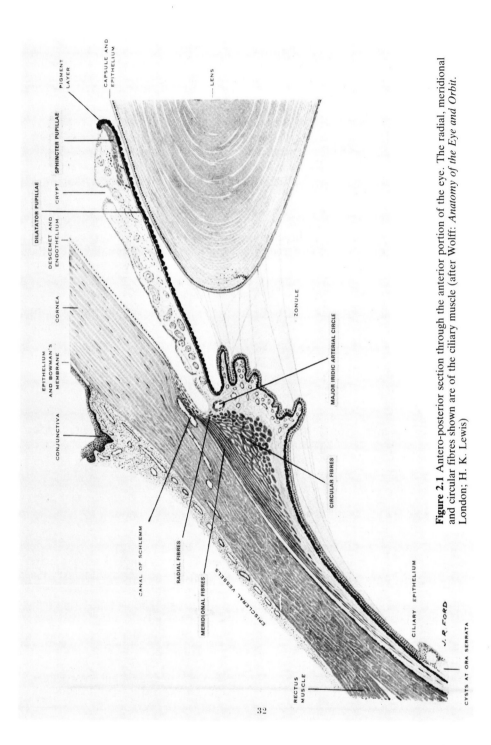

Figure 2.1 Antero-posterior section through the anterior portion of the eye. The radial, meridional and circular fibres shown are of the ciliary muscle (after Wolff: *Anatomy of the Eye and Orbit*. London; H. K. Lewis)

It has been suggested in the past that some sympathetic fibres may supply the ciliary muscle itself (not just its blood vessels), adrenergic impulses affecting receptors on the muscle fibres: the resultant 'negative' accommodation might assist for distance vision. In the past, histochemical and electron microscopical studies have thrown doubt on this theory, although clinical observations appear to support it.

More recently, work by Van Alpen (1976), using material obtained from eye banks, showed that the ciliary muscle has mostly beta-receptors, the dilatator pupillae muscle mostly alpha-receptors, and the sphincter pupillae muscle has both alpha- and beta-receptors. Adrenergic impulses to the intra-ocular muscles should, therefore, simultaneously induce relaxation of the ciliary muscle and contraction of the dilatator pupillae, and have an uncertain response to the sphincter pupillae.

Sphincter pupillae muscle

This is a circular band of smooth muscle fibres 1 mm wide just inside the pupillary border of the iris; innervated by the parasympathetic nervous system.

Dilatator pupillae muscle

This consists of radially arranged smooth muscle fibres, processes of the cells of the anterior layer of the pigment epithelium of the iris; innervated by the sympathetic nervous system.

Sympathetic innervation of the eye and orbit (Colour Plate I)

The pre-ganglionic sympathetic nerve fibres of the dilatator tract supplying the dilatator pupillae muscle probably have their origin in the hypothalamus, not far from the constrictor centre (Edinger–Westphal) to which they are connected, Miller (1978) considers, by an inhibitory pathway, in addition to having connections with the cerebral cortex. The dilatator nerve fibres pass downwards, with partial decussation in the mid-brain, through the medulla oblongata into the lateral columns of the cord. They leave the latter by the anterior roots of the first three thoracic nerves and perhaps the last cervical nerve, passing to the corresponding lateral ganglion chain on each side via the white rami communicantes. These sympathetic nerve fibres then run to the first thoracic or the stellate ganglion (as the frequently found fused first thoracic and inferior cervical ganglion is termed), and from there into the cervical sympathetic chain in the neck, synapsing in the superior cervical ganglion, which is the peripheral ganglion in their path from the central nervous system to the orbit. The non-medullated post-ganglionic fibres enter the cranial cavity in company with the internal carotid artery around which they form networks, the carotid plexus, and a little further on, where this artery lies within the cavernous sinus, the cavernous plexus. It is mainly from the latter that most of the sympathetic nerves to the eye and orbit are derived. The dilatator fibres pass from the cavernous plexus to run over the anterior part of the trigeminal (Gasserian)* ganglion before entering the ophthalmic division of the fifth cranial nerve, the

---

* Current Nomina Anatomica terms are used in this text; the older terms still used in some textbooks are included in brackets.

sympathetic fibres continuing in its naso-ciliary branch. They leave this nerve to enter the long ciliary nerves which enter the eye on either side of the optic nerve. Running forward in the perichoroidal space, the sympathetic fibres then pass through the ciliary body to reach the dilatator pupillae in the iris.

Other post-ganglionic sympathetic fibres from the cavernous plexus form the sympathetic root of the ciliary ganglion, passing through it, without further synapse, to enter the eye via the short ciliary nerves to supply the intra-ocular blood vessels of the uvea. From the cavernous plexus also, further vasomotor sympathetic fibres supply the ophthalmic artery and its branches to the extra-ocular muscles.

Smooth muscles in the orbit (for example, Müller's palpebral muscles in the lids), and the lacrimal gland, also receive sympathetic innervation.

According to Wolff (1976) the post-ganglionic (vasomotor) sympathetic fibres to the lacrimal gland may reach the gland coming from the superior cervical ganglion via: (1) sympathetic nerves along the lacrimal artery from the internal carotid plexus; (2) through the deep petrosal nerve; and (3) those sympathetic fibres that run in the lacrimal nerve with the latter's sensory fibres.

The parasympathetic (secretomotor) fibres to the lacrimal gland have their origin in cells forming a discrete sub-nucleus located very close to the superior salivatory nucleus, which lies lateral to the nucleus of the seventh cranial nerve beneath the floor of the pontine part of the fourth ventricle. Leaving the brain stem in the nervus intermedius, between the pons and inferior cerebellar peduncle, they run with the seventh nerve, fusing with the latter at the geniculate ganglion.

From this ganglion arises the great (superficial) petrosal in which the parasympathetic fibres run to join the deep petrosal (sympathetic) to form the nerve of the pterygoid canal (the Vidian). This nerve joins the pterygopalatine (sphenopalatine; Meckel's) ganglion, where only the parasympathetic component relays, the post-ganglionic parasympathetic fibres then travel via the maxillary nerve to enter its zygomatic branch and reach the lacrimal gland via a connecting branch of this nerve.

It is now thought that the sympathetic lacrimal innervation is to its blood vessels, while the parasympathetic probably controls normal tear secretion. This supposition is supported by the fact that drugs inhibiting the parasympathetic reduce the secretion of the gland, for example, atropine.

Electron microscopic investigations by Ruskell (1969) would appear to confirm this view.

The autonomic nervous system (ANS) includes the two main divisions, sympathetic and parasympathetic, the ocular parts of which have been reviewed above. It should be noted that in a synapse a pre-ganglionic fibre usually makes physiological contact with several post-ganglionic neurones which continue to specific smooth muscles, organs or glands.

The intra-ocular parasympathetic fibres synapse in the ciliary ganglion (short post-ganglionic fibres), and those to the lacrimal gland in the pterygopalatine ganglion.

The sympathetic fibres to the eye and orbit synapse in the superior cervical ganglion (long post-ganglionic fibres).

Efferent fibres, carrying impulses outwards from the central nervous system in somatic nerves, are far in excess of afferent fibres carrying impulses inwards to the CNS; both types of nerve fibre are present in the sympathetic and parasympathetic but little is known regarding the afferent pathways in the autonomic nervous system of the eye.

Antagonistic action of sympathetic and parasympathetic

The autonomic nervous system controls all involuntary actions except reflex actions involving voluntary muscles. Smooth muscle (ciliary, sphincter pupillae and dilatator pupillae muscles, intra-ocularly; Müller's palpebral muscles in the lids), also termed plain, involuntary or unstriped muscle, consists of spindle-shaped fibres $60\mu \times 60\mu$. It has an independent tone, that is, one not dependent on an intact nerve supply. Often sympathetic and parasympathetic fibres innervate the same organ, and then they are usually antagonistic, that is, when one accelerates the other retards, for example, in the heart the sympathetic accelerates and the parasympathetic slows, and vice versa in peristalsis of the gastro-intestinal tract. The salivary glands are an exception, secretion being stimulated by both divisions of the autonomic nervous system. In the eye the sympathetic division dilates the iris pupil and the parasympathetic constricts it. The maintenance of normal pupillary size depends on the balance between these two antagonistic innervations, the superior tone of the sphincter keeping the pupil slightly constricted.

Reciprocal innervation

Sherrington's principle of reciprocal innervation (1893), which indicates that central stimulation of a group of agonist skeletal muscles is accompanied by central inhibition of the opposing antagonist group, the latter even losing their normal dependent tone, has been demonstrated in the extra-ocular muscles of the eye (Björk and Kugelberg, 1953).

Where those intra-ocular smooth muscles of the eye, the sphincter and dilatator pupillae, which control the pupillary diameter, are concerned, both parasympathetic (to the sphincter) and sympathetic (to the dilatator) innervations are active at the same time, with, as already mentioned above, the superior tone of the sphincter pupillae normally dominating. Lowenstein and Loewenfeld (1950) have shown that some inhibition of the Edinger–Westphal nucleus, which controls parasympathetic impulses to the sphincter pupillae, inhibits the tone of the latter in the presence of psycho-sensory reflex dilatation of the pupils. This reflex, precipitated by sensory nerve stimulation (for example, pain), or strong psychical stimuli (for example, extreme fear), appears to be of cortical origin, and to activate the dilatator pupillae through its sympathetic innervation, while at the same time inhibiting the tone of the sphincter pupillae by inhibiting impulses passing to it via the parasympathetic.

Nisida, Okada and Nakano (1960) demonstrated that there was an inhibition of the normal tonic activity of the dilatator pupillae of the cat, the majority of the sympathetic nerve fibres to this muscle being inhibited on stimulation of the animal's pupillo-constrictor mechanism.

From the experimental evidence available, therefore, it would appear, that with regard to the intra-ocular smooth muscles controlling the pupil, a definite reciprocal innervation exists.

Sensory innervation of the eye and orbit (Colour Plate I)

It may not be out of place here, although it is not a part of the ocular autonomic innervation, to mention that the third root (the sensory) of the ciliary ganglion (the other two being the sympathetic and parasympathetic) is a branch of the ophthalmic division of the fifth cranial nerve (the trigeminal), which is the sensory nerve for the whole of the eye and orbit. The short ciliary nerves carry the sensory fibres from the intra-ocular structures of the globe, particularly the cornea. These fibres leave the ciliary ganglion, as its sensory root, to join the nasociliary nerve, which has already received the two long ciliary nerves from the eye, carrying sensory fibres from the ciliary muscle, the iris and the cornea; in addition these two nerves carry sympathetic fibres running in the naso-ciliary forwards to the dilatator pupillae. Proceeding back towards the trigeminal (Gasserian) ganglion the naso-ciliary is joined by the (sensory) frontal and lacrimal nerves (the latter also carries sympathetic fibres), the three branches uniting to form the ophthalmic nerve, the first (or ophthalmic) division of the trigeminal ganglion of the fifth cranial nerve. Drugs, known as local anaesthetics, are used to block the conduction of impulses back along these sensory nerves from the eye and orbit.

Neurohumoral transmission in the autonomic nervous system (Figure 2.2)

The theory of neurohumoral transmission, which is now generally accepted, proposes that nerve fibres (including those of the ANS) act, not by direct electrical stimulation of a muscle, or organ, or second (post-ganglionic) nerve fibre, but by transmitting their impulses across most synapses and neuro-effector junctions by means of specific chemical agents known as neurohumoral transmitters, acetylcholine and noradrenaline (usually known as norepinephrine in the USA), in the case of cholinergic and adrenergic nerve fibres respectively.

Most of the so-called 'autonomic' drugs, affecting smooth muscle and gland cells, act in a manner that mimics or modifies the actions of the 'natural' transmitters, released on stimulation of the autonomic nerves, at either ganglia or effector cells.

Axonal conduction

Axonal conduction is the passage of an impulse along an axon. The currently most acceptable hypothesis on axonal conduction (Hodgkin and Huxley, 1952) is briefly as follows. A stimulus above the threshold level initiates a nerve impulse or nerve action potential (AP) at a local region of the axonal membrane. The internal resting potential of the latter has a negative value and this is reversed through zero, continuing uninterrupted to a positive value. This local reversal is due to a sudden selective increase in the permeability of the membrane to sodium ions, which flow inwards in the direction of their concentration gradient. This occurs because, at rest, sodium and chloride ions are in much higher concentration in the extracellular fluid than in the axoplasm, the axonal membrane then being relatively impermeable to sodium while allowing comparatively easy traverse for other ions. The reverse operates for potassium ions in the resting potential state, when they are approximately 30–50 times more concentrated in the axoplasm than the extracellular fluid, these concentration gradients being maintained by pump and active transport mechanisms, involving an adenosine triphosphatase (ATPase) at the inner surface of the membrane activated by sodium and at its outer surface by potassium (Thomas, 1972). The rapid inflow of sodium ions is immediately followed by increased membrane permeability for potassium ions which flow in the

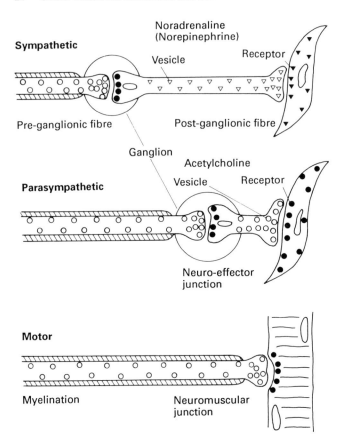

Figure 2.2 Schematic representation of the neurohumoral transmission of autonomic and motor nerves. *Open circles* = acetylcholine storage vesicles; *solid circles* = acetylcholine receptor sites; *open triangles* = noradrenaline (norepinephrine) storage vesicles; *solid triangles* = noradrenaline receptor sites. Only the post-ganglionic sympathetic fibre has noradrenaline vesicles. Transmission at sympathetic neuro-effector junctions is by noradrenaline in contrast to acetylcholine transmission at all ganglia, at the parasympathetic neuro-effectors, and at neuromuscular junctions. It should be noted that this greatly simplified representation of ganglionic transmission has now been superseded by the concept that such transmission is a far more complex process, involving cholinoceptive and adrenoceptive sites (after Drill: *Pharmacology in Medicine*, 3rd edn, 1965. New York; McGraw-Hill)

opposite direction. The local circuit currents around the axon, produced by these transmembrane ionic currents, activate adjacent regions of the axon, propagating the nerve AP along it, the recently activated region remaining momentarily in a refractory state.

Very few drugs in normal therapeutic doses, with the exception of high concentrations of local anaesthetics infiltrated in the immediate vicinity of nerve trunks, modify axonal conduction.

Junctional transmission

Junctional transmission is the passage of an impulse across a synaptic or neuro-effector junction.

The arrival at the axonal terminals of the AP initiates the neurohumoral transmission of an excitatory or inhibitory impulse. The following events occur (Figure 2.3).

(1) *Release of transmitters.* These are probably largely synthesized in the region of the axonal terminals (some in the cell body), and stored there in synaptic vesicles, either in highly concentrated ionic form (as with acetylcholine (ACh)), or as a readily dissociable complex or salt (as with that of noradrenaline with adenosine triphosphate (ATP)) and a specific protein. Slow release of small amounts of these transmitters does take place in the resting state but these are insufficient to initiate a propagated impulse at the post-junctional site. The AP precipitates simultaneous release of larger amounts of transmitter (several hundred quanta). This process is triggered by the depolarization of the axonal terminal. Although the other intermediate steps are uncertain, one step is the mobilization of the calcium ion, which enters the intra-axonal medium and is thought to promote fusion of the vesicular and axoplasmic membranes. The process by which the vesicles' contents are then discharged to the exterior is termed exocytosis.

(2) *Combination of transmitter with post-junctional receptor and production of post-junctional potential.* Diffusing across synaptic or junctional clefts (a distance of 100–500 Å), the transmitter combines with the specialized macromolecular receptors on the post-junctional membrane (second neurone, muscle fibre or gland cell), generally resulting in a localized non-propagated increase in the permeability of this membrane that can be of two types.

(*a*) A general increase for all ions (chiefly Na^+ and K^+) in which case a localized depolarization follows, the excitatory post-synaptic potential (EPSP).

(*b*) A selective permeability increase for smaller ions only (chiefly K^+ or Cl^-) followed by stabilization or actual hyperpolarization of the membrane, the inhibitory post-synaptic potential (IPSP).

(3) *Initiation of post-junctional activity.* A propagated AP in a neurone, or muscle action potential (AP) in most types of skeletal muscle, or secretion in gland cells, is initiated if an EPSP exceeds a certain threshold value. In smooth muscle and certain types of tonic skeletal muscle, propagated impulses do not occur; instead an EPSP activates a localized contractile response. EPSPs initiated by other neuronal sources at the same time and site as an IPSP will be opposed by the latter, the algebraic sum of these effects deciding whether or not a propagated impulse or other response ensues.

The extra-ocular muscles are stimulated in the manner described above for most types of skeletal muscle (Koelle, 1975), but some differences in the structure and reaction of these particular muscles should be noted. It is usual in most skeletal muscle for one motor neurone to innervate between 100 and 200 muscle fibres, whereas in the extra-ocular muscles one neurone may supply one between 5 and 20 fibres. Such small motor units permit a precision of control over extra-ocular muscles not to be found in other skeletal musculature.

This smoothness of ocular movement is further assisted by the exceptionally large amount of elastic connective tissue around the loosely arranged fine extrinsic ocular fibres, not found to the same extent in the dense connective tissue surrounding the bundles of other skeletal muscles.

Vesicles believed to contain acetylcholine are concentrated together with a large number of mitochondria within the axonal terminals of motor nerves. Similar vesicles also occur in the various pre-synaptic terminals or boutons, but unlike the small discrete motor end-plates in skeletal muscle fibres, the pre-synaptic and post-synaptic neuronal processes form complicated patterns of intertwining ramifications amidst the tightly packed cells of the ganglion (for example, approximately 100 000 ganglion cells occur in a cubic millimetre of the superior cervical ganglion). As with the skeletal muscle the transmitter in the autonomic ganglia has proved to be acetylcholine, which has been obtained from the perfusate of isolated ganglia after stimulation of the pre-ganglionic fibres. The superior cervical ganglion of the cat is often used in such experiments.

Eccles (1964, 1973), Katz (1966), McLennan (1970) and Krnjevic (1974) are only a few of the many research scientists who have contributed much to our understanding of synaptic transmission. Koelle (1975), referring to the work of Katz and Miledi (1972), stated that this demonstrated that immediate post-junctional response (of skeletal muscle) to acetylcholine liberated by stimulation of the motor nerve is the development of a localized depolarization at the motor end-plate, the EPP (end-plate potential), equivalent to EPSP at post-synaptic sites, which on reaching a critical level generates a propagated muscle AP, leading to a contraction.

Smooth muscle (and cardiac), in contrast to cholinergically innervated skeletal muscle, exhibits an inherent activity that is independent of a nerve supply, although this quality probably does not apply to all smooth muscles equally.

This activity may be modified but is not initiated by nerve impulses, and though it is less sensitive to electrical stimuli than striped, smooth muscle is more sensitive to chemical stimulation. It has been suggested that the inherent activity of smooth muscle may be regulated by acetylcholine synthesized and released by the muscle fibres. Spikes or waves of reversed membrane polarization travel from cell to cell at rates considerably slower than the action potentials of axons or of skeletal muscle. Rhythmic fluctuations in the membrane resting potential in smooth muscle seem to initiate spikes which, as in skeletal muscle, in turn initiate contractions, which in some tissues pass as a wave along the muscle sheet, for example, peristalsis in the small intestine.

Experiments have demonstrated that depolarization of the smooth muscle fibres of the rabbit's colon, occurring after a delay of 400 ms after stimulation of the cholinergic post-ganglionic fibres to this tissue, produces a spike which persists for approximately 600 ms. As the response occurred simultaneously in all the muscle fibres and the rate of depolarization is proportional to the stimulus, Gillespie (1962) concluded that each muscle fibre is probably innervated by more than one nerve fibre.

Membrane potential changes of single smooth muscle cells of the guinea-pig vas deferens, where the excitatory fibres from the hypogastric nerve are adrenergic, show a somewhat similar state of affairs, although, on stimulation of the nerve, the delay in depolarization is much briefer. The actions of acetylcholine and adrenaline at membrane level have been described by Bulbring (1958). Burnstock and Holman (1961) also found in the vas deferens of the guinea-pig miniature potentials similar to those at motor end-plates of skeletal muscles, in the absence of nerve stimulation, probably due to spontaneous release of small amounts of noradrenaline (Figure 2.3). Burnstock and Holman (1961) include among their conclusions the remark: 'Our results have shown that the mechanism of transmission of excitation from sympathetic nerve to smooth muscle is essentially similar to that of transmission at other neuro-effector junctions, stimulation of the effector nerve producing depolarization of the post-junctional membrane.' As in skeletal muscle, the spike initiates a contraction (Figure 2.4).

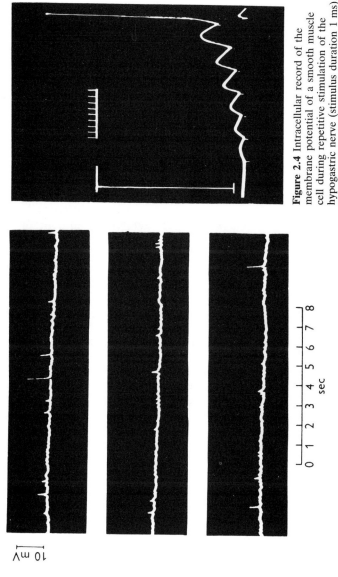

Figure 2.4 Intracellular record of the membrane potential of a smooth muscle cell during repetitive stimulation of the hypogastric nerve (stimulus duration 1 ms). Vertical calibration 50 mV; the horizontal trace = 0 mV; time marker, 100 ms (reproduced by courtesy of the Editor of the *Journal of Physiology*, 1961, **155**, 115–133)

Figure 2.3 Continuous record of membrane potential in the absence of nervous stimulation showing a spontaneous discharge of 'miniature junction potentials' (reproduced by courtesy of the Editor of the *Journal of Physiology*, 1961, **155**, 115–133)

Although to the author's knowledge similar potential changes, involving this slow build-up of graded potentials to an action potential, have not been recorded from ocular smooth muscle, it would appear probable that they are applicable to smooth muscle in general, including ocular.

(4) *Destruction or dissipation of the transmitter.* As Koelle (1975) remarks, when impulses can be transmitted across junctions at frequencies ranging from a few to several hundred a second an efficient means of disposing of the transmitter subsequent to each impulse is essential. Acetylcholinesterase (AChE) is the highly specialized enzyme available at most cholinergic junctions for disposing of ACh released there as the transmitter. It is abundantly present in skeletal muscle tissue and is concentrated in the region of the motor end-plates. Diffusion may account for the termination of action of acetylcholine at some synapses, and it seems likely that this contributes to the method, which is mainly uptake by the axon terminals themselves and by other cells, of ending the activity of the adrenergic transmitter, noradrenaline. There are two enzymes capable of metabolizing noradrenaline and adrenaline, catechol-O-methyltransferase (COMT) found in practically all tissues, and monoamine oxidose (MAO), which is present in nervous tissue and the liver. These enzymes have not the importance or speed of action of acetylcholinesterase in cholinergic transmission.

Effector cells are cells which respond characteristically to a stimulus (*see* Figure 2.2).

Neuro-effector junctions are those junctions where two cells are in more or less close physical relationship, the term being confined to nerve and effector cells of cardiac muscle, smooth muscle and gland.

A *synapse* is the area of proximity between two neurones where impulses are transmitted from one nerve cell to another across an ultra-microscopic gap (20 nm) called the synaptic cleft. Ganglia contain many such synapses.

Ganglionic transmission is a highly complex process, incorporating many of the elements of transmission at the myoneural junctions of both skeletal and smooth muscles. It is now considered that interneurones and additional transmitters may also be involved. In addition to the primary pathway involving ACh depolarization of post-synaptic sites (described above) secondary pathways for the transmission of excitatory and inhibitory impulses have also been described. Specific non-depolarizing ganglion blocking drugs effect the primary pathway but the secondary pathways are insensitive to these agents (Volle and Koelle, 1975). There is some evidence indicating the participation of a catecholamine (dopamine or noradrenaline, from a catecholamine containing cell or interneurone within the ganglion) acting on the ganglion to cause hyperpolarization (IPSP) (Eccles and Libet, 1961. It has been suggested that multiple cholinoceptive and adrenoceptive sites exist in the mammalian superior cervical ganglion (Greengard and Kebabian, 1974).

Neuro-muscular junctions are the spaces that occur between motor nerve fibre endings and skeletal muscle motor end-plates, and are comparable to synaptic clefts at synapses.

Myo-neural junction is a term that embraces neuro-effector junctions with smooth muscle and neuromuscular junctions, that is, it includes all types of motor nerve endings.

Evidence for neurohumoral transmission

Evidence for neurohumoral transmission may be deduced from the following experimental data.

(1) The demonstration, at appropriate sites, of the presence of a physiologically active compound and of the enzymes involved in its metabolism.

(2) Recovery of the compound from the perfusate during stimulation of an innervated organ, the substance not being present (or only in vastly reduced amounts) in the absence of such stimulation.

(3) Appropriate administration of the compound produces the same responses as nerve stimulation.

(4) The demonstration that these responses to nerve stimulation and administration of the compound are modified in the same way by various drugs.

This evidence is further supported by that important feature of junctional transmission, the irreducible latent period, that is, the time lag between the arrival of an impulse at the axonal terminal and the manifestation of the post-junctional potential.

The evidence for the existence of neurohumoral transmitters is well substantiated by Otto Loewi's classical experiment in 1921 to demonstrate the release of a vagus substance ('vagustoff') on stimulation of the cardiac nerve to the frog's heart. He stimulated the vagus fibres, whilst this heart (the donor) was perfused with a balanced salt solution, the perfusion fluid then being perfused through a second isolated, denervated, frog's heart (the recipient). Recordings of the rates of contraction of both hearts were made. A substance was liberated from the donor heart that dissolved in the perfusion fluid and slowed the rate of contraction of the recipient heart. This 'vagustoff' was later identified as acetylcholine. Loewi also discovered that an accelerator substance similar to adrenaline (at first called sympathin—later identified as noradrenaline) was liberated into the perfusion fluid (accelerating the rate of contraction of the recipient heart), when the action of the sympathetic fibres in the cardiac nerve of the frog's vagus predominated over that of the inhibitory parasympathetic vagus fibres.

As the cardiac branch of the frog's vagus contains a sympathetic accelerator component, the accelerens, as well as parasympathetic fibres, it is a mixed nerve, and its stimulation at times causes inhibition, and at other times acceleration. The particular result varies with the frog and the time of the year; in winter inhibition dominates and in summer acceleration.

Further substantiation has been produced by identification by various pharmacological, chemical and physiological tests of the substance present in perfusate from an innervated structure during the period of nerve stimulation, that is not present in the absence of stimulation. In addition, it has been demonstrated that the substance so obtained is capable of producing responses identical to those of nerve stimulation and that both responses are modified in the same manner by various drugs. Most of the general principles concerning the physiology and pharmacology of the autonomic nervous system and its effector organs are applicable, with some reservations, to the neuromuscular junctions (for example, those of extra-ocular voluntary muscles), and in some respects to the central nervous system, although here knowledge of the transmitters involved is far from complete.

The autonomic nervous system (involuntary, visceral or vegetative nervous system) consists of nerves, ganglia and plexuses that innervate the heart, blood vessels, glands, viscera and smooth muscles throughout the body (*see Colour Plate*

II). The motor nerves of this system supply all structures of the body except skeletal muscle. Somatic nerves with their synapses occurring entirely in the central nervous system supply the latter, whereas the most distal synaptic junctions in the autonomic system are in ganglia occurring outside the spinal cord, for example, the superior cervical ganglion (SCG) and ciliary ganglion (CG) (Figure 2.5) which are the final relay stations for the sympathetic and parasympathetic autonomic innervation, respectively, of the eye. The motor nerves to skeletal muscle, including the extra-ocular muscles, are medullated (myelinated), where the post-ganglionic autonomic nerves are non-myelinated, with the exception of the short ciliary nerves.

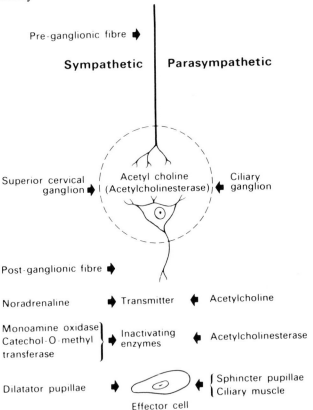

Figure 2.5 Diagrammatic representation of the neuro-effector mechanism of the ANS to the eye (drawn by J. B. Davey)

Acetylcholine

Acetylcholine is the neurohumoral transmitter of all pre-ganglionic autonomic nerve fibres, all parasympathetic post-ganglionic fibres, and a few post-ganglionic sympathetic fibres (as previously mentioned, those which innervate the sweat glands, vasodilator fibres to skeletal muscle arteries, and post-ganglionic fibres to the adrenal medulla).

The complex sequence of enzymatic reactions in the formation of acetylcholine (ACh) may be outlined as follows (Moses, 1975).

acetate + adenosine triphosphate (ATP)
$$\downarrow$$
adenylacetate + coenzyme A
$$\downarrow \text{ (acetylkinase)}$$
acetylcoenzyme A + choline
$$\downarrow \text{ (choline acetylase)}$$
acetylcholine (ACh)

Choline present in the extracellular fluid is taken up, by active transport, into the axoplasm. Choline acetylase (choline-acetyltransferase) which occurs in all cholinergic nerves, is synthesized within the perikaryon and then transported, by unknown means, along the axon to its terminal. The axonal terminals, in addition to their vesicles, contain the large number of mitochondria in which the acetyl coenzyme A is synthesized. The final step in the synthesis of ACh probably takes place within the cytoplasm, and subsequently most of this transmitter is stored within synaptic vesicles. These are mostly concentrated at the synaptic and neuro-effector junctions (Figures 2.6 and 2.7), and are spherical structures approximately 400–500 Å in diameter.

It has been estimated that each synaptic vesicle contains from 1000 to over 50 000 molecules of ACh, and a single motor-nerve terminal contains 300 000 or more vesicles (Koelle, 1975).

The simultaneous discharge of 100 or more quanta (vesicles), following a latent period of 0.75 ms, occurs when an AP arrives at the motor-nerve terminal (Katz and Miledi, 1965). The action potential appears to depolarize the terminal, increasing the permeability of the terminal axoplasmic membrane, permitting the inflow of calcium ions. This causes the liberation of ACh into the synaptic cleft by the process of exocytosis, that is, the membranes of the vesicles (ACh is found in clear and noradrenaline in granulated vesicles) fuse to the nerve cell membrane and the area of fusion breaks down, extruding the contents on the outside of the cell, the membrane of the latter remaining intact (Ganong, 1979).

Combination of the transmitter with post-junctional receptors and subsequent effects of this have already been discussed, the effects of this mediator being rapidly terminated by (*a*) diffusion and/or (*b*) the antagonistic enzyme AChE. The storage, release and disposal of ACh at synaptic and other cholinergic neuro-effector sites is considered to be essentially the same at neuromuscular junctions.

Acetylcholinesterase

Acetylcholinesterase (AChE) is an enzyme present at neuromuscular junctions and in the neurones of cholinergic nerves throughout their entire lengths. It is also found in large amounts in erythrocytes. Also called specific, or true cholinesterase (ChE), this enzyme is capable of rapidly hydrolysing acetylcholine liberated in the process of cholinergic transmission, to choline and acetic acid (the latter has no action, and the choline very little, on cholinergic receptors), in time periods as little as a millisecond. The transmitter acetylcholine is its preferred or only substrate. Butyro-cholinesterase is another type of enzyme found in the body tissues and fluids (nerves, plasma, liver and other organs), and is also capable of hydrolysing acetylcholine, but at a slower rate. It is known as non-specific, or pseudocholinesterase, but its physiological function is unknown as its experimental inhibition with certain drugs produces no apparent functional derangement at most sites.

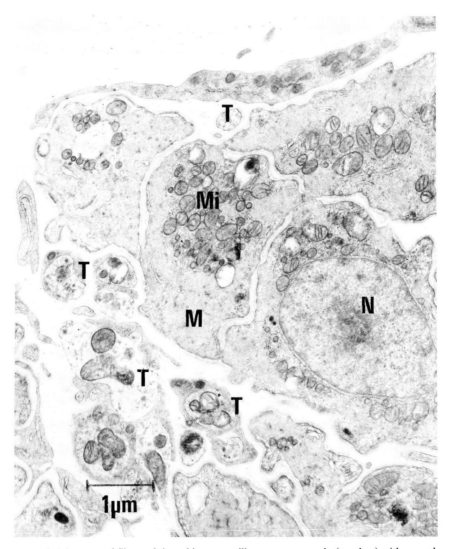

Figure 2.6 A group of fibres of the sphincter pupillae cut transversely (monkey) with several nerve fibre terminals. *M* = myofilaments; *Mi* = mitochondria; *N* = nucleus; *T* = nerve fibre terminals with agranular vesicles (electron micrograph reproduced by courtesy of G. L. Ruskell)

Some drugs, known as anticholinesterases (for example, physostigmine) neutralize acetylcholinesterase, and then the liberated acetylcholine continues to act until it diffuses away, for example, after physostigmine has been instilled in the eye, the constriction of the ciliary and sphincter pupillae muscles continues long after parasympathetic stimulation of these muscles has ceased.

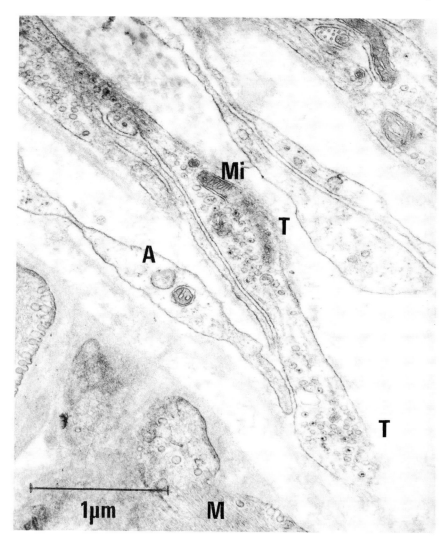

Figure 2.7 Vasomotor nerve terminals adjacent to smooth muscle cells of a choroidal arteriole (monkey). Swellings of varicosities occur at intervals along the terminal axons, those of the sympathetic system containing many small vesicles, some of which have central granules; these identify the axons as sympathetic. *A* = adventitial cell process; *M* = myofilaments; *Mi* = mitochondria; *T* = nerve fibre terminals with small agranular and small granular vesicles (electron micrograph reproduced by courtesy of G. L. Ruskell)

Noradrenaline

Noradrenaline is the neurohumoral transmitter for the great majority of post-ganglionic sympathetic fibres, and these latter are termed adrenergic. Sir Henry Dale (1934) was the original proposer of the terms 'cholinergic' and 'adrenergic' to describe neurones that liberated acetylcholine and noradrenaline respectively.

Elliott (1905) suggested that post-ganglionic sympathetic fibres might transmit their impulses to autonomic effector cells by liberation of an adrenaline-like substance, later called sympathin. Euler in the 1940s conclusively identified sympathin as noradrenaline. This transmitter is released from all stimulated post-ganglionic sympathetic fibres except those to certain sweat glands and vasodilator fibres in man, which were discovered to be cholinergic (Dale and Feldberg, 1934).

The steps in the enzymatic synthesis of noradrenaline and adrenaline (known in the USA as norepinephrine and epinephrine, respectively), proposed by Blaschko (1939) and confirmed by demonstration (using radioactive labelled phenylalanine in rats) by Gurin and Delluva (1947), are as follows.

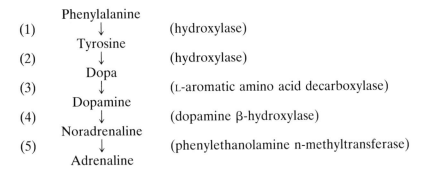

	Phenylalanine	
(1)	↓	(hydroxylase)
	Tyrosine	
(2)	↓	(hydroxylase)
	Dopa	
(3)	↓	(L-aromatic amino acid decarboxylase)
	Dopamine	
(4)	↓	(dopamine β-hydroxylase)
	Noradrenaline	
(5)	↓	(phenylethanolamine n-methyltransferase)
	Adrenaline	

Tyrosine is taken up into the neurone from the extracellular fluid the other steps of the enzymatic synthesis occurring within the neurone, steps (2) and (3) taking place in the cytoplasm. Dopamine then enters the granules to be converted into noradrenaline (step 4).

Most of the noradrenaline in the adrenal medulla leaves the granules and is converted in the cytoplasm to adrenaline (step 5), re-entering another group of granules for storage until released. Adrenaline accounts for approximately 80 per cent of the catecholamines in the adult human adrenal medulla, noradrenaline contributing most of the remainder.

Under very high magnification (electron micrographs) varicosities can be seen on adrenergic nerve fibres which contain noradrenaline stored in granular vesicles (Ruskell, 1967, 1969) (Figure 2.7).

The Falk–Hillorp fluorescein technique for the demonstration of catecholamines may be used to show these. Briefly, this involves treating the neurones with formaldehyde vapour and examining the resultant histochemical stain under ultra-violet light. The noradrenaline can be seen within the vesicles as fluorescent material.

Adrenergic fibres can sustain the output of noradrenaline for long periods of stimulation, but the maintenance of adequate reserves to allow this is dependent on an unimpaired synthesis and re-uptake of the transmitter, by active transport, into the adrenergic neurone terminals. Cocaine inhibits the re-uptake of catecholamines by adrenergic nerve endings, which temporarily prolongs the activity of noradrenaline, and instillation of cocaine in the eye results in mydriasis, as an additional effect to its local anaesthetic property.

It is considered that some of the noradrenaline within the granules is in a smaller mobile pool in equilibrium with some held in reserve as a salt of ATP (four molecules of the catecholamine to one of ATP) along with a specific protein. A much larger mobile pool of noradrenaline exists in the cytoplasm within the nerve terminal. The cytoplasmic and intragranular mobile pools are kept in equilibria by active transport mechanisms, passive diffusion, enzymatic synthesis, and destruction (by mitochondrial monoamine oxidase (MAO) (Figure 2.8).

The noradrenaline is discharged rapidly from the neurone terminal by the nerve action potential, the latter requiring the presence of calcium ions (Burn and Gibbons, 1965).

The possible involvement of acetylcholine, contained in the sympathetic neurone, as an essential or facilitatory step in the release of noradrenaline, the Burn and Rand hypothesis (1965), is still controversial.

In the adrenal medulla, according to Koelle (1975), ACh, liberated by the pre-ganglionic fibres, combines with the receptors on the chromaffin cells to produce a localized depolarization, which is followed by the entrance of calcium

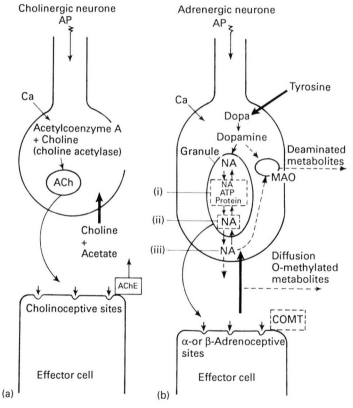

Figure 2.8 Diagrammatic representation of sequence of events occurring at **a** cholinergic and **b** adrenergic neuro-effector junctions, showing synthesis, storage and release of transmitters, and subsequent disposal of the last named after interaction with post-junctional receptor sites on effector cells. Active transport is depicted by *heavy* arrows; passive diffusion by *dash* arrows; enzymatic synthesis by *light* arrows; and active release of transmitter by *curved* arrows. Noradrenaline (*NA*) within the granules forms (in a complex with ATP and a specific protein) a reserve pool (*i*); a smaller mobile pool (*ii*), and, in the cytoplasm, a much larger mobile pool (*iii*), see **b**; the NA released by the AP comes from the intragranular pools of storage vesicles

ions into these cells. This results in their granular content (adrenaline, ATP, chromogranin, dopamine β-hydroxylase) being extruded by exocytosis into the extracellular fluid and thus into the circulation.

In the release of noradrenaline at adrenergic terminals calcium ions again appear to play an essential role in conjunction with the nerve impulse, but the sequence of steps in this case is not fully understood.

The termination of the effects of noradrenaline, released at adrenergic terminals, at the adrenoceptive sites of effector cells, other than those in blood vessels, is mostly by active reabsorption into the adrenergic nerve terminal, and partly by diffusion and subsequent enzymatic inactivation by extraneuronal catechol-O-methyl-transferase.

Although much slower acting than AChE, catechol-O-methyltransferase (COMT) and monoamine oxidase, are of major importance in the initial metabolic transformation of noradrenaline, adrenaline and other catecholamines in humans. Both enzymes are widely distributed in tissues, including the brain, throughout the body, their highest concentrations being found in the liver and the kidney.

MAO is associated chiefly with the mitochondria, including those within the adrenergic fibre terminals and is concerned with the metabolism of intraneuronal catecholamines, by such processes as oxidative deamination. COMT, on the other hand, is mainly concerned with extra-neural degradation of catecholamines by way of 3-O-methylation to 3-methyoxy compounds (Figure 2.8) (Penn, 1980).

Alpha- and Beta-Receptors (Table 2.1)

Noradrenaline, adrenaline and other members (for example, dopamine) of the catecholamines acting as neurohumoral transmitters can cause either excitation or inhibition of smooth muscles, depending on the site and amount of catecholamine present. Catecholamines are a group of chemical compounds (catechol is dihydroxybenzene) distributed throughout the tissue of the body in cells called chromaffin cells, due to the brown colour of the latter produced when they are treated with dichromate. Today the Falck–Hillorp fluorescein techniques more eloquently demonstrate their presence. The actual percentage of these catecholamines in various tissues depends on the site in the body, for example, the adrenal medulla secretes 80 % adrenaline, the remainder of its secretion being noradrenaline, very little dopamine being present. On the other hand, the transmitter liberated from adrenergic nerve fibres is noradrenaline with perhaps a little adrenaline.

The most potent excitatory catecholamine is noradrenaline, which has a correspondingly low activity as an inhibitor, whereas adrenaline is relatively potent in both excitatory and inhibitory activities.

Ahlquist (1948) studied the excitatory and inhibitory actions of various catecholamines (including *l*-adrenaline, *dl*-adrenaline, noradrenaline, methyl-noradrenaline, methyl-adrenaline, and isopropyl noradrenaline [isoprenaline]), using vascular, bronchial, stomach and intestinal, uterine and ureter smooth muscle, cardiac muscle and the smooth muscle in the nictitating membrane of the cat. He proposed the terms alpha- and beta-receptors for adrenoreceptive sites on smooth muscles where catecholamines produce excitation or inhibition, respectively. Both types may be present in the same tissue. This occurs in blood vessels, where with the usual amounts of physiologically circulating adrenaline, beta-receptor response (vasodilatation) predominates in the blood vessels of the skeletal muscle and the liver; alpha-receptor response (vasoconstriction) occurs in blood

Table 2.1 — Effector Organ Responses to Autonomic Impulses*

Effector organs	Adrenergic impulses		Cholinergic impulses
	Receptor type	Response	Response
Eye**			
Dilator pupillae	mainly α (very few β)	Contraction (mydriasis)	—
Sphincter pupillae	α and β in equal amounts	—	Contraction (miosis)
Ciliary muscle	mainly β (very few α)	Relaxation for far vision (slight effect)	Contraction for near vision (accommodation)
Heart			
S-A node	β†	Increase in heart rate	Decrease in heart rate; vagal arrest
Atria	β†	Increase in contractility and conduction velocity	Decrease in contractility and (usually) increase in conduction velocity
A-V node and conduction system	β†	Increase in conduction velocity	Decrease in conduction velocity; A-V block
Ventricles	β†	Increase in contractility, conduction velocity, automaticity and rate of idiopathic pacemakers	—
Blood vessels			
Coronary	α	Constriction	Dilatation
	β	Dilatation	
Skin and mucosa	α	Constriction	—
Skeletal	α	Constriction	Dilatation
	β	Dilatation	
Cerebral	α	Constriction (slight)	—
Pulmonary	α	Constriction	—
Abdominal viscera	α	Constriction	—
	β	Dilatation	
Renal	α	Constriction	—
Salivary glands	α	Constriction	Dilatation
Lung			
Bronchial muscle	β	Relaxation	Contraction
Bronchial glands		Inhibition (?)	Stimulation
Stomach			
Motility and tone	β	Decrease (usually)	Increase
Sphincters	α	Contraction (usually)	Relaxation (usually)
Secretion		Inhibition (?)	Stimulation
Intestine			
Motility and tone	α, β	Decrease	Increase
Sphincters	α	Contraction (usually)	Relaxation (usually)
Secretion		Inhibition (?)	Stimulation
Gall bladder and bile ducts		Relaxation	Contraction
Urinary bladder			
Detrusor	β	Relaxation (usually)	Contraction
Trigone and sphincter	α	Contraction	Relaxation

Table 2.1 (*cont.*)

Effector organs	Adrenergic impulses		Cholinergic impulses
	Receptor type	*Response*	*Response*
Ureter			
Motility and tone		Increase (usually)	Increase (?)
Uterus	α, β	Variable‡	Variable‡
Male sex organs		Ejaculation	Erection
Skin	α	Contraction	—
Pilomotor muscles			
Sweat glands	α	Slight, localized secretion	Generalized secretion
Spleen capsule	α, β	Contraction Relaxation	—
Adrenal medulla		—	Secretion of adrenaline and noradrenaline
Liver	β	Glycogenolysis	—
Pancreas			
Acini		Decreased secretion	Secretion
Islets	α	Inhibition of insulin and glucagon secretion	Insulin and glucagon secretion
	β	Insulin and glucagon secretion	
Salivary glands	α	Thick, viscous secretion	Profuse, watery secretion
Lacrimal glands	—	Secretion	
Nasopharyngeal glands	—	Secretion	

*Modified from Goodman and Gilman: *The Pharmacological Basis of Therapeutics*, 5th ed., 1975. New York; Macmillan: and Ganong, W. F.: *Review of Medical Physiology*. 9th ed., Lange Medical Publications.
**According to Van Alpen (1976).
β† The receptors of the heart producing excitatory responses have been classified as β_1-receptors, and most of the other β-receptors producing inhibitory responses as β_2 receptors.
‡Depends on presence or absence of pregnancy, stage of menstrual cycle, amount of circulating oestrogen and progesterone and other factors.

vessels of the abdominal viscera, skin and mucosa (including the conjunctival vessels).

Exceptions to the general proposal associating alpha-receptors with excitation and beta-receptors with inhibition are recognized. An inhibitory response is mediated by both alpha- and beta-receptors in the intestine, the latter being generally relaxed by catecholamines.

Lands *et al.* (1967) have shown on the basis of relative selectivity of effects of both excitatory and antagonist agents that there are at least two different types of beta-receptors.

As excitatory responses, positive chronotropic and inotropic effects (increased rate and force respectively) are the response of cardiac nodes and muscle which have beta-receptors, these latter in the heart have been classified as beta₁. Most of the other beta-receptors, where inhibition is produced, are termed beta₂.

Adrenergic receptor-blocking drugs may be of the alpha-adrenergic blocking type (for example, tolazoline, phentolamine, ergotamine and thymoxamine; the last of these is of use in eyedrops for reversing pupillary blockage caused by

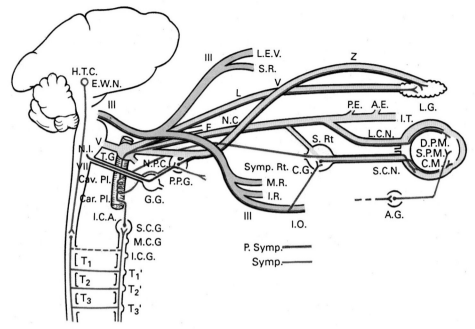

Plate 1 Autonomic and sensory nerve supply of the eye (schematic) (drawn by J. B. Davey)

KEY

III	Oculomotor nerve	L.G.	Lacrimal gland
V	Trigeminal nerve	M.R.	Nerve to the medial rectus muscle
VII	Facial nerve	N.C.	Naso-ciliary nerve
A.E.	Anterior ethmoidal nerve	N.P.C.	Nerve of pterygoid canal
A.G.	Accessory episcleral ganglion of Axenfeld	N.I.	Nervus intermedius
		P.E.	Posterior ethmoidal nerve
Car. Pl.	Carotid plexus	P.P.G.	Pterygo-palatine (sphenopalatine) ganglion
Cav. Pl.	Cavernous plexus		
C.G.	Ciliary ganglion	P. Symp.	Parasympathetic nerves
C.M.	Ciliary muscle	P.Symp.Rt.	Parasympathetic root to ciliary ganglion
D.P.M.	Dilatator pupillae muscle		
E.W.N.	Edinger—Westphal nucleus	S.C.N.	Short ciliary nerves
F.	Frontal nerve	S.P.M.	Sphincter pupillae muscle
G.G.	Geniculate ganglion	S.R.	Nerve to superior rectus muscle
H.T.C.	Hypothalamic centre	S.Rt.	Sensory root from ciliary ganglion
I.C.A.	Internal carotid artery	Symp.	Sympathetic nerves
I.C.G.	Internal carotid ganglion	Symp. Rt.	Sympathetic root to ciliary ganglion
I.O.	Nerve to the inferior oblique muscle	T1, T2, T3	1st, 2nd and 3rd thoracic nerves respectively
I.R.	Nerve to the inferior rectus muscle		
I.T.	Infratrochlear nerve	T1', T2', T3'	1st, 2nd and 3rd thoracic ganglia respectively
L.	Lacrimal nerve		
L.C.N.	Long ciliary nerves	T.G.	Trigeminal ganglion
LEV.	Nerve to levator palpebrae superioris	Z	Zygomatic nerve

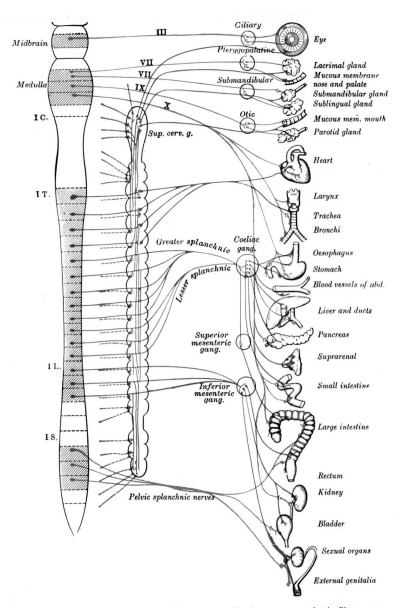

Midbrain

Medulla

I C.

I T.

1 L.

I S.

III

Ciliary

Eye

Pterygopalatine

VII
VII
IX

X

Sup. cerv. g.

Submandibular

Otic

Lacrimal gland
Mucous membrane
nose and palate
Submandibular gland
Sublingual gland
Mucous mem. mouth
Parotid gland

Heart

Larynx

Trachea

Bronchi

Greater splanchnic
Lesser splanchnic

Coeliac
gang.

Oesophagus
Stomach
Blood vessels of abd.

Liver and ducts

Superior
mesenteric
gang.

Inferior
mesenteric
gang.

Pancreas

Suprarenal

Small intestine

Large intestine

Pelvic splanchnic nerves

Rectum
Kidney

Bladder

Sexual organs

External genitalia

Plate II—Diagram of the autonomic nervous system. The pre-ganglionic parasympathetic fibres use certain cranial and sacral nerves for their distribution. The pre-ganglionic sympathetic fibres leave the spinal cord by the anterior roots of the twelve thoracic nerves and the first two or three lumbar nerves. The parasympathetic fibres are represented by blue, and the sympathetic fibres by red. The interrupted red lines indicate sympathetic post-ganglionic fibres to the cerebral and spinal nerves. (after Gray's Anatomy, 35th ed., 1973. London: Longmans Green). Note: There is now considerable doubt concerning the existence of the accessory ganglion.

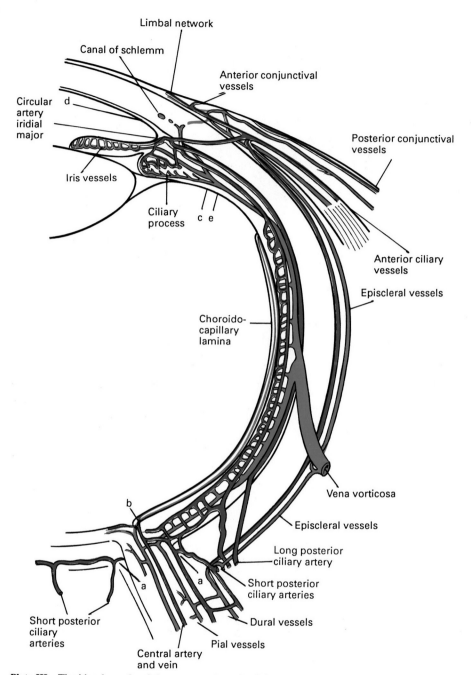

Limbal network

Canal of schlemm

Anterior conjunctival vessels

Circular artery iridial major

d

Posterior conjunctival vessels

Iris vessels

Ciliary process

c e

Anterior ciliary vessels

Episcleral vessels

Choroido-capillary lamina

Vena vorticosa

b

Episcleral vessels

Long posterior ciliary artery

Short posterior ciliary arteries

Short posterior ciliary arteries

a

a

Dural vessels

Pial vessels

Central artery and vein

Plate III—The blood supply of the eye: a = branch of short posterior ciliary artery to the optic nerve; b = anastomoses between choroidal and central vessels. In the case of the artery this is capillary only; c = vein from ciliary muscle to vena vorticosa; d = branch of anterior ciliary vein from ciliary muscle; e = recurrent artery (after Wolff, Anatomy of the Eye and Orbit (1976). London: Lewis)

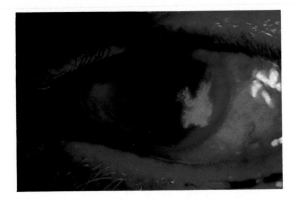

Plate IV—Geographical ulceration (Courtesy of Mr A. Elkington)

Plate V—A tetra-curve corneal lens C5/8.10:7.00/ 8.60:7.60/9.60: 8.20/10.80:8.80/12.25:9.20. The fluorescein pattern shows the central flat fit with bearing on the apex of the cornea and a slight epithelial abrasion as a result. The lens is riding lower temporarily. The lens periphery also appears to have excessive clearance, partially due to the central flat fit. (Courtesy of M. Wilson)

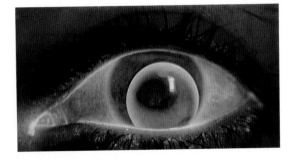

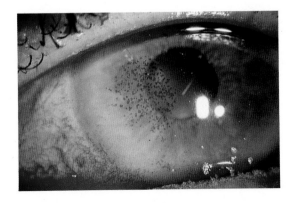

Plate VI—Rose bengal staining of a dry eye (Courtesy of A. J. Phillips)

sympathomimetic mydriatics), or beta-adrenergic blocking agents (for example, propranolol, oxprenolol; both of these drugs are non-selective blockers of beta$_1$- and beta$_2$-receptors).

Non-selective beta-receptor blocking drugs, some of which have a mild initial intrinsic sympathomimetic activity (for example, oxprenolol) reduce cardiac output (by inhibiting sympathetic cardiac stimulation), increase airways resistance (by blocking sympathetically induced bronchodilation), and reduce tremor (by inhibiting beta-receptor activity in skeletal muscle). They are therapeutically effective in the treatment of angina, arrhythmias, hypertension, anxiety (to control excessive sympathomimetic effect, for example, tachycardia, sweating) and hyperthyroidism.

Autonomic drugs

The humoral mode of transmission provides numerous opportunities to influence the functioning of the autonomic nervous system by the use of other chemicals (drugs). Drugs can be used to modify the release of transmitter, the transmitter-receptor interaction or transmitter breakdown. As most agents are normally foreign to the body, specific enzymes for their destruction are absent and the duration of action is prolonged. An exception is the presence of the enzyme atropinesterase, which is capable of inactivating atropine in rabbits. The action of this drug is correspondingly short in these animals.

There are three principal sites at which transmission can be influenced.
(1) Autonomic ganglia;
(2) Parasympathetic neuro-effector junctions;
(3) Sympathetic neuro-effector junctions.

Autonomic ganglia

At first sight, influencing transmission across the synapse would not appear to be a useful method of modifying the action of effector cells because the dual innervation of such structures would mean that both systems would be equally affected. However, for some tissues, one system is far more important than the other. Most blood vessels are only innervated by the sympathetic system and so interfering with ganglion transmission will have a significant effect on peripheral vascular resistance and hence on blood pressure.

The sympathetic nerves on the other hand have very little effect on the ciliary muscle and thus modifying transmission will alter accommodation.

Ganglion stimulants
These are chemicals which are similar to acetylcholine in that they will have the same effect on nicotinic receptors. Nicotine itself can be considered as a ganglion stimulant, and this effect is responsible for some of the pleasurable effects of smoking. Ganglion stimulants have little or no use in general medicine.

Ganglion blocking agents
Ganglionic blocking agents react with the nicotinic receptors at ganglia without producing a stimulus for the generation of an impulse in the post-ganglionic nerve. While they occupy the receptor, acetylcholine is unable to react and thus the ganglion is blocked. Transmission from the CNS to the periphery via the ANS is

prevented. Such drugs were developed for the treatment of systemic hypertension. Ganglion blockade of the sympathetic system inhibits the vasoconstrictor nerve fibres serving blood vessels and vasodilation results. One of the many side effects is a blurring of vision caused by paralysis of accommodation resulting from the effects on the ciliary ganglion.

Examples of ganglion blocking agents are hexamethonium and mecamylamine. This form of treatment for hypertension has, to a large extent, lost favour because of the many side effects.

Nicotinic receptors are also found in the skeletal neuromuscular junction but the two types of nicotinic receptor appear to have different sensitivities. It is possible to produce drugs which act preferentially in ganglia and others which affect nicotinic receptors on skeletal muscles (neuromuscular blocking drugs), for example curare.

Parasympathetic neuroeffector junction

Direct parasympathomimetics
Chemicals which produce the same effect as acetylcholine on muscarinic receptors or the nicotinic receptors of the neuroeffector junction are termed direct parasympathomimetic agents because they mimic the action of stimulating the parasympathetic nervous system. They can be divided into two groups:
  (i) Choline esters;
  (ii) Cholinomimetic alkaloids.

Choline esters.   These are synthetic drugs which are derivatives of acetylcholine. Principal examples of this group are methacholine, carbachol and bethanecol.

Synthetic acetylcholine can also be used as a parasympathomimetic, but the action is very short because of its destruction by cholinesterase. Methacholine is slowly broken down by true cholinesterase, while carbachol and bethanechol are resistant to the action of this enzyme.

Cholinomimetic alkaloids.   As for all alkaloids, plants provide the source of the following examples of this group: muscarine, arecoline and pilocarpine.

Parasympathomimetics, when given systemically, produce the effects of stimulating the parasympathetic system. Their principal use in medicine today is as miotics for the treatment of glaucoma and reversing mydriatics.

Miosis is produced by stimulation of the pupil sphincter muscle. In addition, there is a small amount of dilator inhibition but this is not so important. The light reflex will be maintained unless the dilation is maximal. The effect on the ciliary muscle is manifested as a spasm of accommodation and a reduction in AC/A ratio, even in presbyopic eyes.

Intraocular pressure is reduced due to a reduction in the resistance to outflow, brought about by the stimulation of the ciliary muscle opening up the trabecular spaces. Secretion is also reduced slightly, but the mechanism for this is not clear.

Even if blood vessels are not innervated they will contain muscarinic receptors, and topical application of a parasympathomimetic will cause vasodilatation and conjunctival hyperaemia. Dilation of deeper vessels can sometimes lead to an initial rise in intraocular pressure before a more persistent fall. The permeability of the blood/aqueous barrier may be increased, allowing larger molecules to pass into the aqueous humour. Although they do not normally reach the retina in sufficient quantities after topical instillation, parasympathomimetics have the ability to cause a significant and lengthy reduction in the electroretinogram.

The lacrimal gland is innervated by the parasympathetic nervous system and topical drugs such as pilocarpine can produce increased secretion.

Indirect parasympathomimetics

Some parasympathomimetics owe at least a part of their action to an indirect effect. As well as stimulating the receptors directly, they can also stimulate the nerve ending to release natural acetylcholine.

Anticholinesterases

There is a natural background release of acetylcholine from cholinergic terminals which is broken down by cholinesterase before it can accumulate in physiologically active quantities. Anticholinesterases are compounds which bind to cholinesterase in a similar manner to acetylcholine. The difference between the two is that acetylcholine can be broken down very quickly while anticholinesterases are only slowly metabolized. While anticholinesterases are occupying the cholinesterase site they are not available to hydrolyse acetylcholine, and the transmitter can build up to pharmacologically active levels.

Anticholinesterases vary greatly in duration of action and can be divided into two groups:

(i) Reversible anticholinesterases;
(ii) Irreversible anticholinesterases.

Reversible anticholinesterases.   The best known example of these compounds is physostigmine from the calabar bean, while neostigmine is a more modern synthetic copy which has the advantage of greater stability.

Irreversible anticholinesterases.   Originally developed as nerve gases and insecticides, the organophosphorus compounds produce an inhibition of cholinesterase which is so prolonged that it is thought that the body produces new enzyme before the original has been regenerated.

The effects of anticholinesterases are similar to those of parasympathomimetics, with additional effects due to the nicotinic actions of acetylcholine. Anticholinesterase agents produce effects at the neuromuscular junction, causing enhanced transmission which is sometimes evident as muscle fasciculation or twitching.

Anticholinesterases, in addition to their ophthalmic application, are used in the treatment of myasthenia gravis.

Anticholinesterases produce similar effects to parasympathomimetics on the pupil, ciliary body and lacrimal gland. An intense miosis will be produced which may be sufficient to abolish the pupil light reflex. The effect on the ciliary muscle is slower in onset and of shorter duration than the miotic effect. However, even when accommodation has apparently returned to normal, the ciliary muscle still remains 'irritable' and cyclospasm can return if close work is attempted. Like parasympathomimetics, anticholinesterases reduce intraocular pressure by increasing outflow.

Dilatation of blood vessels in the conjunctiva and ciliary body occurs and an increase in the permeability of the blood/aqueous barrier will cause a rise in the level of protein in the aqueous humour which in turn will increase the viscosity of the medium, resulting in a small rise in intraocular pressure.

Unlike most parasympathomimetics, which have only muscarinic effects, all anticholinesterases have nicotinic actions because of their mode of action. Nicotinic receptors are found in extraocular muscle fibres of both types. Stimulation of the slow fibres will bring about contracture, while that of fast fibres will lead to muscle fasciculation, manifested in the eye as lid twitching.

Drugs which interfere with the transmission of impulses by effects on the post-ganglionic nerve ending
These are drugs which prevent the release of acetylcholine from the postganglionic nerve terminal when the nerve is stimulated. Hemicholinium prevents the synthesis of the transmitter, while the very toxic substance botulinum toxin prevents its release. The compounds have very limited application due to their high toxicity. Botulinum toxin has been used to paralyse extraocular muscles for the treatment of squint.

Antimuscarinic agents
Antimuscarinic agents react with the muscarinic receptor but do not produce the normal stimulus that results when acetylcholine or a directly acting parasympatho-mimetic drug reacts with it. While they occupy the site, acetylcholine cannot produce its effects and transmission is prevented. These drugs are also referred to as anticholinergic, parasympatholytic, antispasmodic, or atropine-like drugs.

The first example of these compounds was atropine but now many compounds with an antimuscarinic action have been prepared. Until the advent of the histamine-2 receptor blocking drugs such as cimetidine, they were important in the treatment of gastric ulcers. Their effects on the gut are usually quite marked and this leads to their use in the treatment of travel sickness and in anti-diarrhoeal preparations. They also cause relaxation of the bronchi and have been used to treat asthma. Throughout the body they are notable for drying up secretions from exocrine glands, and one of the first symptoms of poisoning is a dry mouth resulting from inhibition of the salivary glands.

Antimuscarinics produce a mydriasis which is accompanied by a loss of pupil light reflex resulting from paralysis of the pupil sphincter muscle. There is little effect on the pupil dilator muscle. Depending on the strength of the antimuscarinic agent employed, cycloplegia will be produced with a residual accommodation varying from nothing to a significant amount. As regards to intraocular pressure, these agents produce an effect opposite to that of parasympathomimetics, with a rise in pressure being noted due to relaxation of the ciliary muscle.

There will be no direct effect on blood vessels as the muscarinic receptors are not normally innervated, but a reflex vasodilation can sometimes occur due to the release of histamine. The lacrimal gland will be inhibited and tear production will be reduced.

Sympathetic neuro-effector junction

Because of the influence of the sympathetic system on vascular tone and blood pressure and the high incidence of systemic hypertension, drugs acting on these structures have received much attention.

Directly acting sympathomimetic agents
These drugs produce the same effects as noradrenaline on the adrenergic receptors. Some drugs have more effects on alpha-receptors while others are more active on beta. Their effects are similar to those of stimulating the sympathomimetic system. Blood pressure is raised, the bronchi are dilated and the gut is inhibited.

Sympathomimetics are used as local vasoconstrictors (they are sometimes administered with a local anaesthetic for dental work) and cardiac stimulants. Beta-stimulant sympathomimetics have an important role to play in the relief of some obstructive airway diseases such as asthma.

Sympathomimetics produce mydriasis by stimulating the pupil dilator muscle. The mydriasis is less than that produced by antimuscarinics and the pupil light reflex is not normally abolished. The sympathetic nervous system has little influence on accommodation and so these drugs produce little or no cycloplegia. Blood vessels are constricted even when the drugs are applied at very low concentrations, especially in the conjunctiva. Sympathomimetics produce increased uveal vascular resistance but have little effect on retinal blood vessels.

Sympathomimetics produce a reduction in the intraocular pressure by a complex series of events. The alpha-mediated vasoconstriction of uveal blood vessels produces a reduction in secretion which is to some extent reversed by an increase in the secretion of chloride ions, a beta-mediated effect. The level of chloride ions requires an increased level of sodium to maintain neutrality and these together increase the osmotic pressure, drawing water into the aqueous humour.

Beta-receptors are also present in the outflow channels, stimulation of which brings about increased outflow, further reducing the intraocular pressure. It is interesting to note that the effects on the intraocular pressure follow a completely different time course to the mydriatic response of the pupil.

Smooth muscle present in the upper lid can be affected by sympathomimetics, leading to retraction of the eyelids and widening of the palpebral fissure.

Indirectly acting sympathomimetic agents
These produce similar actions to the directly acting sympathomimetics but produce their effect by causing the release of noradrenaline from the sympathetic nerve terminals rather than by reacting with the receptor directly. They, of course, require the presence of a functioning nerve terminal to produce their effect, unlike a direct agent which only requires the appropriate receptor.

Drugs which interfere with the re-uptake of noradrenaline
The re-uptake process is responsible for limiting the action of noradrenaline. If it is inhibited, then noradrenaline released from the nerve terminals will have enhanced effects. Cocaine is an example of a drug which produces its effects in this way.

Adrenergic receptor blocking drugs
These are agents which block adrenergic receptors in the same way that atropine blocks cholinergic receptors. As there are alpha- and beta-receptors, there are alpha-blocking drugs and beta-blocking drugs. Beta-blocking drugs are further divided into $beta_1$- and $beta_2$-blocking drugs according to which subtype of receptor they affect.

Adrenergic receptor blockers produce a depression of sympathetic tone. Alpha-blockers will cause vasodilation while beta-blockers slow the heart and cause broncho-constriction.

Alpha-receptor blocking drugs are notable for their effect on the ocular musculature, while beta-blockers have more effect on aqueous humour dynamics.

Alpha-blockers.   The pupil dilator is paralysed and a miosis occurs. This can be produced even if the iris is pretreated with a sympathomimetic or an antimuscarinic. The smooth muscle of the eyelid is paralysed and slight ptosis occurs.

Beta-blockers.   By blocking the secretion of chloride ions mediated by beta-receptors, these agents are potent reducers of intraocular pressure. They have no effect on outflow facility.

Adrenergic neurone blocking drugs
These agents, instead of acting on the receptor, interfere with the sympathetic nerve terminal. By a variety of mechanisms they prevent the release of noradrenaline from adrenergic nerve endings. Reserpine causes a depletion of noradrenaline from the vesicles in the nerve ending so that there is no transmitter to release when the nerve is stimulated. Guanethidine causes an initial release of noradrenaline but prevents new transmitter being produced. Bretyllium stabilizes the nerve membrane, preventing the release of transmitter.

All these agents produce a pharmacological denervation syndrome and have been used with varying degrees of success in the treatment of hypertension.

Denervation supersensitivity

When the nerve to an effector cell is cut or destroyed, the cell becomes supersensitive to the transmitter normally supplied by the nerve or to any drug capable of mimicking its effects. This supersensitivity is brought about by the lack of a neurotropic factor, which is present when the nerve is functioning.

The mechanism of supersensitivity is due to an increased number of receptors and an absence of the re-uptake mechanism in the case of sympathetic nerves. It can be produced chemically using 6-hydroxydopamine or pharmacologically with guanethidine, as well as surgically. It also, of course, occurs spontaneously in Horner's and Adie's syndromes, in which the sympathetic and parasympathetic systems are affected, respectively.

When the nerve returns to normal (regenerates), the effector cell loses its supersensitivity.

References

Ahlquist, R. P. (1948) A study of the adrenotropic receptors. *Am. J. Physiol.*, **153**, 586–600
Bjork, A. and Kugelberg, E. (1953) Motor unit activity in the human extraocular muscles. *E.E.G. clin. Neurophysiol.*, **5**, 271–278
Blashko, H. (1939) The specific action of L-dopa decarboxylase. *J. Physiol., Lond.*, **96**, 50–51
Bulbring, E. (1958) Physiology and pharmacology of intestinal smooth muscle. *Lect. scient. Basis Med.*, **7**, 374–397.
Burn, J. H. and Rand, M. J. (1965) Acetylcholine in adrenergic transmission. *A Rev. Pharmac.*, **5**, 163–182
Burnstock, G. and Holman, M. E. (1961) The transmission of excitation from autonomic nerve to smooth muscle. *J. Physiol., Lond.*, **155**, 115–133

Dale, H. H. (1934) Chemical transmission of the effects of nerve impulses. *Br. Med. J.*, **I**, 835–841

Dale, H. H. and Feldberg, W. (1934) Chemical transmitter of vagus effects to stomach. *J. Physiol., Lond.*, **81**, 32–334

Eccles, J. C. (1964) *The Physiology of Synapses*, Springer-Verlag, Berlin; Academic Press, New York

Eccles, J. C. (1973) *The Understanding of the Brain*, McGraw-Hill, New York

Eccles, R. M. and Libet, B. (1961) Origin and blockade of the synaptic responses of curarised sympathetic ganglia. *J. Physiol., Lond.*, **157**, 484–503

Elliot, T. R. (1905) The action of adrenaline. *J. Physiol., Lond.*, **32**, 401–467

Ganong, W. F. (1979) *Review of Medical Physiology*, 9th ed, Lange Medical Publications, Los Altos, p. 57

Gillespie, J. S. (1962) The electrical and mechanical responses of intestinal smooth muscle cells to stimulation of their extrinsic parasympathetic nerves. *J. Physiol.*, Lond., **162**, 76–92

Greengard, P. and Kebabian, J. W. (1974) Role of cyclic AMP in synaptic transmission in mammalian peripheral nervous system. *Fedn. Proc. Fedn. Am. Socs. exp. Biol.*, **33**, 1059–1067

Gurin, S. and Delluva, A. (1947) The biological synthesis of radioactive adrenaline from phenylalanine. *J. biol. Chem.*, **170**, 545–550

Hodgkin, A. L. and Huxley, A. F. (1952) A quantitative description of membrane current and its application to conduction and excitation in nerves. *J. Physiol., Lond.*, **117**, 500–544

Katz, B. (1966) *Nerve, Muscle and Synapse*, McGraw-Hill, New York

Katz, B. and Miledi, R. (1965) The measurement of synaptic delay, and the time course of acetylcholine release at the neuromuscular junction. *Proc. R. Soc. B.*, **161**, 483–495

Katz, B. and Miledi, R. (1972) The statistical nature of acetylcholine potential and its molecular components. *J. Physiol., Lond.*, **224**, 665–699

Koelle, G. B. (1975) In Goodman and Gilman's *The Pharmacological Basis of Therapeutics*, 5th ed, Macmillan, New York, pp. 404–444

Krnjevic, K. (1974) Chemical nature of synaptic transmission in vertebrates. *Physiol. Rev.*, **54**, 418–540

Lands, A. M., Arnold, A., McAnliff, J. P., Luduena, F. P. and Brown, R. G., Jr. (1967) Differentiation of receptor system activated by sympathomimetic amines. *Nature, London.*, **214**, 597–598

Lowenstein, O. and Loewenfield, I. E. (1950) Role of sympathetic and parasympathetic systems in reflex dilatation of the pupil. *Archs. Neurol. Psychiatr.*, **64**, 313–340

McLennan, H. (1970) *Synaptic Transmission*, 2nd ed, Saunders, Philadelphia

Miller, J. H. S. (1978) *Parsons' Diseases of the Eye*, 16th ed, Churchill Livingstone, London, pp. 34–36

Moses, R. A. (1975) *Adler's Physiology of the Eye—Clinical application*, 6th ed, Mosby, St Louis, p. 326

Nickerson, M. and Collier, B. (1975) In Goodman and Gilman's *The Pharmacological Basis of Therapeutics*, 5th ed, Macmillan, New York, pp. 533–564

Nisida, I. P., Okada, H. and Nakano, O. (1960) The activity of the ciliospinal centres and the inhibition in pupillary light reflex. *Jap. J. Physiol.*, **10**, 73–84

Penn, R. G. (1980) *Pharmacology*, 3rd ed, Baillière Tindall, London, pp. 42–79

Ruskell, G. L. (1967) Vasomotor axons of the lacrimal gland of monkeys and the ultrastructural identification of sympathetic terminals. *Z. Zellforsch. microsk. Anat.*, **83**, 321–333

Ruskell, G. L. (1969) Changes in nerve terminals and action of the lacrimal gland and changes in secretion induced by autonomic denervation. *Z. Zellforsch. microsk. Anat.*, **94**, 261–281

Sherrington, C. S. (1893) Further experimental note on the correlation of action of antagonist muscles. *Proc. Roy. Soc., Lond.*, **53**, 407–420

Thomas, R. C. (1972) Electrogenic sodium pump in nerve and muscle cells. *Physiol. Rev.*, **52**, 563–594

Van Alpen, G. W. H. M. (1976) The adrenergic receptors of the intraocular muscles of the human eye. *Invest. Ophthal.*, **15**, 502

Volle, R. L. and Koelle, G. B. (1975) In Goodman and Gilman's *The Pharmacological Basis of Therapeutics*, 5th ed, Macmillan, New York, pp. 565–566

Wolff, E. (1976) *Anatomy of the Eye and Orbit*, 7th ed, Lewis, London, p. 226

Chapter 3

Basic microbiology

An understanding of the basic science of microbiology is essential for the optometrist. It will help him deal with matters such as:

(a) patients with 'red eye';
(b) contact lens solutions and the claims made for them by manufacturers;
(c) preventive measures following contact tonometry and foreign body removal;
(d) the constituents of eye drops and the maintenance of sterility.

The science of microbiology covers organisms invisible to the naked eye. Micro-organisms include protozoa, fungi, bacteria, rickettsia, chlamydia and viruses.

Protozoa and fungi are the only micro-organisms which have eukaryotic cells similar in structure to those of higher organisms. Such cells have inclusions like nuclei and an endoplasmic reticulum. Fungi and protozoa can be either parasitic or free-living. Bacteria are simpler cells (procaryotic cells) but some species are capable of an independent existence. However, many bacteria are parasitic or saprophytic but there are others which can exist in very simple environments. Rickettsia and chlamydiae are more simple and are obligate intracellular parasites. Viruses are the simplest and can only multiply by utilizing the host cell's biochemical systems. Of the above, it is the bacteria that have received most attention.

Bacteria

Bacteria are important because of their ubiquity, the capability of some types to cause disease and their ability to infect and multiply in varied environments such as eyebrows. In order to avoid problems caused by bacteria, it is important to understand something of their structure, growth, environmental and metabolic requirements, classification, relationship with disease and the particular problems they can cause in the eye.

Structure (Figures 3.1 and 3.2)

The cytoplasm of bacterial cells is notable because of the absence of discrete structures normally found in eucaryotic cells. There are no mitochondria; the respiratory enzymes are instead located on the cell membrane.

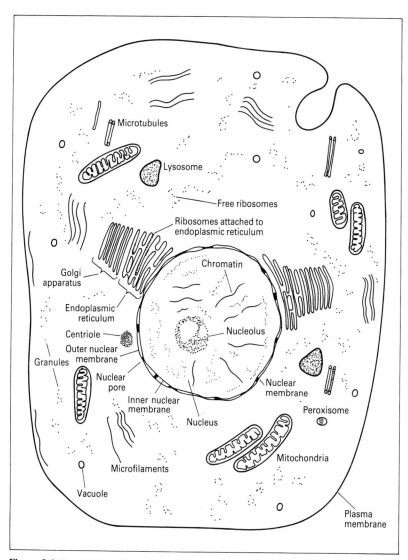

Figure 3.1 Eucaryotic cell

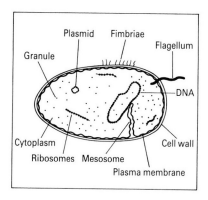

Figure 3.2 Protocaryotic cell

There is no endoplasmic reticulum and the ribosomes are found free in the cytoplasm. There is also no nucleus and no nuclear membrane, and when the cell divides there is no mitosis. Genetic material is carried on a single strand of DNA.

Surrounding the cytoplasm is a thin, selectively permeable, lipoprotein, elastic membrane — the plasma membrane. It is the site of action of many of the bacterial enzymes and controls entry of substances into the cell.

Being elastic, the cell membrane does not determine the shape of the bacterial cell. This is the function of the cell wall, a rigid, permeable structure principally composed of a substance called murein. Because of the osmotic pressure of the cytoplasm, the cell membrane is usually pushed hard against the inside of the cell wall by a pressure of up to 20 atmospheres. The cell wall is relatively thick, especially in Gram positive bacteria.

In some bacteria the cell wall is surrounded by the capsule or slime layer. This is a poorly organized layer of large molecules such as polysaccharides or polypeptides. The effect of this layer is to impede the ingress of substances (useful and harmful) into the cell wall. The result is that the cells tend to grow and divide at a slower rate but are more resistant to antibacterial chemicals, viruses (bacteriophages), phagocytes and other adverse agents. It may also inhibit antibody formation against the bacteria, thereby rendering the bacteria more harmful to the body. Such a bacterium is *Mycobacterium tuberculosum*, the causative organism of tuberculosis.

On the outside of some types of bacteria are found flagella. The number of flagella per cell is constant for each species. Flagella are long filamentous structures containing a contractile protein, flagellin, which is similar to muscle myosin. The presence of flagella normally confers the ability or motion which it is assumed allows the bacterium to migrate to better environments.

Other bacteria have the ability to move without possessing flagella. These are the spiral forms which move by twisting the whole body.

Environmental and metabolic requirements

Bacteria are ubiquitous and can exist in many environments that are far too hostile for the cells of higher organisms. More fastidious bacteria have requirements closer to those of the internal environment of animals and hence are more likely to be parasitic and pathogenic.

Nutritional requirements
All organisms have a requirement for carbon hydrogen, oxygen and nitrogen. Since hydrogen and oxygen can be obtained from water, it is the requirement for the other elements that is most critical. Some bacterial species can obtain their nutrient requirements from inorganic sources. They obtain energy from other sources, e.g. bacterial chlorophyll. Others have the ability to utilize inorganic nitrogen providing they are supplied with an organic source of carbon. Such organisms are found in soil and are responsible for maintaining its fertility.

Others require both organic carbon and nitrogen to survive. Pathogenic bacteria need other complicated growth factors and minerals.

Oxygen requirement
Although oxygen can be obtained from water, some types of bacteria have a need for atmospheric oxygen and cannot exist without it. These bacteria are termed

obligate aerobes. Others are the exact opposite and cannot exist in the presence of oxygen, requiring anaerobic situations. The majority, however, are facultative anaerobes, which means they can exist in either the absence or presence of oxygen.

Physical conditions

For both pH and temperature different bacteria can exist at both high and low extremes. Pathogens prefer the medium state of pH7 and 37°C. Acidophilic bacteria prefer a low pH, while basophiles like a high one. Thermophilic bacteria grow best at between 55 and 80°C, while the spores of *Bacillus stearothermophilus* can withstand boiling. Psychrophilic bacteria grow at 0°C.

Growth

Reproduction of bacteria is by binary fission. The cell divides and two equal daughter cells are formed. As there is no nucleus there is no mitosis. The time between a daughter cell being formed and itself dividing to form two new cells is called the generation time and varies greatly between species. It also varies with environmental conditions and the supply of nutrients. Some bacteria multiply very quickly and divide every 20 minutes. Others, like *M. tuberculosus*, take hours or even days.

When a new sterile environment with finite limits is colonized the bacterial cell population goes through four phases (Figure 3.3):

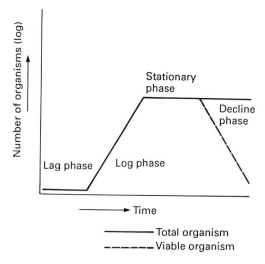

Figure 3.3 Bacterial growth

(a) Lag phase, when the original innoculum remains dormant and no increase in numbers is seen.

(b) Log phase, during which there is an exponential growth in the number of organisms and the logarithm of the number of cells is directly proportional to time. It is during the early stages of this phase that the bacterial population is most susceptible to antibacterial agents.

(c) Stationary phase represents a time when the number of viable organisms remains constant because the number of new organisms is equal to the number dying. This phase can be brought about by a depletion of essential nutrients, a change in the oxygen level or an accumulation of metabolites which regulate the growth.

(d) Decline phase, in which the number of viable organisms declines.

Sporulation
It is the property of certain bacteria to produce endospores. They are produced inside the vegetative cell as compact masses with a very resistant coat. Once formed, the rest of the cell disintegrates releasing the spore.

Spores have the ability to withstand adverse environments which would be lethal to the vegetative cell. When the conditions are right the spore germinates into one vegetative cell (sporulation is not a form of multiplication).

Classification

Once a pure colony of an organism has been isolated by successive culturing, it is often necessary to find out which organism is present. Not only genus and species require elucidation but also the particular strain. To elicit this information the following techniques can be used:

(a) Microscopy and staining;
(b) Differential media and biochemical tests;
(c) Serological testing;
(d) Bacteriophage typing.

Microscopy and differential staining
Gram's stain divides bacteria into Gram positive and Gram negative bacteria. Bacteria are fixed onto a microscopy slide and stained with a dark purple stain. The slide is then covered with an iodine solution to act as a mordant, i.e. to fix the stain onto the organisms. The next step is the decolourizing process in which the slide is treated with a solvent. A counterstain completes the process and the slide is viewed under the microscope. If the organism has resisted decolourization it is termed Gram positive and will appear purple under the microscope. If the original stain has been lost the colour of the counterstain will show through and the organism will be deemed Gram negative. This is a fundamental method of classifying bacteria.

Other differential stains have been used, e.g. acid fast staining, in which the organisms are subjected to a decolourizing process using acid. Specific stains can be used to show the presence of spore-forming bacteria.

Examination under the microscope not only gives information about the organisms' staining characteristics but, of course, about the shape. Basically, bacteria can be spherical (cocci), rod-shaped (bacilli) or spiral. Cocci can be divided according to their form of aggregation. Some bacteria appear in just one direction and form chains (Streptococci) while others give the appearance of a bunch of grapes (Staphylococci). However, the appearance of aggregations under the microscope can sometimes be deceptive and other tests are necessary to differentiate between Streptococci and Staphylococci.

Differential media and biochemical tests
Special media which can be designed to support the growth of some types of bacteria and not others can be useful in bacterial typing. Other tests examine the

organisms's ability to break down hydrogen peroxide, to liquify protein and to ferment certain sugars. Media containing blood are useful in differentiating Streptococci.

Serological testing
Bacteria possess many potentially antigenic substances and one of the body's defences against bacterial invasion is to produce antibodies to these antigens. These antibodies are specific to the antigens and this specificity can assist in the determination not only of the genus and species but also the strain of bacteria present.

Bacteriophage typing
Bacteriophages are viruses that attack bacteria. They invade the bacterial cell just like any other host cell. Once inside they combine with the bacterial DNA and change the genetic material. This effect can be destructive and the whole cell is taken over, producing new phage particles. Bacteriophages are species specific to the bacterium they invade.

Viruses

Viruses are much smaller than bacteria (18–300 nm). All known bacteria will be trapped by a 0.22 μm filter (sterilizing filter). Many viruses will pass through, hence the term filtrable viruses. Viruses can infect any form of higher organism and are usually divided into: animal viruses; plant viruses; and bacteriophages.

Viruses consist of either RNA or DNA (never both), surrounded by a layer of protein or capsid (Figure 3.4). The nucleic acid may be single strand or double strand. They contain few if any enzymes and are entirely reliant on the host cell to bring about replication. They vary greatly in size and in the number of genes they carry (from three to several hundred).

Virus reproduction

Virus reproduction does not take place by binary fission. It generally takes the following pattern:

(a) The virus particle (virion) becomes adsorbed onto the surface of the cell. There are usually specific receptors involved and this leads to the viral preference for certain cells within the host. For example, the HIV (AIDS) virus binds to CD4 receptors which are found on T cells.

(b) The virus particle passes into the cell either with or without its capsid.

(c) The viral RNA (RNA viruses) brings about the production of certain essential enzymes such as RNA-replicase.

(d) These enzymes in turn bring about the production of new nucleic acid and new protein sheaths. The host cell's DNA is unaffected.

(e) Assembly of new virus particles takes place within the host cell and these are then released. The release may bring about disruption of the host cell. The new virus particles are available to infect new cells.

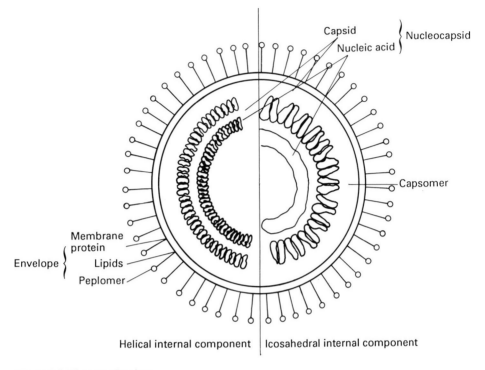

Figure 3.4 Diagram of a virus

Classification of viruses

The classification of viruses is more difficult than that of bacteria. Many criteria are used in classifying viruses.

(a) Morphology
(b) Nucleic acid type
(c) Immunological properties
(d) Transmission methods
(e) Host and cell tropisms
(f) Symptomatology and pathology.

The following are the main groups of animal viruses:

Single strand DNA viruses
    Parvo viruses

Double strand DNA viruses
    Papova viruses, e.g. papilloma (wart virus)
    Adeno viruses, e.g. adeno virus 8 -epidemic
                          keratoconjunctivitis
    Herpes viruses, e.g. Herpes simplex
    Pox viruses

Single strand RNA viruses
  Picorna, e.g. poliomyelitis

Double strand RNA viruses
  Toga viruses, e.g. human respiratory disease
  Arena viruses, e.g. Lassa fever
  Corona viruses, e.g. human respiratory disease
  Retro viruses, e.g. HIV (AIDS)
  Bunya viruses, e.g. insect borne diseases
  Orthomyxo viruses, e.g. influenza
  Paramyxo viruses, e.g. measles, mumps
  Rhabdo viruses, e.g. rabies

Chlamydiae

These organisms are more complex than viruses but less complex than bacteria. They can only multiply in susceptible cells but unlike viruses contain both DNA and RNA. They multiply by binary fission and are susceptible to certain antibiotics.

They exist in two forms: (a) as an elementary body (300 nm) which can exist outside the body and is the infectious unit; and (b) as a reticulate body (1000 nm) which only exists inside the cell and is not infectious.

Chlamydiae attack mucous membranes and inhibit host cell protein synthesis. They rely on the host to provide ATP, which they cannot generate. They synthesize their own nucleic acids and proteins. There are two species, *C. trachomatis* (trachoma, inclusion conjunctivitis) and *C. psittaci* (psittacosis).

Fungi

As causative organisms of disease, fungi are less important than bacteria and viruses. Out of the tens of thousands of species probably only about 100 are pathogenic. Some of these, however, are capable of producing very severe infections as well as the more trivial, such as athlete's foot. Fungi have the ability to colonize non-living structures and lead to spoilation, e.g. contact lenses.

Fungi are composed of eucaryotic cells with the normal inclusions, e.g. a nucleus and mitochondria. They can be divided into four groups according to their structure.

Moulds

These grow as a mycelium, which is composed of filamentous multi-cellular structures called hyphae. The mycelium is divided into the vegetative mycelium, which grows into the substrate and assimilates nutrients, and the aerial mycelium, which produces the spores either asexually by budding or sexually by the fusion of two cells.

Yeasts

These fungi occur as single cells and reproduce by budding.

Yeast-like fungi

Both hyphae and yeast cells exist together.

Dimorphic fungi

Dimorphic fungi exist either as yeasts or filaments. If they are grown on artificial media they appear as hyphae. When they inhabit a living host they occur as yeast cells.

Micro-organisms and disease

The human plays host to a large number of bacteria which normally do no harm and to varying degrees contribute to the body's well-being. For example, bacteria live on the dead surface of the skin and prevent other more potentially dangerous organisms from occupying the site. In the gut, bacteria in exchange for nutrients provide the body with vitamin K essential for the production of prothrombin. These commensal organisms only maintain this mutually advantageous relationship providing they remain in their proper place. One tissue's commensal is another's pathogen.

It is not always the micro-organism itself that causes the harm, but substances that the organism produces. Some bacteria live and multiply in food, producing toxins as they do so. When the food is ingested the toxins produce adverse effects. *Clostridium botulinum* is such an organism and the toxin it produces, botulinum toxin, is fatal in minute quantities. *Staphylococcus aureus* is also capable of bringing about food intoxication.

Most micro-organisms, however, cause disease by acting as parasites on the body, gaining access by a variety of routes.

Direct contact. This normally means sexual contact and the disease is classed as a venereal one. This method of transmission favours the very fastidious bacteria which exist only with difficulty outside the human body. *Treponema pallidum* (syphilis) is so fastidious that it cannot be grown on lifeless media.

Indirect transmission. Infection is passed from one person to another by an inanimate object (fomite), e.g. bedclothes, used dressings, etc.

Dust-borne infection. Dust contains discarded human cells and dried water droplets. These are likely to carry bacteria, especially spores.

Droplet infection. Bacteria are present in the fine spray that is exhaled with forced expirations such as coughing and sneezing.

Water borne infection. Water is an excellent medium for transmitting infection. Public health and sanitation prevent this until a disaster interrupts the supply of clean drinking water.

Insect borne infection. Biting and sucking insects have the ability to take organisms from an infected host and transfer them to a new one.

Maternal transmission. In addition to the route mentioned above, infections can also be passed from mother to child either while the child is still in the womb or during birth.

Microbiology of the eye

The eye is at risk from infection by opportunistic and invasive organisms via a variety of routes. In addition to congenital ocular infections, micro-organisms can gain access as a result of:

(a) Direct contact e.g. Herpes simplex;
(b) Airborne infections;
(c) Insect-borne infections, e.g. trachoma;
(d) Migration of bacteria from the nasopharynx;
(e) Metastatic infection from other loci in the body;
(f) Trauma, especially penetrating injuries;
(g) Infected contact lenses;
(h) Infected eyedrops and lotions;
(i) Infected instruments.

Obviously the lids, cornea and conjunctiva are the most exposed and hence the most at risk from infection. Infections of these tissues are far more common than those of deeper tissues. They are also less serious.

The eye is covered with a medium which contains a number of antimicrobial agents in order to reduce the incidence of infections. The result is a fairly low level of microbial contamination in the fornices. Tears contain immunoglobulins A, G and M (IgA, IgG and IgM) (Reim, 1985) in different proportions to those found in plasma, suggesting that their origin is secretory rather than just the result of filtration.

There are also two agents with marked antibacterial properties, lysozyme and beta-lysin.

Lysozyme is an enzyme capable of dissolving the cell wall of bacteria, especially Gram positive bacteria. The level of lysozyme decreases with age and is reduced in patients with dry eye syndrome (Mackie and Seal, 1976). Beta-lysin, on the other hand, acts principally on the cell membrane (Ford, Delarge and Petty, 1976) and works in concert with lysozyme. Since the cell membrane is the site of action of the bacterial enzymes, the effect is quite marked. Beta-lysin is also present in aqueous humour.

Some common ocular pathogens

Gram positive cocci

Staphylococcus aureus
Some Staphylococci are normal inhabitants of the skin and mucous membranes, whilst other species are capable of producing conditions such as boils, abscesses and even a fatal septicaemia. They are capable of bringing about a form of food poisoning by the liberation of an enterotoxin. Resistance to certain antibiotics develops easily and the term 'hospital Staph' is applied to some resistant forms.

Staphylococci are differentiated from Streptococci by the presence of an enzyme capable of breaking down hydrogen peroxide (catalase). Pathogenic Staphylococci possess coagulase, which clots blood plasma.

In the eye Staphylococci can cause infections of the lids, lacrimal apparatus, conjunctiva and cornea (Davis, Sarff and Hyndiuk, 1978). Infections of the lash follicle lead to the formation of a stye (hordeolum). Staphylococci can also produce acute or chronic blepharitis. This is sometimes associated with acute conjunctivitis (Brook, 1980; Brook *et al.*, 1979; Brown, 1978). This organism has also been found to be present in a large number of cases of ophthalmia neonatorum in one study (Jarvis, Levine and Askell, 1987). Following septicaemia Staphylococci have caused endophthalmitis (Bloomfield *et al.*, 1978).

Because *Staphylococcus aureus* is so common, it is often employed in the efficiency testing of preservative systems. *Staphylococcus epidermis* is normally considered to be a commensal and is a normal inhabitant of the skin. Unlike *Staph. aureus* it produces white colonies. Maske, Hill and Oliver (1986) found a higher than normal incidence in a group of patients with bacterial corneal ulcers. It has been suggested that *Staph. epidermis* releases a toxin to cause some of the signs of blepharitis and keratophy (McGill *et al.*, 1982).

Streptococci
Streptococci lack the enzyme catalase and are characterized by their ability to cause haemolysis. Complete haemolysis is brought about by beta-haemolytic Streptococci while the haemolysis produced by alpha-haemolytic species is incomplete and leads to the formation of a green pigment. There are also non-haemolytic Streptococci.

Streptococci are capable of producing local and general infections. One of the most common local infections of beta-haemolytic Streptococci is the Streptococcal sore throat which in young children can extend into the middle ear to cause otitis media. On the skin they can cause impetigo.

Beta-haemolytic Strept. infections give rise to puerperal fever, wound sepsis and endocarditis. It is fortunate that penicillin continues to be effective against many strains of Streptococci.

In the eye, infections may cause conjunctivitis, dacryoadenitis, dacryocystitis and blepharitis (Brook, 1980).

Gram negative cocci

Neisseriae
The Neisseriae are a group of Gram negative bacteria which include the normal flora of the respiratory system and the pathogens which cause meningitis (*N. meningitidis*), and gonorrhoea (*N. gonorrhoeae*).

In the eye Neisseriae can infect the lids, lacrimal apparatus and conjunctiva but *N. gonorrhoea* is best known as the one-time principal cause of ophthalmia neonatorum, an infection which occurs as the infant passes down the birth canal. The disease becomes manifest between the second and fifth day after birth. The lids become swollen and there is a bilaterial purulent discharge. The lids are tightly closed and difficult to open and the acute phase lasts for 4–6 weeks. The condition is treated with topical and systemic antibacterials. If treatment is not carried out, the cornea may become involved and the eye lost. However other causative organisms and causes are more important today (Jarvis, Levine and Asbell, 1987).

Gram positive rods

Corynebacterium diphtheriae

Corynebacteria are non-motile Gram positive rods which do not form spores. Species are found normally resident in the human respiratory tract. *C. diphtheriae* when infected with the appropriate bacteriophage produces a powerful exotoxin which causes the pathology of diphtheria. The disease results in the growth of a membrane across the throat, leading to suffocation. It can similarly affect the eyelids, with the appearance of such membranes on the inner surface of the lids. The conjunctiva may become involved in the same way. Diphtheroids have been isolated in a proportion of infected conjunctivae (Brooke *et al.*, 1979; Brown *et al.*, 1978).

Clostridia spp.

The Clostridia are a group of obligate anaerobes notorious for their pathogenicity. In particular, they include *Cl. botulinum*, which when it infects food produces botulinum toxin. Although botulinum toxin ingestion is potentially fatal, this substance has been used to paralyse the antagonist muscles in cases of paralytic strabismus (Cole and Lee, 1985; Elston and Lee, 1985) and other ocular disorders (Alpar, 1987). *Cl. tetani* is a possible infectant of deep wounds and prophylaxis against the effects of its toxin is routine. Other Clostridia such as *Cl. perfringens*, *Cl. welchii* and *Cl. oedematiens* cause gangrene. Gas gangrene of the lids has been reported (Crock *et al.*, 1985).

Gram negative rods

This is by far the biggest group of pathogens, most of which are facultative anaerobes.

Pseudomonas aeruginosa

Pseudomonas aeruginosa is perhaps the most notorious of bacteria for causing ocular problems and is normally found in small numbers in the gut and on the skin. It is a common contaminant of water and has been cultured from jacuzzis (Brett 1985). Its numbers are kept in check by the presence of other organisms, but since it is resistant to many antibiotics it can gain dominance if the surrounding organisms are suppressed. *Pseudomonas aeruginosa* produces a bluish green colour when grown on media with a characteristic odour, and is pyogenic, the presence of green pus suggesting the presence of a *Pseudomonas* infection.

Pseudomonas aeruginosa is an opportunistic organism and is normally kept at bay by the body's defence mechanisms. Once these are breached a serious infection often results. It can infect burns, especially if of large area, and can also gain hold in patients who are immuno-compromised.

Ps. aeruginosa is an extremely versatile organism in that it can metabolize fluorescein and hydroxybenzoates as carbon sources for energy, which means that it can survive in conditions which are alien to most other organisms. This organism is only susceptible to antibiotics such as gentamicin and polymixin.

In the eye, *Ps. aeruginosa* can produce meibomitis, conjunctivitis and corneal ulcers and is one of the causes of ophthalmia neonatorum (Cole, Davies and Austin, 1980). Should access be gained to the sterile interior of the eye, then panophthalmitis may result and indeed has been responsible for causing more than one serious case of hospital acquired disease leading to the loss of an eye (Crompton, 1978). It is an important test organism for contact lens solutions and eyedrop preservative systems.

Haemophilus spp.

These are small aerobic organisms which get their name from their requirement for enriched media containing blood for culturing *in vitro*. They include certain important human pathogenic organisms. *H. influenzae* is a secondary invader which helps to produce some of the symptoms of influenza and can produce inflammation in most parts of the respiratory tract. *Bordetella pertussis* is another of this group to affect the respiratory system, causing whooping cough which is transmitted by airborne infections from one person to another. It cannot exist for long periods outside the body. Similarly, *H. ducreyi* is so fastidious in its requirements that it can only be transmitted sexually and consequently is the causative organism of chancroid, a form of venereal disease.

   H. influenzae and *H. ducreyi* are capable of infecting ocular tissues. There are two members of this group which are particularly noted for their ability to cause conjunctivitis. *H. aegyptius* (*H. conjunctivitidis*, Koch–Weeks bacillus) is often the cause of acute epidemic conjunctivitis, especially in school children. *Moraxella lacunata* (Morax–Axenfeld bacillus) is another well-known causative organism of conjunctivitis.

Viruses

Herpes viruses

The most important members of the Herpes group as far as the eye is concerned are H. zoster, H. simplex and Cytomegalovirus.

   H. zoster (varicella) virus leads to chickenpox in children. This is a mild highly contagious disease characterized by a vesicular rash. The disease leaves the patient with a continuing immunity to the disease. In the adult a reactivation of the virus leads to shingles, in which an area of the body becomes covered with a painful rash. Evidently the virus becomes stored in a sensory ganglion, the attack being caused by a migration of the virus along the nerve root. When the nerve affected is the ophthalmic division of the trigeminal nerve, the area served by it exhibits signs, i.e. the eye, the orbit and surrounding areas. This is known as Herpes zoster ophthalmicus, in which the cornea becomes inflamed and oedematous, and sensitivity may be impaired permanently. Secondary infection can occur, leading to ulceration and scarring.

   Herpes simplex can be differentiated into Types I and II. Type II is associated with genital herpes and neonatal herpes. Transplacental infection with Type II virus has led to the development of neonatal cataract (Cibis and Burge, 1971). Type I causes cold sores, inflammation of the oral cavity, encephalitis and dendritic ulcers.

   Dendritic ulcers are so called because of their branching pattern. As the ulcer extends it may lose this appearance and become amoeboid or geographic. The patient complains of pain, photophobia, blurring of vision and a watery discharge (unlike that from bacterial conjunctivitis). In the early stages infection only affects the epithelium, later progressing to the superficial stroma. The cornea becomes oedematous and there is further loss of stroma and possible vascularization.

The condition is treated with intense local anti-viral therapy. Herpes simplex can also produce a keratoconjunctivitis similar to that caused by adenovirus 8 (Darougar *et al.*, 1978) (see below).

The third virus in this group is Cytomegalovirus, which normally inhabits the female reproductive tract giving rise to congenital infections. Congenital infections can give rise to chorioretinitis, optic atrophy and cataract.

Adenovirus 8

Adenovirus 8 gives rise to epidemic kerato-conjunctivitis sometimes called 'eye hospital eye' because of its possible transmission by contaminated instruments. The infection produces severe acute conjunctivitis, which can spread leading to keratitis. Marked discomfort can last for months. Adenovirus was the cause of 8% of cases of acute conjunctivitis in one study (Wishart *et al.*, 1984).

Pox viruses

This group of viruses includes smallpox and cowpox. There is a relatively uncommon skin condition affecting young adults and children, Molluscum contagiosum, which is caused by a pox virus. Transparent nodules (2–3 mm in diameter) appear on the skin of the arm, legs, back and face, with possible involvement of the lid margins and conjunctiva. This condition is sometimes seen in patients with AIDS and AIDS-related complex (ARC).

Toga viruses

The best known member of this group is rubella (German measles), which can be passed from mother to baby in the uterus, leading to congenital defects in 30% of the children of mothers suffering rubella in the first trimester of pregnancy. Particularly affected are the heart, ears and eyes. Ophthalmic defects lead to microphthalmia, cataracts and congenital glaucoma.

Retroviruses

The Human Immunodeficiency Virus (HIV) is present in many of the body fluids of affected individuals, including tears. Although there has been no recorded case of transmission via infected contact lenses, it has become a point of concern of contact lens practitioners. The virus has also been recovered from contact lenses worn by patients with AIDS and ARC (AIDS related complex) (Tervo *et al.*, 1986).

AIDS can have certain ocular manifestations, partially because the patients are from the very nature of the disease more likely to develop opportunistic infections such as Cytomegalovirus retinitis. Conjunctival Kaposi's sarcoma is another ocular complication (Kanski, 1987).

Fungi

Candida albicans

This is a dimorphic opportunistic fungus which is normally found in the mucous membranes of the mouth, vagina, gut and eye (Liotet *et al.*, 1980). It causes oral thrush in newborn infants and terminally ill patients. In the eye it can cause corneal ulcers, conjunctivitis and severe uveitis.

Aspergillus niger
This fungus, which is not dimorphic, grows in the form of mycelia. Often found in vegetable matter, it can cause bronchial problems. This fungus is also capable of producing severe local infection in the eye, especially following the injudicious use of local corticosteroids, which tend to mask the clinical signs of the infection, allowing it to get a stronger foothold. *A. niger*, which also can be found in the healthy eye (Liotet *et al.*, 1980), has the ability to infect contact lenses and destroy them. Other species of *Aspergillus* have been implicated in contact lens contamination. For example, Yamaguchi (1984) reported growth on contact lens of *A. flavus* and Filppi, Pfister and Hill (1973) found that *A. fumagatus* penetrated soft contact lenses. Aspergillus species are not the only ones to infect contact lenses. Yamamoto *et al.* (1979) found *Cephalosporium acremonium* growing on a contact lens worn for the treatment of metaherpetic keratitis.

Chlamydia

Trachoma (C. trachomatis)
Trachoma affects a large proportion of the world's population, being endemic in many areas. Where it is endemic, it affects over 90% of the population. Associated with poor living conditions, this organism is passed on by insects and contaminated objects such as bedclothes. It is sometimes a resident of the female genital tract (Barton *et al.*, 1989) and can produce a form of ophthalmia neonatorum (Markham, 1979). The incidence of Chlamydial ophthalmia neonatorum varies. In one study in America, 1.4% of all newborn babies acquired chlamydial conjunctivitis (Schacter *et al.*, 1979) and similar findings were reported in Sweden (Persson *et al.*, 1983). This condition starts as a mild inflammation of the conjunctiva with the development of small follicles which become larger. The cornea is invaded and vascularized, resulting in pannus which can lead to severe scarring and contraction which causes deformity of eyelids. Symblepharon and trichiasis are also seen.

In temperate climates, the organism results in inclusion conjunctivitis.

Amoebae

As well as the free living forms that are studied by every student of biology, Amoebae have been known for a long time as disease causing organisms. *Entamoeba histolytica* is the causative organism of amoebic dysentery. Amoebic keratitis has been reported as a result of infection with *Acanthamoebae* (Moore *et al.*, 1986). The patients in the report were myopes corrected with soft contact lenses who had used salt tablets dissolved in distilled water during disinfection procedures. This infection has so far proved to be difficult to treat.

Antimicrobial agents

There are many 'agents' which have the ability to kill or inactivate microorganisms. Within this broad term we encompass the body's defence mechanisms, i.e. the white blood cells and circulating antibodies of the blood, the gastric hydrochloric acid and the lyzosyme and beta-lysin of tears, whilst other microorganisms such as bacteriophages must also be considered as antimicrobial agents. Here we are concerned with three basic groups:

(a) Physical agents capable of rendering objects and chemicals free of contamination.

(b) Antimicrobial preservatives which are incorporated into solutions to maintain sterility.

(c) Chemotherapeutic agents used either to treat or prevent an infection in the body.

It is important to define certain terms which are relevant to this subject and are sometimes used incorrectly.

Sterilization means the killing or removal of all viable organisms (including bacterial spores) from an object or pharmaceutical product by the use of chemical or physical agents.

Disinfection is a lesser process by which the capacity of an object to cause infection is removed. A disinfected product may not be 'sterile'. *Antisepsis* is a similar degree of decontamination, but refers to solutions and chemicals that are safe to apply to surfaces of the body.

Chemotherapeutic agents are described as bacteriocidal or bacteriostatic; the former are actually capable of killing the bacteria (although not necessarily bacterial spores) while bacteriostatic agents prevent bacteria from growing and rely on the body's own defence mechanism to get rid of the organisms.

Physical agents

All physical agents are forms of energy and the antimicrobial action is dependent on supplying sufficient to cause disruption to the cell. Bacteria and other micro-organisms are far more resistant to adverse situations than animal cells and can withstand environments which would be quickly lethal to us. The effect of antimicrobial agents follows a first order reaction in which the log number of survivors is inversely proportional to the time. The time for 1 log cycle reduction, i.e. the time taken for 90% of the bacteria to be killed, is called the D value or decimal death time, this value reducing as the antimicrobial effect of the antimicrobial increases.

Heat

Heat is one of the best known sterilizing agents. It is used for sterilizing solutions (providing that the substances are thermostable), dressings and some instruments. The effectiveness of heat is increased by the presence of water, especially if the pH is raised, the use of moist heat bringing hydrolysis to bear on the organisms as well as pyrolysis.

Temperatures of around 60°C will kill most viruses as well as the vegetative cells of pathogenic bacteria and fungi, whereas boiling brings about the demise of spores of pathogenic bacteria.

However, there are organisms whose spores will withstand boiling for lengthy periods. Therefore to obtain sterility without compromising the product, autoclaves are used. These work on the 'pressure cooker' principle by heating the product in steam (not air) to a defined temperature and specified time, which is usually 121°C for 15 minutes.

The use of dry heat is far less efficient and temperatures of up to 160°C for 1 hour are needed to kill spores.

Disinfection, as opposed to sterilization, can be brought about by boiling for 10–15 minutes.

Temperatures below boiling can reduce the number of micro-organisms present and are used for materials which cannot withstand heating at high temperatures. Milk is pasteurized at 60–70°C for example. The temperature inside a soft lens storage case, subjected to heating by steam, will not reach boiling but the temperature attained (95°C) is very bacteriocidal. Thermal disinfection of contact lenses is discussed in Chapter 12. With the current concern over AIDS, it is comforting to know that the causative virus is killed at 60°C.

Freezing
Freezing the cultures of bacteria will markedly reduce the number of bacteria, as a proportion may be damaged by the formation of ice crystals, but the rest will survive in a dormant state even at temperatures as low as that of liquid nitrogen. Indeed this process is used to store cultures of bacteria.

Ionizing radiation
This technique is used for disposable plastic items and for paper products like Fluorets. All types of rays are lethal to micro-organisms (alpha, beta, and gamma rays). Usually it is gamma rays that are used at a dosage of 2.5–3.5 MRad.

Ultraviolet radiation
Light is only markedly bacteriocidal at low wavelengths (240–280 nm — the UVC region) and at this level it does not penetrate well, making it suitable only for surface and aerial disinfection.

Filtration
Solutions of thermolabile drugs can be sterilized by passing the solution through a 0.22 μm filter which retains all bacteria (the smallest bacterium is about 0.5 μm). The filters, which are sterilized before use, will not remove viral contamination.

Ultrasonics
Sound will kill bacteria but high power inputs are required. Ultrasonic cleaners with antibacterial cleaners have been used on contact lenses. Studies on the antimicrobial effectiveness of such devices have yet to be published.

Antimicrobial preservatives

There are a whole range of substances incorporated into products to prevent the growth of micro-organisms. These are used in foods and drinks and cosmetics but are most important in multi-dose sterile pharmaceutical solutions to ensure that the product is protected from microbial attack while it is in use.

These compounds are selected for their ability to kill or inhibit the growth of micro-organisms, particularly bacteria and fungi. The rate of kill represented by the D value is dependent upon the concentration of the preservative, but is not always a simple inverse relationship, i.e. with the D value inversely proportional to the concentration of the preservative compound. With some compounds the effect is exponential, with a reduction of concentration to half of the original leading to an increase in D value of a factor of 2^8 or 256. Such compounds are thus quickly inactivated by dilution.

These agents are capable of producing damage to human cells, and it is necessary to use them in as low a concentration as possible to reduce toxicity, the final concentration therefore representing a compromise between safety and efficacy. In order to achieve greater efficacy without increasing the toxic effects, mixtures of preservatives are often used.

Many such agents have been used in the past; the following are those in common use.

Benzalkonium chloride
Benzalkonium chloride has a detergent action which causes disruption of the cell membrane, and it is by far the most commonly used preservative for eye drops. Benzalkonium chloride has a disruptive effect on the tear film when used in concentrations of 0.01% and greater (Wilson, Duncan and Jay, 1975). This preservative is often found combined with EDTA (ethylene diamine tetra acetic acid, sodium edetate). EDTA is a chelating agent which combines with divalent ions (normally calcium) to form a non-ionizable complex. This agent has a slight antibacterial action of its own but is principally used to enhance the bacteriocidal action of benzalkonium chloride.

Mercury compounds
Mercurial compounds include thiomersal and phenylmercuric nitrate. They produce mercury ions which react with sulphydryl groups of essential enzymes. They are slower in action against certain organisms but are less quickly inactivated by dilution than other compounds. Unlike benzalkonium chloride, mercury compounds are not potentiated by the addition of EDTA (Richards and Reary, 1972). In fact, Morton (1985) found that EDTA actually reduces the antimicrobial efficacy of thiomersal. Significant penetration of mercury-containing compounds into the aqueous humour following their use has been recorded by Winder *et al.* (1980). These compounds have been demonstrated to have cytotoxic effects which are time and concentration dependent (Takahashi, 1982), but which are less than those of benzalkonium chloride (Gasset, 1974), and their use in many contact lens solutions has led to the increasing incidence of allergic reactions (Gold, 1983).

Chlorhexidine gluconate
Chlorhexidine is a useful alternative to benzalkonium chloride and is used when the latter is incompatible with the active ingredient. It is very toxic to the endothelium of the cornea in concentrations of 20 μg/ml and if the epithelium is perfused the result is a sloughing of the cells without corneal swelling (Green *et al.*, 1980).

Other compounds
Other compounds that have been used include chlorbutol, cetrimide, phenylethanol, hydroxybenzoates and chlorocresol.

Chemotherapeutic agents

The treatment of infections has evolved somewhat since the treatment of syphilis with mercurial compounds. Developments have led to the introduction of agents which are more effective against the infecting organism and less toxic to the host. Agents to treat infections which are used routinely in ophthalmology are discussed in Chapter 15.

Anti-infectives tend to be specific against groups of organisms, e.g. antibacterials, antifungals, although there is some overlap. Certain antibacterials are effective against chlamydiae.

The mode of action of antibacterial agents varies greatly. Some agents cause disruption to the cell wall, leaving the protoplast at the mercy of phagocytes and to osmotic lysis. The mode of action of penicillin is to prevent the building of the cell wall.

Sulphonamides produce their action by acting as false substrates, interfering with the uptake of essential metabolites.

Many antibiotics work by gene function suppression, interfering with the production of enzymes and other essential proteins.

The administration of antimicrobial agents for the treatment of infection requires the achievement of adequate levels of the antimicrobial agent as quickly as possible. Many antibacterials compete for sites with other compounds. The higher the concentration of the agent the greater will be the effect on the organism.

Failure to achieve these levels may lead to the development of resistant strains. In any population there will be a proportion of organisms which are resistant to the agent. In the presence of the agent these will be selected and will form the majority of the population.

Some bacteria develop resistance by altering their metabolic pathways to avoid those with which the antimicrobial interacts. Other bacteria produce enzymes capable of destroying the chemical, e.g. penicillinase, which is an enzyme produced by certain strains of Staphylococci and is capable of breaking down penicillin.

Hygiene in practice

Whilst there has been no recorded case of a patient contracting AIDS from a contaminated contact lens, this condition has highlighted the necessity for good practice hygiene. The AIDS virus is not the only organism (opportunist or invasive) that could be transmitted in an optometrist's practice and simple disinfection procedures should be employed in order to protect both practitioner and patient.

The first consideration is one of cleanliness, since clean objects and surfaces are easier to disinfect and will remain uncontaminated for longer. Normal contaminants will harbour bacteria, protect them from antibacterial agents, provide them with nutrients and inactivate disinfectants.

Jacobs (1986) has laid down simple infection control guidelines for optometrists and contact lens practitioners. Basically, anything that can be boiled without adversely affecting its performance should be, e.g. bowls, soft contact lenses. Items of equipment that will touch the eye should be swabbed with 70% alcohol, e.g. tonometer heads, chin rests, trial frames. Working surfaces should be treated with 1% sodium hypochlorite solution, which is effective against bacteria and viruses. At levels as low as 500 ppm (0.05%) it destroys Herpes simplex, Adenovirus 8 and Enterovirus 70 within 10 minutes (Naginton, Satehall and Whipps, 1983). Such procedures will protect the patient more than will a prophylactic eye drop.

In the interests of self protection the practitioner should have no open cuts uncovered, but the added precaution of wearing gloves is only necessary for high risk patients, e.g. patients who are HIV positive.

References

Alpar, A. I. (1987) Botulinum toxin and its uses in the treatment of ocular disorders. *Am. J. Optometry Physiol. Optics*, **64**, 79–82

Barton, S. E., Thomas, B. J., Taylor-Robinson, D. and Goldmeier, D. (1985) Detection of *Chlamydia trachomatis* in the vaginal vault of women who have had hysterectomies. *Br. Med. J.*, **27**, 250

Bloomfield, S. E., David, D. S., Cheigh, J. S., Kim, Y., White, R. P., Stengel, K. H. and Rubin, A. L. (1978) Endophthalmitis following staphylococcal sepsis in renal failure patients. *Arch. Int. Med.*, **138**, 706–708

Brett, J. (1985) Pseudomonas aeruginosa and whirlpools. *Br. Med. J.*, **April 6**, 1024–1025

Brook, I. (1980) Anaerobic and aerobic bacterial flora of acute conjunctivitis in children. *Arch. Ophthalmol.*, **98**, 833–835,

Brook, I. Pettit, T. H., Martin, W. J. and Finegold, S. M. (1979) Anaerobic and aerobic bacteriology of acute conjunctivitis. *Ann. Ophthalmol.*, **11**, 389–393

Brown, D. H. (1978) The conjunctival flora of nursing home patients and staff. *Ann. Ophthalmol.*, **10**, 333–334

Cibis, A. and Burge, R. M. (1971) Herpes simplex virus induced cataracts. *Arch. Ophthalmol.*, **85**, 220–223

Cole, G. F., Davies, D. P. and Austin D. J. (1980) Pseudomonas ophthalmia neonatorum: a cause of blindness. *Br. Med. J.*, **August 9**, 440–441

Crock, G. W., Heriot, W. J., Janakiraman, P. and Weiner, J. M. (1985) Gas gangrene infection of the eye and orbit. *Br. J. Ophthalmol.*, **69**, 143–148

Crompton, D. O. (1978) Medical ethics and hospital-acquired disease. *Lancet*, **July 15**, 146

Darougar, S., Hunter, P. A., Viswalingam, M., Gibson, J. A., and Jones, B. R. (1978) Acute follicular conjunctivitis and keratoconjunctivitis due to Herpes simplex virus in London. *Br. J. Ophthalmol.*, **62**, 843–849

Davis, S. D. Sarff, L. D. and Hyndiuk, R. A. (1978) Staphylococcal keratitis. *Arch. Ophthalmol.*, **96**, 2114–2116

Elston, J. S. and Lee, J. P. (1985) Paralytic strabismus: the role of botulinum toxin. *Br. J. Ophthalmol.*, **69**, 891–896

Filppi, J. A., Pfister, R. M. and Hill, R. M. (1973) Penetration of hydrophilic contact lenses by *Aspergillus Fumagatus*. *Am. J. Optometry Physiol. Optics*, **50**, 553–557

Ford, L. C., DeLange, R. J. and Petty, R. W. (1976). Identification of a nonlysozymal bacteriocidal factor (beta lysin) in human tears and aqueous humour. *Am. J. Ophthalmol.*, **81**, 30–33

Gasset, A. R., Ishii, Y., Kaufman, H. E. and Miller, l. (1974) Cytotoxicity of ophthalmic preservatives. *Am. J. Ophthalmol.*, **78**, 98–105

Gold, R. M. (1983) The war on thiomersal. *Contemporary Optometry*, **2**, 7–10

Green, K., Livingston, V., Bowman, K. and Hull, D. S. (1980) Chlorhexidine effects on corneal epithelium and endothelium. *Arch. Ophthalmol.*, **98**, 1273–1278

Jarvis, V. N., Levine, R., and Asbell, P. A. (1987) Ophthalmia neonatorum. Study of a decade of experience at the Mount Sinai Hospital. *Br. J. Ophthalmol.*, **71**, 295–300

Jacobs, R. J. (1986) Infection control guidelines for optometrists and contact lens practitioners. *Clin. Exp. Optometry*, **69/2**, 40–45

Kanski, J. J. (1987) Ocular manifestation of AIDS. *The Optician*, **2 March**, 24–25

Liotet, S., Krzywkowski, J. C., Warret, V. N. and Jacqui, C. (1980) Conjunctival flora of healthy people. *J. Francais Ophthalmol.*, **103**, 557–560

Mackie, I. A. and Seal, D. V. (1976) Quantitative tear lysozyme essay in units of activity per microlitre. *Br. J. Ophthalmol.*, **60**, 70–74

Markham, J. G. (1979) Genital tract to eye infection — tissue culture of *Chlamydia trachomatis*. *NZ Med. J.*, **90**, 186–188.

Maske, R., Hill, J. C. and Oliver, S. P. (1986) Management of bacterial corneal ulcers. *Br. J. Ophthalmol.*, **70**, 199–201

Moore, M. B., McCulley, J. P., Kaufman, H. E. and Robin, J. B. (1986) Radial keratoneuritis as a presenting sign in acanthamoeba keratitis. *Ophthalmology*, **93**, 1310–1315

Morton, D. J. (1985) EDTA reduces the antimicrobial efficacy of thiomersal. *Int. J. Pharm.*, **23**, 357–358

McGill, J., Goulding, N. J., Liakos, G., Jacobs, P. and Seal, D. V. (1982) Pathophysiology of bacterial infection in the external eye. *Transact. Ophthalmol. Soc. UK*, **102**, 7–10

Naginton, J., Sutehall, G. M. and Whipp, A. (1983) Tonometer disinfection and viruses. *Br. J. Ophthalmol.*, **67**, 674–676

Persson, K., Ronnerstam, R., Svanberg, L. and Pohla, M-A. (1983) Neonatal chlamydial eye infection: an epidemiological and clinical study. *Br. J. Ophthalmol.*, **67**, 700–704

Reim, M. (1983) Normal and pathological components of tears and conjunctival secretion. *The Ophthalmic Optician*, **May 21**, 346–350

Richards, R. M. E. and Reary, J. M. E. (1972) Changes in antibacterial activity of thiomersal and PMN on autoclaving with certain adjuvants. *J. Pharm. Pharmacol.*, **24**, 84P–85P

Schacter, J., Holt, J., Goodmer, E., Grossman, M., Sweet, R. and Mills, J. (1979). Prospective study of chlamydial infection in neonates. *Lancet*, **August 25**, 377–379

Takahashi, N. (1982) Cytotoxicity of mercurial preservatives in cell culture. *Ophthalmic Research*, **14**, 63–69

Tervo, T., Lahdevirto, J., Vaheria, A., Valle, S. L. and Suni, J. (1986) Recovery of HTLV-III from contact lenses. *Lancet*, **February 15**, 379–380

Wilson, W. S., Duncan, A. J. and Jay, J. (1975) Effect of benzalkonium chloride on the stability of the precorneal tear film in rabbit and man. *Br. J. Ophthalmol.*, **59**, 667–669

Winder, A. F., Astbury, N. J., Sheraidah, G. A. K. and Ruben, M. (1980) Penetration of mercury from ophthalmic preservatives into the human eye. *Lancet*, **2**, 237–239

Wishart, P. K., James, C., Wishart, M. S. and Darougar, S. (1984) Prevalence of acute conjunctivtis caused by chlamydia adenovirus, and Herpes simplex virus in an ophthalmic casualty department. *Br. J. Ophthalmol.*, **68**, 653–655

Yamaguchi, T. (1984) Fungus growth on soft contact lenses with different water contents. *Contact Lens J.*, **10**, 166–171

Yamamoto, G. K., Pavan-Langston, D., Stowe, G. C. and Albert, D. M. (1979) Fungal invasion of a therapeutic soft contact lens and cornea. *Ann. Ophthalmol.*, **11**, 1731–1735

Further reading

Coster, D. J. (1979) Treacher Collins Prize Essay. Inflammatory diseases of the outer eye. Transactions of the Ophthalmological Societies of the United Kingdom, **99**, 463–480

Coster, D. J. (1978) Herpetic keratitis and corneal destruction. Transactions of the Ophthalmological Societies of the United Kingdom, **98**, 372–376.

Chapter 4

Introduction to ophthalmic drugs

Drugs will only produce their desired action if they are present at the site of action in sufficient quantities, and the design and choice of the route of administration must take this into account. Certain parts of the eye are more accessible to drugs given by one route than they would be by another. Drugs also vary in their ability to cross capillary and mucous membrane barriers.

Basically, there are three routes by which drugs can be administered to the eye.

Direct injection

This can be either periocular (subconjunctival or retrobulbar) or intravitreal. These routes are used when relatively large doses of drug are required at a site very quickly. Antibiotics such as gentamicin are poorly absorbed and for deep infections intravitreal injection may be the only possible route.

In the treatment of serious corneal and anterior segment infections, subconjunctival injections of 500 000 units or more of crystalline penicillin with adrenaline may be repeated every 3 hours. In desperate cases of intro-ocular suppuration an absolutely pure penicillin solution injection may be given directly into the anterior chamber or the vitreous (Miller, 1978). A Tenon's capsule injection should result in more effective penetration of the drug than a subconjunctival one in Havener's opinion (1978).

Local anaesthesia of the eye may be produced by retrobulbar injection of local anaesthetics.

Systemic administration

This route makes use of the ocular blood supply to carry drugs to the eye (see Plate III). While some parts of the eye are richly supplied with blood vessels, others are not. The systemic route, of course, means that the rest of the body receives a dose of the drug which may not be desirable. Drugs may gain access to the systemic blood supply by a variety of routes but for opthalmic treatment, they are given either orally or parenterally. Acetazolamide (a diuretic for the treatment of glaucoma) is not effective topically and is administered as tablets for the emergency treatment of chronic open angle glaucoma or by injection for the emergency treatment of closed angle glaucoma. Antibiotics are sometimes given orally to supplement their topical use. Fluorescein is injected intravenously for diagnostic purposes in fluorescein angiography.

Topical application

This is by far the most common route of administration of drugs for the eye. Topically applied agents produce effective levels mainly in the anterior segment. However, if the lens capsule is removed during intracapsular cataract extraction drugs can gain access to deeper layers.

As far as the optometrist is concerned, the topical route is the only one that is applicable.

Dosage forms for ophthalmic use

The following is a list of dosage forms that have been used for ophthalmic drugs.

    (a) Aqueous Eye Drops
    (b) Oily Eye Drops
    (c) Eye Ointments
    (d) Eye Lotions
    (e) Paper Strips
    (f) Lamellae
    (g) Ocuserts
    (h) Iontophoresis
    (i) Contact Lenses

Eye drops (Figure 4.1)

Aqueous eye drops
Aqueous eye drops have the advantage of quick absorption and effect and there is little or no interference with viewing the media, the fundus or its reflex in such examination procedures as ophthalmoscopy, slit-lamp microscopy and retinoscopy. The effects of eye drops are briefer than those of eye ointments, which constitutes an advantage in their diagnostic application but a disadvantage in their therapeutic or prophylactic use. Aqueous eye drops carry the risk of systemic toxicity due to their absorption by the alimentary tract following drainage through the naso-lacrimal duct.

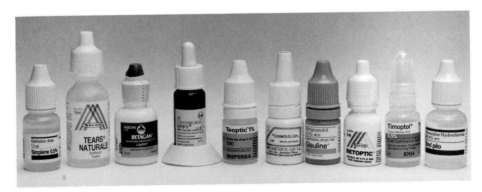

Figure 4.1 Eyedrops

Viscous or oily eye drops reduce this possibility, while eye ointments allow for even less drainage. Retention of the medicament in the conjunctival sac will give better therapeutic results and fewer systemic toxic effects.

Although eye drops may appear to be an efficient method of drug application, their effects are subject to many variables. In spite of these, reproducible results may nevertheless be obtained from their use. For example, it is calculated that only 1.5% of topically applied pilocarpine is absorbed (Patton and Francoeur, 1978).

The volume of the drop varies and so does that of the conjunctival sac into which it is instilled, a problem which is exacerbated by multiple instillations of eye drops. At least 10 minutes should be allowed between drops to allow absorption. Normally the volume of the drop exceeds the volume of the conjunctival sac, leading to an immediate loss of some of the drug. There is some controversy about the volume of a drop delivered by a dropper bottle, Brown, Hotchkiss and Davies (1985) finding volumes of between 50 and 70 µl, whereas Akers (1983) reported a normal drop size of 25–50 µl. Both investigators agreed that the conjunctival sac volume is between 7 and 10 µl. The excess is mostly lost into the nasolacrimal system, where it poses the risk of possible systemic toxicity. Virtually all eye drops sting on instillation and thus will cause reflex tearing, resulting in further loss of drug. Some of the compound will be absorbed by the conjunctival blood vessels and be unavailable for absorption by the cornea.

The state of the corneal epithelium will have a great influence on the rate at which drugs will be absorbed, especially water soluble (polar) drugs (Akers, 1983). Furthermore, the level of pigmentation of the eye, the state of health of the eye and concomitant systemic medication will also influence the response. If the eye is inflamed then the increased blood flow will serve to carry drugs away from the eye.

Aqueous eye drops are solutions of the drug in water, often with other ingredients.

Preservatives   All multi-dose containers contain a preservative (*see* Chapter 3) to prevent bacterial growth during use. As an additional safeguard against infection, multidose drop bottles should be discarded after 28 days if used on one patient or 7 days if used on several patients.

The level of preservative in eye drops is important and is often higher than that in those contact lens solutions that come in contact with the eye. Adverse reactions to preservatives may develop after chronic use of drops, e.g. in glaucoma or dry eye patients who require continuing therapy. In many eye drops, benzalkonium chloride is the chosen preservative and these should not be administered to patients wearing soft contact lenses because it binds to hydrogel materials. When soft lens patients require such an eye drop, the lens should be removed and not re-inserted until at least an hour after instillation.

With some drugs the choice of preservative is determined by the limited compatibility of some drugs and preservatives.

Preservatives will only cope with small innocula of micro-organisms. Good hygiene is still necessary to prevent contaminated eye drops. Harte, O'Hanrahan and Timoney (1978) found contamination in 44% of the residues of eye drops returned to the pharmacy after use in hospitals. This figure is very high and should not be encountered routinely. Aslund, Olson and Sandell (1978), however, found a much lower level of contamination in eye drops. In their study only 10 out of 436 containers produced positive cultures. In a laboratory test they found that contamination was likely to be much higher when untrained personnel used eye drops.

pH adjusters   Some drops are buffered while others contain small amounts of acid or alkali to adjust the pH. The correct pH is necessary to avoid adverse effects, to produce adequate therapeutic effect, to stabilize the preparation and to allow the preservative the correct conditions for action.

Unfortunately, some of these desirable effects have conflicting demands on pH and the value chosen for any particular eye drop may be a compromise. Adrenaline, for example, is most active at a high pH but stable at a lower one. A pH of around neutral is normally chosen. However, for pilocarpine there was no difference in ocular hypotensive effect and stability between solutions of pH 4.1 and pH 5.8 (David, Goldberg and Luntz, 1978) and it was concluded that because of enhanced comfort, near neutral solutions should be used. Buffers are used when the pH is critical and cannot be allowed to vary widely.

Viscosity agents   The dwell time of a drop in the conjunctival sac is very short and the fall off in the tear concentration reduces the amount available for absorption. Any modification of the drop which will increase the dwell time will therefore increase the therapeutic effect and reduce the potential for adverse effect. Hardberger, Hanna and Boyd (1975) found the following half-lives* for radioactive sodium pentechnate when instilled into human eyes in different vehicles.

Ointment   — 9.7 minutes
Polyvinyl alcohol — 7.2 minutes
Methylcellulose   — 4.2 minutes
Saline   — 4.6 minutes

Haas and Merrill (1962) demonstrated a much greater effect from pilocarpine in reducing intraocular pressure and causing miosis when the solution was made viscous with methylcellulose, compared with an aqueous solution and Davies *et al.* (1977) found a similar effect from polyvinyl alcohol.

Similar dramatic increases in activity were seen when pilocarpine was made viscous with carbomer gel (Schoenwald *et al.*, 1978), but there is a level at which a viscous eye drop stops being an eye drop and becomes a gel.

Mattila, Idanpaan and Takki (1968) found varying modifications of response to drugs made viscous with methylcellulose, which modified the cycloplegic effect of tropicamide but not the mydriatic effect. Conversely, it quickened the onset of miosis from physostigmine but had less effect on the resulting cyclospasm. The results would seem to demonstrate the variability of drug response rather than the lack of effect from methylcellulose.

Viscosity agents such as polyvinyl alcohol, methylcellulose or hydroxy ethyl cellulose are added to drops, particularly therapeutic drops, to retard the loss of drugs down the nasolacrimal duct. Viscous drops may also be more comfortable.

Antioxidants   Antioxidants such as sodium metabisulphite or N-acetyl cysteine are incorporated into eye drops containing oxygen sensitive chemicals such as adre-

---

* The half-life is the time taken for half of the concentration to disappear. Thus one half-life after instillation, half of the original concentration will remain, after two half-lives a quarter, after three an eighth, and so on.

naline. Anti-oxidants are reducing agents which are preferentially attacked by the oxygen, leaving the active ingredient unaffected.

Tonicity agents   At one time, tonicity was thought to be all important and hypotonic drops were made isotonic by the addition of solutes such as sodium chloride. In practice problems are only really encountered with hypertonic drops which, of course, cannot be adjusted. Hypotonic drops are well tolerated and only for products such as artificial tears is isotonicity important.

Oily eye drops

Oily eye drops can be used for three reasons: to produce an emollient effect, to protect a compound liable to hydrolysis and to obtain an enhanced effect.

Liquid paraffin and castor oil eye drops are used to form a protective film over the eye following trauma or for an unconscious patient. They can also be used prior to making an eye impression for scleral contact lens fitting.

Some drugs such as DFP are broken down in an aqueous solution and are supplied in arachis oil to prevent this.

Since lipophilic substances cross the epithelial barrier more easily than hydrophilic ones, it would appear logical to provide drugs in the former state rather than the latter. Smith, Smith and Lazare (1978) found that pilocarpine in oil had a greater and longer miosis than a similar amount given in aqueous solution.

Containers for eye drops

The containers for eye drops are very important because not only do they hold the solution and protect them from the potentially destructive effects of air, light and micro-organisms but they also act as a method of application.

For many of the drops the optometrist may wish to use in practice, there is the choice of using a multidose or single dose container.

Multidose containers (Figure 4.2)   The British Standard (BS 1679:1974) amber ribbed dropper bottle made of neutral glass is now becoming less frequently used,

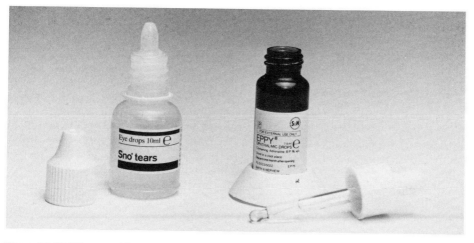

Figure 4.2 Multidose containers

but has the advantage that the eye drops can be autoclaved in the final container. In modern pharmaceutical manufacturing methods, the plastic container into which the dropper is incorporated is favoured. Sterilization of the container is by means of gamma irradiation and the solution is sterilized by filtration, with the two being brought together under aseptic conditions. This type of container usually has an inbuilt tamper evident seal while the glass dropper bottle has a plastic sleeve around the cap. Tamper evidence is now very important for all pharmaceutical preparations and in the case of eye drops constitutes a guarantee of sterility.

The integral plastic dropper is much easier to use for both patient and optometrist than the separate pipette found in the glass bottle.

Single use containers (Figure 4.3)   Unit dosing of eye drops has been available for a long time and has been recommended since the mid 1960s as the most appropriate container for use where patients are likely to be treated, e.g. hospital outpatient departments, operating theatres, accident and emergency departments.

Two types of single use units are available in the United Kingdom — *Minims*, manufactured by Smith & Nephew Pharmaceuticals, Ltd and *Opulets* by Alcon Laboratories UK, Ltd.

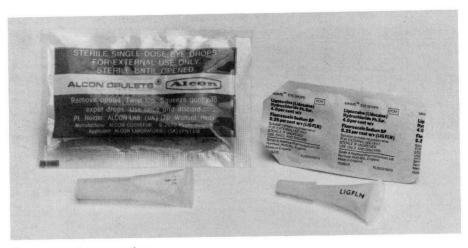

Figure 4.3 Single use containers

Single use containers have the following advantages:

(i) The drop is always sterile — there is no possibility of cross-contamination. Claoue (1986) subjected single use containers to extreme challenges of contamination and found that under conditions likely to be encountered in practice the contents remained sterile.

(ii) The units contain no preservative so that patients with preservative allergies may be safely treated.

(iii) There are cost savings because there is no need to discard a partly used container at the end of the week.

Single use containers are ideal for use in optometric practice and should be selected whenever possible.

Instillation of eyedrops

Eyedrops are normally instilled, one or two on each occasion, into the lower conjunctival sac. The patient's head should be tilted backwards, almost horizontal and slightly to the temporal side of the eye concerned, with the eyes looking back over his head, and the lower lid pulled gently away by the examiner. The end of the eye-dropper must be held just clear of the sweep of the lashes, being less than an inch or so above the sac, before releasing the drop. The sterile glass tube of the eye-dropper must not be allowed to touch the lashes, eye or cheek of the patient or the examiner's hand in order to avoid as far as possible, contamination of the eyedrops. The dropper must be firmly screwed back in place immediately after use. The patient is instructed previously that as soon as the drop has fallen (below the cornea, to minimize the force of the blink reflex, and directly into the sac) he must close his eyes gently, with no lid squeezing. A small pad of cotton wool or fresh paper tissue (held ready between the fingers of the same hand that holds the bottle, or the other hand when employing a sterile single-dose eyedrops unit) is used to control any tearing. Only one or two drops are instilled at a time as any in excess of this amount will only be expelled on closure of the lids (Figure 4.4). Pressure should be applied over the canaliculi by the examiner using the tips of his thumb and forefinger on either side of the bridge of the patient's nose, pressing backwards and inwards for about a half of a minute or so.

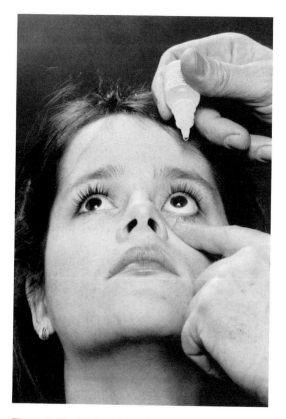

Figure 4.4 Installation of eyedrops

Except when checking the patency of the lacrimal ducts (with fluorescein), immediately following instillation of any eyedrops routine occlusion of the canaliculi should be regarded as highly desirable, even when not mandatory. Such a procedure is admittedly not essential in healthy individuals receiving no systemic medication when ophthalmic drugs which have a wide margin of safety (a relatively high maximum therapeutic dose) are involved. Nevertheless, routine canaliculi occlusion appears to be a commendable clinical practice, as on the not infrequent occasions when it is necessary, occlusion will not then be overlooked. It reduces, as far as is practicable, the possibilities of rapid systemic absorption of drugs through the mucous membranes of the canaliculi, nasopharynx, oesophagus and stomach, and reduces the possibility of interaction between an ophthalmic drug and any systemic medication the patient may be taking (and possibly inadvertently has not disclosed). Ophthalmic drugs, not significantly potent on their own, may be contra-indicated when a patient has certain medical conditions and/or is receiving certain systemic therapy associated with particular agents.

The intra-ocular penetration of a drug via the cornea does not contribute appreciably to any rapid systemic concentration following instillation of eyedrops because of the relatively slow diffusion of any unchanged drug from the eye via its blood or aqueous drainage. Occlusion of the canaliculi, therefore, only leaves that fraction of the drug not absorbed via the cornea to enter the systemic system via the conjunctival membrane. Normally this amount is not sufficient to produce undesirable systemic effects as long as due observance is given to the contra-indications for certain drugs where particular medical conditions exist, or the patient is receiving specific systemic medication: for example, pilocarpine, carbachol and bethanechol are contra-indicated in asthmatics; sympathomimetic drugs are contra-indicated in patients receiving MAO inhibitors, tricyclic antidepressives and antihypertensive drugs.

Eye ointments (Figure 4.5)

Eye ointments have the advantage that they may be instilled by an adult in the home, and they are far safer when poisonous alkaloids are involved. For example, atropine eye ointment is the preparation of choice for domiciliary use, when an atropine cycloplegic refraction of a child is considered necessary. It is standard dosage recommendation that this ointment should not be used on the day of refraction because the greasy film can interfere with the retinoscopic reflex. Cable, Hendrickson and Hanna (1978) employed ointments of cyclopentolate and tropicamide for cycloplegia and mydriasis and found that if small volumes of ointment were applied then, there was minimal irritation and interference with the subsequent ocular examination.

Eye ointments are also useful as protective agents following trauma. They do not adversely affect corneal wound healing (Hanna *et al.*, 1973). As well as being fairly safe and well tolerated, eye ointments have the advantage of prolonged contact with the ocular conjunctival membrane with slow but continued absorption of the medicament (Robin and Ellis, 1978). This continuous absorption necessitates less frequent application and can give comfort to inflamed tissues. Hanna, Hof and Smith (1985) found that four times daily administration of sulphacetamide eye ointment was sufficient to maintain a minimum inhibitory concentration in tear flow. Of course, this advantage of prolonged action becomes a disadvantage when ointments are used diagnostically as opposed to therapeutically or prophylactically.

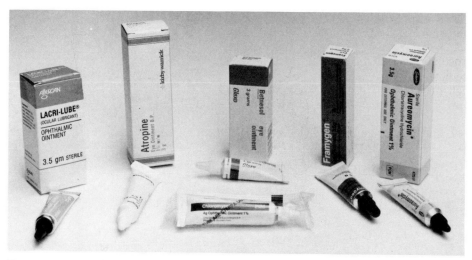

Figure 4.5 Eye ointments

Eye ointments drain from the lacrimal sac by the same route as eye drops, namely through the nasolacrimal duct into the oral cavity (Scruggs, Wallace and Hanna, 1978).

Eye ointments, like eye drops are susceptible to contamination (Harte, O'Hanrahan and Timoney, 1978) and are also subject to variations in formulation leading to differences in consistency and drug release patterns (Ford *et al.*, 1982).

Instillation of eye ointments
Eye ointments are instilled, again into the lower conjunctival sac, a grape-pip size amount being applied on the end of a clean glass eye rod. The patient is instructed to hold his head more upright than for the instillation of eyedrops, and the examiner again pulls the lower lid gently away, placing the ointment on the end of the rod into the lower conjunctival sac. On instruction the patient closes his eyes, the examiner, or parent in domiciliary cases, holds the upper lid gently, but firmly closed, while the glass rod is given a gentle twirl and smoothly withdrawn horizontally via the outer canthus, leaving the eye ointment behind (Figure 4.6). Gentle massage for a few moments, by the examiner or parent with the lids remaining closed, is followed by removal of any excess ointment from their outer edges with cotton wool. Alternatively, the eye ointment can be applied directly from a tube without the aid of a glass ointment rod, and this is the recommended practice, in the consulting room or clinic, when using sterile single-dose application packs. The practitioner applying an eye ointment in his own consulting rooms, if using a glass rod, should disinfect immediately beforehand. This can be done by wiping it with a cotton-wool pad soaked in a solution of 1 in 6 Savlon Liquid Antiseptic (ICI) in Surgical Spirit (*BPC*), then, rinsing the rod in sterile saline solution (a suitable preserved proprietary 'rinsing' solution), and drying with a fresh paper tissue.

For domiciliary use, where a glass rod is being used, the patient (or parent when a child is involved) should be cautioned to avoid contaminating the medicament by observing good hygiene; a clean glass rod should be used and hands and rod washed

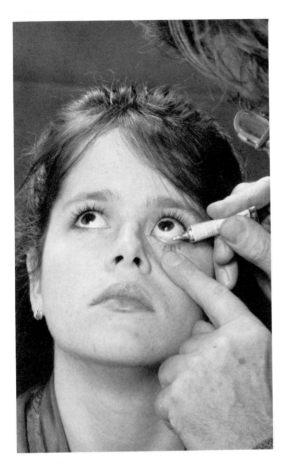

Figure 4.6 Instillation of eye ointment

and dried on a clean towel. In hospital out-patient clinics and ophthalmic wards either single-dose containers should be used (whenever available), or a separate multiple-dose tube of eye ointment should be reserved for each patient. The ointment should be applied with a sterile applicator used for one application only (recommendation of *Codex* 1979), a small portion of ointment being discarded on each occasion, before squeezing the material on to the applicator (H.M. (69) 86), The *BPC* (1973) recommended that eye ointment for domiciliary use, after the 'sterile' seal or plastic envelope has been broken, should be discarded after 1 month, but the *Pharmaceutical Codex* (1979) does not stipulate a time factor.

When eye ointments are used in the practice by an optometrist a small amount of ointment should be squeezed out and discarded each time, before applying any to a freshly disinfected eye ointment rod when administering to each new patient. Opened tubes should be discarded after 1 week.

Ocuserts

A method of continuous release of pilocarpine to control the intra-ocular pressure of glaucomatous patients responsive to this therapy is the Ocusert (May & Baker).

This is an elliptically shaped unit (approximately) 5.5 mm (vertical axis) by 13.5 mm (horizontal axis) by 0.3 mm thick depending on the dosage of pilocarpine enclosed in the permeable outer membrane. The former thickness represents 5 mg and the latter 11 mg of the drug, the 5 mg reservoir possibly being suitable for patients previously on pilocarpine 1 or 2% eyedrops, and the 11 mg may be required for those previously on higher concentrations of the eyedrops. The slow release of the pilocarpine in both strength Ocuserts is by diffusion into the tears fluid over a period of 1 week after the Ocusert has been placed in the lower conjunctival sac. The strength of the Ocusert system chosen by the ophthalmologist will be that which achieves adequate reduction of the intra-ocular pressure. Each individual sterile unit is replaced by the patient every 7 days, and the inconvenience of three or four daily instillations of pilocarpine eyedrops is obviated. This system is in some regards a modern more sophisticated prolonged (depot) version of the older lamellae.

Drug classification

Ophthalmic drugs may be conveniently, if somewhat arbitrarily, classified into two main groups: (1) therapeutic and (2) diagnostic.

Many ophthalmic drugs are used for both therapeutic and diagnostic purposes (for example, atropine, homatropine, physostigmine, pilocarpine, etc.), but if their main interest for the optometrist is as a diagnostic agent, they will be discussed in the second grouping with appropriate references to their therapeutic applications.

Therapeutic ophthalmic drugs are those used in the treatment of ocular injury and disease. In the United Kingdom they are therefore normally in the province of the medical practitioner to whom such cases must be referred by the optometrist 'unless he is acting on the advice or instructions of a registered medical practitioner' (Rule 3),* in accordance with the Rules laid down by the General Optical Council, by virtue of the powers conferred on it by the Opticians Act, 1958, Section 25 (3). This regulation applies, except in an emergency, when 'Nothing in these rules shall operate to prevent a registered optician from rendering in an emergency whatever services are, having regard to the circumstances, in the best interest of the person consulting him.' (Rule 6).* Thus, in special circumstances where it 'is impracticable or inexpedient' to refer, the optometrist may find it necessary to use ophthalmic drugs as a therapeutic rather than a diagnostic measure, if this is in the best interests of his patient. His authority, albeit in a somewhat negative form, to do so is given under this exemption clause in the General Optical Council Rules, which applies to emergencies and first-aid treatment.

Diagnostic and prophylactic drugs

Diagnostic ophthalmic drugs may be subdivided as follows.

(1) Cycloplegics: used to inhibit or paralyse the accommodation.
(2) Mydriatics: used to produce dilatation of the pupil.
(3) Miotics: used to constrict the pupil.
(4) Topical local anaesthetics: drugs applied to the surface of the mucous membrane of the eye to produce local insensitivity in this area.

* See General Optical Council's *Notice for the Guidance of the Profession*, No. 22, Section IX.

(5) Staining agents: used to stain corneal or conjunctival abrasions, in applanation tonometry and contact lens fitting procedures.

(6) Decongestants: used as vasoconstrictors of congested conjunctival blood vessels.

(7) Prophylactic anti-infective preparations: these are therapeutic anti-infective drugs used to prevent pathological conditions developing after minor abrasions of the ocular epithelial tissues, that may occur in many situations, including certain diagnostic procedures and contact lens practice.

Therapeutic drugs

The principal groups of therapeutic drugs are:

(1) Anti-infective drugs;
(2) Anti-inflammatory and anti-allergic drugs;
(3) Anti-glaucoma drugs;
(4) Miscellaneous drugs and drugs used in surgery.

References

Akers, M. J. (1983) Ocular bioavailability of topically applied drugs. *Am. Pharm.*, **NS23**, 33–36

Aslund, B., Oslund, O. T. and Sandell, E. (1978) Studies on the in use microbial contamination of eye drops. *Acta. Pharm. Suec.*, **45**, 389–394

Brown, R. H., Hotchkiss, M. L. and Davis, E. B. (1985) Creating smaller eye drops by reducing the eyedropper tip dimension. *Am. J. Ophthalmol.*, **99**, 460–464

Cable, M. K., Hendrickson, R. D. and Hanna, C. (1978) Evaluation of drugs in ointment for mydriasis and cycloplegia. *Arch. Ophthalmol.*, **96**, 84–86

Claoue, C. (1986) Experimental contamination of Minims of fluorescein by *Pseudomonas aeruginosa*. *Br. J. Ophthalmol.*, **70**, 507–509

David, R., Goldberg, L. and Luntx, M. H. (1978) Influence of pH on the efficacy of pilocarpine. *Br. J. Ophthalmol.*, **62**, 318–339

Davies, D. J. G., Jones, D. E. P., Meakin, B. J. and Norton, D. A. (1977) The effect of polyvinyl alcohol on the degree of miosis and intraocular pressure reduction induced by pilocarpine. *Ophthalmol. Dig.*, **39**, 13–26

Ford, J. L., Rubinstein, M. H., Duffy, T. D., and Ireland, D. S. (1982) A comparison of the physical properties of some sulphacetamide eye ointments commercially available in the U.K. *Int. J. Pharm.*, **12**, 11–18

Haas, J. S. and Merrill, D. L. (1962) The effect of methylcellulose on response to solutions of pilocarpine. *Am. J. Ophthalmol.*, **54**, 21–27

Hanna, C., Fraunfelder, F. T., Cable, M., and Hardberger, R. E (1973) The effect of ophthalmic ointments on corneal wound healing. *Am. J. Ophthalmol.*, **76**, 193–200

Hanna, C., Hof, W. C. and Smith, W. G. (1985) Influence of drug vehicle on ocular contact time of sulphacetamide sodium. *Ann. Ophthalmol.*, **17**, 560–564

Hardberger, R., Hanna, C. and Boya, C. M. (1975) Effects of drug vehicles on ocular contact time. *Arch. Ophthalmol.*, **93**, 42–45

Harte, V. J., O'Hanrahan, M. T. and Timoney, R. F. (1978) Microbial contamination in residues of ophthalmic preparations. *Int. J. Pharm.*, **1**, 165–171

Havener, H. W. (1978) *Ocular Pharmacology*, 4th edn, Mosby, St Louis

Mattila, M. J., Idapaan-Heikkila, J. E. and Takki, S. (1968) Effect of eyedrop adjuvants on the response of the human eye to some autonomic drugs. *Farmaseuttinen Aikakausleti*, **10**, 205–213

Miller, S. J. H. (1978) *Parson's Diseases of the Eye*, 16th ed, Churchill Livingstone, London, pp. 141–150

Robin, J. S. and Ellis, P. P. (1978) Ophthalmic ointments. *Surv. Ophthalmol.*, **22**, 335–340

Patton, T. F. and Francoeur, M. (1978). *Am. J. Ophthalmol.*, **85**, 225

Schoenwald, R. D., Ward, R. L., De Santis, L. M. and Roehus, R. E. (1978) Influence of high viscosity vehicles on miotic effect of pilocarpine. *J. Pharm. Sci.*, **67**, 1280–1283

Scruggs, J., Wallace, T. and Hanna, C. (1978) Route of absorption of drug and ointment after application to the eye. *Ann. Ophthalmol.*, **10**, 267–271

Smith, S. A., Smith, S. E. and Lazare, R. (1978) An increased effect of pilocarpine on the pupil by application of the drug in oil. *Br. J. Ophthalmol.*, **68**, 314–317

Chapter 5

Cycloplegics

Cycloplegics are drugs that paralyse the ciliary muscle by blocking the muscarinic receptors normally stimulated by the release of acetylcholine from the nerve endings of the parasympathetic system. Since the parasympathetic nervous system also innervates the pupil sphincter pupillae muscle, cycloplegia is always accompanied by mydriasis (mydriasis is not always accompanied by cycloplegia however!). They are used to prevent or reduce accommodation during refraction, thus making latent refractive errors manifest (Table 5.1).

Ideal properties of cycloplegics

   (i) Quick in onset (the delayed onset of atropine puts special requirements on its dosing).
  (ii) Adquate depth of cycloplegia.
 (iii) Adequate duration of cycloplegia (a static level of cycloplegia must be achieved).
  (iv) No mydriasis (although this is unattainable — see above — the mydriasis that invariably accompanies cycloplegia must be considered an unwanted side effect).
   (v) No other pharmacological effect.
  (vi) No local toxicity.
 (vii) No systemic toxicity.
(viii) Stable.
  (ix) Capable of presentation in single use eye drops.

Advantages of cycloplegic refraction

Full static refraction can, under cycloplegia, be estimated without interference from a tonic or clonic (fluctuating) contraction of the ciliary muscle. This is particularly important in the very young because of their very strong accommodation, the latency resulting from this masking a large part of their full refractive error, if it is of the hypermetropic type. The unreliability of subjective findings in the very young makes the retinoscopy results of paramount importance.

   The full cycloplegic correction found is not necessarily given in any subsequent prescription deemed necessary, but especially in these young people, particularly

Table 5.1 Cycloplegics*

Official Name	Trade Name	Strengths % w/v	Single dose	Cycloplegic onset	Cycloplegic duration	Residual accom	Adverse effects	Notes
Atropine sulphate	—	1.0	Yes	36 h	Up to 7 days	NIL	Allergic reactions general antimuscarinic side-effects	Used as ointment
Cyclopentolate hydrochloride	Mydrilate	0.5 1.0	Yes	60 min	24 h	1.00D	CNS effects such as hallucinations	
Homatropine hydrobromide	—	1.0 2.0	2.0% only	90 min	24 h	1.00D	As for atropine	
Tropicamide	Mydriacyl	1.0	Yes	30 min	6 h	2.00D	Occasional hallucination	
Lachesine	—	1.0	No	60 min	24 h	?	—	Little used today

*Since all cycloplegics produce mydriasis, they pose the threat of precipitating angle closure glaucoma in susceptible patients where manifest (intermittent or constant) strabismus, medium to high heteropho-ria, pseudo-myopia, or marked accommodative asthenopic symptoms exist, this knowledge is of primary importance. Amos (1978) considered cycloplegia necess-ary for mentally retarded and uncooperative patients.

Disadvantages of cycloplegic refraction

Refraction under cycloplegia is unnatural because the shape of the lens has been changed and as this will resume its normal shape when the effects of the drug have worn off, a post-cycloplegic test is preferable wherever possible. The optical aberrations, present with the widely dilated pupil, are then very much reduced. This procedure, of course, necessitates the inconvenience of a further visit. Additional disadvantages include making an allowance for the dependent tone of the ciliary muscle, and the dangers of cycloplegia, but as these can be successfully overcome (*see later*) the advantages of cycloplegic refraction, when it is called for, far outweigh the disadvantages.

Precycloplegic examination

The following tests include those recommended by Bartlett (1978) before the use of a cycloplegic:

(1) Visual acuity at distance and near.
(2) History, paying particular attention to drugs and allergy.
(3) Pupillary function.
(4) Manifest refraction.
(5) Accommodation function.
(6) Cover test at distance and near.
(7) Slit-lamp microscope examination.
(8) Tonometry.

Perform an external examination (using focal illumination and a 10 × monocular loupe), and brief internal ocular examination. If a normal fundus reflex is observed, a detailed intra-ocular examination may then be left to the cycloplegic visit, but only as long as no suspicious pathological symptoms or signs have been detected. Not all the above tests will be applicable to every child and, with children under the age of 4 or 5 years, vision may only be estimated approximately.

Cycloplegic examination

Thorough ophthalmoscopy and retinoscopy are carried out at this visit. Such objective tests, especially with the young, are of the utmost importance; the prescription, if any, in young children under the age of 6 years is based almost entirely on the retinoscopy. With older children the power and axis of high cylinders may be checked subjectively at a post-cycloplegic visit, but it must never be forgotten that retinoscopy (with or without cycloplegia) is the main objective method of estimating total astigmatic and spherical errors that may be present, and a refractionist who can depend on the accuracy of his retinoscopy has a sure foundation on which to base any optical treatment found necessary. As they cannot always be relied upon, especially in children, the mentally tardy and the aged (in the case of the latter, who fatigue easily, a cycloplegic refraction is, of course, obviously contra-indicated), subjective methods should be applied, whenever possible, principally as a confirmation of the retinoscopic results. Even in adults only small subjective alterations to the spherical or cylindrical power or the axis of the latter, should be necessary, following the skilled use of the retinoscope. Most patients (especially children) are not trained observers, and their ability to interpret subjective differences in visual acuity with the application of lenses may not always be acceptable. Too much reliance should not be placed on subjective findings of even those in the 10–12 year age-group, although, of course, there is a great variation in standards of observation and intelligence in all age-groups. An expert retinoscopist will avoid many mistakes from undue reliance on subjective refraction. The student, in particular, cannot spend too much time practising retinoscopy; it is an art which requires continuous exacting effort and much practice is needed before the results can be relied upon to indicate the refractive error with a consistent degree of accuracy.

During retinoscopy carried out under cycloplegia, because of the pronounced mydriasis present, it is essential to observe the movement of the light reflex in the central 3–4 mm pupillary area only, ignoring the light movement in the periphery, which may be in the same or reverse direction to that in the centre. When a cycloplegic is used the child is encouraged to look directly at the retinoscopy light, this not being a difficult request to obey in the darkened consulting room. Thus, retinoscopy is carried out along the visual axis, but in strabismus, it is necessary to occlude the fixing eye.

In very young children, under the age of 3 years or so, the most satisfactory arrangement is to have the yong patient sitting on the mother's lap. No trial frame is used and, where a squint is present, but not otherwise, the mother occludes each eye of the child separately with the palm of her hand, while the lenses are held up in quick succession, before the unoccluded eye, during the progress of the retinoscopy. The use of spheres only is preferred by some optometrists, as then only the movement of the 'light' (once its direction has been ascertained—and thus the axes of the two main meridians) in the pupillary aperture central area needs to be observed carefully. Older children, say those aged 4 years and over, who will not be upset by a trial frame, may then have the spherocylinder correction (if astigmatism is present) put up and checked objectively. Even those too young for this procedure can have a spherocylinder combination held before the eye for checking of the axis; reasonable accuracy (with reference to the axis estimated for the cylinder) may be attained by this latter method, with practice and experience.

Objective checking of the cylinder axis

The following method is described by Duke-Elder (1978).

Undercorrect (preferably by 0.50 DC) when using plus cylinders or overcorrect (by the same amount) when using negative cylinders, in order to create a 'with' movement. Move the retinoscopy light exactly at right-angles to the cylinder axis in the trial frame. If the cylinder axis, as set in the trial frame, is correct, the edge of the retinoscopic light reflex will move exactly parallel with this axis, across the central pupil. Alternatively, if the cylinder axis in the trial frame has been set in error, the edge of the light reflex in the pupil will move along a different axis, not parallel to the cylinder axis in the trial frame, but making an angle (with the cylinder axis) which is approximately six times greater than the angle of error in the setting of the cylinder axis in the trial frame. For example, if the correct cylinder axis is 85 degrees, but the cylinder in the trial frame has been set in error with its axis at 90 degrees, the edge of the light reflex will then lie very neatly along the 60 degrees meridian, as it gives a 'with' movement. The cylinder axis in the trial frame should be reset, tilting it approximately one-sixth of the difference between its original position and the position occupied by the edge of the light reflex, and towards the latter position. This adjustment is repeated until light edge reflex and cylinder axis are parallel as the retinoscopy light is tilted. In the author's opinion, the use of a streak retinoscope greatly facilitates accurate axis location.

Another objective method of checking the cylinder axis, which is preferred by some practitioners, is that of Lindner, which has been described by Hodd (1955) as follows.

Observation is made along the meridians approximately 45° to either side of the axis of the trial cylinder. If the trial cylinder is slightly off axis, a 'with' shadow movement will be noted in one oblique meridian and an 'against' shadow movement will be noted in the other oblique meridian. To correct the error in setting, locate the meridian showing the 'with' shadow movement and turn the trial cylinder axes slightly towards this position. This procedure is repeated until the oblique movements are eliminated. If the 'with' movement is difficult to locate it may be accentuated by moving forward slightly or by adding 0.12D or −0.25 sphere. The addition should be just sufficient to neutralize the 'against' movement in the other oblique meridian: the refractive error in the first oblique meridian will then be doubled.

Interpretation of refractive results under cycloplegia

Positive and negative aberration
Movement of the light reflex in the peripheral parts of the dilated pupil may show positive or negative aberrations due to the differing refractive conditions in this area as compared to the central 'axial' region.

In *positive aberration* (four or five times more common than negative aberration) the peripheral area is more myopic or less hypermetropic than the central area, and thus an 'against' movement still persists in the periphery when the central axial zone is neutralized.

A *negative aberration* causes the opposite effect. Regardless of any peripheral movement the central 3 or 4 mm diameter zone alone must be neutralized and the outer area reflex ignored.

Due to peripheral aberrations a scissor movement of the light reflex may be observed on occasion, usually near the neutralization point. Movement of the refractionist's head forwards and backwards over a range of about 25 cm, giving first a 'with' then an 'against' movement, is a useful check that neutralization has been attained. It can readily be seen that, with positive aberration, if the peripheral zone is erroneously corrected, too little plus or too much minus power will be recorded and vice versa when negative aberration is present.

These retinoscopy rules (concerning peripheral aberrations) apply, of course, in all cases of dilated pupils whether drugs have caused the mydriasis or not. With too bright a light source when performing a retinoscopy with dilated pupils it is difficult to differentiate clearly the central from the peripheral light reflex and, therefore, the minimum light retinoscopic reflex that can be seen easily is desirable.

Only when the stronger cycloplegics have been used is it ideal for the patient to look constantly directly at the light. With weaker cycloplegics, a final check on neutralization should be taken with the patient looking in the distance, when any slight (unparalysed) ciliary activity should be detected.

Subjective verification

If this is carried out immediately following the cycloplegic retinoscopy, because of the presence of spherical aberration, it must be expected that the sphere power will vary somewhat from that estimated objectively and also that accepted at a post-cycloplegic visit. Usually (as positive spherical aberration is more common) less plus sphere will be accepted in hypermetropia and more minus sphere in myopia. A further discrepancy under these conditions, also attributable to this aberration, will frequently be the loss of a line or so in the visual activity (VA), that is, in the corrected vision.

In older children (usually aged over 7 or 8 years) it should be possible to verify with a crossed cylinder (0.50D) the cylinder axis. The cylinder power, where a moderately good standard of visual acuity exists, can be verified with an 0.25D crossed cylinder. These details should remain constant after the cycloplegia has worn off.

Post-cycloplegic subjective verifications, necessary on occasion (for example, doubtful cycloplegic retinoscopy or high-power cylindrical lenses), are not obligatory in all cases, but where some doubt about the accuracy of the original cycloplegic retinoscopy result exists, they should be undertaken, and are probably preferable in all cases, if possible, in view of the age. When, during the cycloplegic retinoscopy, fluctuating neutrals are obtained, if the child is old enough +3.00D lenses should be put up and the monocular accommodation should be measured. A reading much in excess of 3.00D would indicate that full cycloplegia has not been attained. Another method of proving that such is the case is to note if a further 'with' movement occurs, once neutralization has been obtained, when the child is asked to look away from the retinoscopy light into the distance. Where these results are positive the parent should then be questioned further as to whether or not the full applications of the atropine eye ointment had been made. If more than 1.0D of accommodation is still active further applications of atropine are called for, and when even under this amount is recorded no tonus allowance (*see later*) should be made, and the child must be instructed not to watch the retinoscope light but instead a distant fixation light. Where squint is present full cycloplegia must be obtained before proceeding with the retinoscopy.

A fully dilated, immobile pupil with absence of pupillary reflexes is not proof of full cycloplegia; this condition only indicates with certainty a paralysed sphincter pupillae muscle.

Choice of cycloplegic

Many antimuscarinic agents have been used in the past but today only three are used regularly. Arranged alphabetically, (and in descending order of efficacy) they are: atropine, cyclopentolate and tropicamide.

Of the others, homatropine is still used in smaller and smaller amounts, while hyoscine is hardly ever employed at all.

The principle of 'as little as possible but as much as necessary' should apply to the use of drugs by doctors, optometrists and patients alike. Having decided that a particular patient will benefit from a cycloplegic refraction, it is encumbent on the optometrist to use as weak an agent as possible. Antimuscarinic drugs can affect the whole body and the stronger the cycloplegic, the stronger will be the side effects. Additionally, stronger agents will produce longer effects and the inconvenience to the patient of dilated pupils and the inability to read or do close work will be prolonged.

There are many opinions as to the indications for atropine. Some authorities advocate its use in many situations, while others consider it to be of limited value. Where cycloplegic refraction is appropriate, Duke-Elder (1978) recommends that atropine should be used on all children below the age of 7 and on older children with accommodative squints. They would appear to be in agreement with Whittington (1958), who recommended atropine for all young children. Martin-Doyle (1967) also believed that atropine should be used on children up to 10 years old. It must be remembered that children of this age will be attending school and prolonged cycloplegia will make life difficult for them and their teachers. Amos (1978) considers 5 years to be the maximum age for the use of atropine.

It is difficult to be rigid about which drug should be used on which patient. One cannot just rely on age as the only determining factor. For example, heavily pigmented eyes may require a stronger cycloplegic than light coloured ones of the same age. The following are just recommendations, not hard and fast rules. Atropine cycloplegia is only normally required for young preschool children with constant esotropia.

The use of atropine cycloplegic refraction in cases of intermittent squints and high heterophorias has been rejected by Mallett (1970) and a number of other optometrists on the grounds that there is a possible danger of converting these conditions into constant squints. The shorter acting, but less complete, effects of cyclopentolate are preferable in these conditions, regardless of age.

Ingram and Barr (1979) consider that atropine is absolutely contra-indicated in the first 3 months of life because of the danger of amblyopia.

Cyclopentolate will suffice for all children without concomitant esotropia and all children of school age irrespective of refractive and binocular states. Up to the age of 12 years, 1% is the recommended strength and 0.5% for older children.

Tropicamide may be used as an alternative cycloplegic for the older patient, especially when a quick reversal of the cycloplegia is desirable. In the main only 1% is suitable as a cycloplegic; the results with 0.5% are too variable.

Whittington (1958) describes an excellent routine to be followed, prior to deciding on whether or not a full refractive examination is necessary in a young child, and indicates the approximate monocular and binocular vision to be expected at various ages.

He also includes the sound advice that the refractionist should always keep in mind the fact that poor vision may have a very important effect on the mental and physical health of the developing child.

Children aged under 3 years:
(1) Parent's history of the child.
(2) Presence or not of full ocular movements. A small light or toy may be used in this motility test.

(3) Cover test. Note any heterophoria or heterotropia, and speed of recovery of former. (*Note:* dislike of 'thumb' occluder over one eye may indicate an amblyopia or reduced vision in the other (uncovered) eye.)

(4) Simultaneously observe the ocular media to ensure a healthy pink fundus reflex. Also examine the lids, tear sac and external eyeball of each eye for signs of abnormality or disease.

If the history, fixation, motility, cover test, external appearance and fundus reflex are all normal, there is no need to proceed further to cycloplegic refraction. If not, an atropine (preferably the 1% ointment) cycloplegic refraction is advisable.

Children aged 3–4 years: In addition to the above procedures, at this stage it is now usually possible to check the vision with Sheridan-Gardiner, Landolt 'C', or illiterate 'E' tests.

Myopia is rare in infancy and young children, but is occasionally found: pseudo-myopia will be revealed under cycloplegic refraction. Children rarely complain of eye symptoms and are most frequently brought by their mother because she suspects periodic squint, or notices her child screwing up his eyes, or holding a book very close. This latter condition is quite often caused by excessive effort to overcome hypermetropia, but more usually by myopia.

Atropine

Atropine is an alkaloid extracted from a variety of plant species such as *Atropa belladonna*, and *Hyoscyamus niger*. It was the first antimuscarinic agent used in medicine and is the most toxic substance available for use by optometrists. It is available as 1% eyedrops, both in multi-dose and single use units. Because of the systemic toxic reactions that can occur, the ointment form is most often favoured.

The ointment is applied twice a day for 3 days prior to refraction (Sowden 1974) but not on the day of refraction because the unabsorbed ointment may interfere with refractive procedures.

Time scale

With the usual 1% strength, after one instillation mydriasis commences in 10–15 minutes, and is maximal in 30–40 minutes. Recovery from mydriasis following a single instillation may take as much as 3–7 days, but as it is usual to require complete cycloplegia when atropine is used in children, and this necessitates twice daily application for 3 days, pupillary recovery then usually takes from 10 to 14 days. Cycloplegia commences in half an hour, the action is slow and full recovery may take 7–10 days, although usually adequate accommodation for near work has returned within 4–5 days (after the usual six applications). Even with one application full ciliary muscle recovery may take 3–7 days, the resulting cycloplegia reached in 1–3 hours, although marked, is not complete.

Because of the different times courses of mydriasis and cycloplegia, the size of the pupil is a poor indicator of cycloplegic effect (Amos, 1978). Wide dilatation of the pupil causes photophobia and sometimes the patient complains of micropsia. Normal pupillary reflex constrictions to light and to accommodation-convergence are completely abolished.

Very powerful miotics (for example dyflos 0.1% or ecothiopate 0.3%) will overcome the mydriatic effects of atropine 1% but these drugs are not available to the optometrist in the United Kingdom.

Tonus allowance

The ciliary muscle, like all other smooth muscles in the body, has both a dependent and an independent tone, the former being conditional on an intact nerve supply, while the latter is not. The independent tone in the ciliary muscle is very small and does not give rise to symptoms, neither is it affected by cycloplegics. On the other hand, the dependent tone of the ciliary muscle is totally abolished by complete atropine cycloplegia, but not by the full effects of other cycloplegics.

An allowance, therefore, has to be made in the case of complete atropine cycloplegia only, for the return of the dependent tone of the ciliary muscle on its recovery from the effects of atropine paralysis. This tonus allowance is an adjustment of the spherical element only of the retinoscopic findings in such cases, to take into account the fact that the eyes, when fully returned to normal, will once more usually have their overall refractive power increased slightly in a positive direction by the constant effect of the (dependent) tone of the recovered ciliary muscle. The quantitative effect of this tone will vary slightly depending on the nature of the refractive condition of the eye being considered. In hypermetropic, emmetropic, and myopic eyes (up to about $-1.00D$), the result of full recovery of the ciliary muscle is to add approximately 1.00D of positive power to the refractive power of the eye found under cycloplegic retinoscopy. Experience has shown that in higher degrees of myopia, as might be expected, less dependent tone is exhibited by the ciliary muscle, and the positive power added back to these myopic eyes by the recovered muscle is usually less (say, about 0.50D for myopes over $-1.00D$ and up to $-2.00D$, with probably 0.0D for eyes with over a $-3.00D$ correction). This explains why, if at the post-cycloplegic examination the exact atropine retinoscopy results are put up in the trial frame, the patient's visual acuity is usually below the maximum that can be attained after adding the tonus allowance. The latter, when given, always means adding a negative amount, whether the refractive error is positive or negative. Mitchell (1965) comments 'in myopes it is found to be unnecessary to add as much as one dioptre, the amount required being decided by a comparison of the cycloplegic and pre-cycloplegic or post-cycloplegic findings'. It is usually possible, even with children as young as 3 or 4 years, by using the Sheridan–Gardiner or other simple tests described earlier in this chapter, to see whether or not a 0.0D–0.50D, or $-1.00D$ tonus allowance should be given in these cases, expecting an alteration of 0.50D to improve the visual acuity by a few further letters or symbols from the next smaller line. No increase of minus lens power should be prescribed in a myopic correction unless there is reason to believe a corresponding increase in visual acuity has been obtained.

As already mentioned, any tonus allowance is only made to the spherical element of the cycloplegic retinoscopic results, and any subsequent modification of a cylindrical element (found under cycloplegia) at a post-cycloplegic examination follows the usual rules relating to the correction of astigmatic errors, and is not influenced by the use of the cycloplegic.

The refractionist should always enquire of the parent, before commencing the cycloplegic examination, whether or not the full number (six) of applications of atropine eye ointment has been instilled into each eye as directed. The author's reason for stipulating 'both right and left eyes' (rather than just 'both eyes') in his prescription directions for labelling is an endeavour, especially in cases of strabismus, to ensure that eye ointment is instilled in both eyes, and not just the squinting or non-squinting eye. Unfortunately, this mistake happens occasionally, even after the most emphatic verbal and written instructions to the parent.

Often in hypermetropic children, where convergent squint is also present, somewhat less than the usual tonus allowance of 1.00D may be given, and when this binocular anomaly is accompanied by small refractive errors of this type, even no allowance may be made in an endeavour to gain relaxation of the accommodation for distance.

On the other hand, as Duke-Elder (1978) suggests, when referring to deductions (over and above normal tonus allowances) for non-squinting young hypermetropes, 'in younger children, below the age of 6 years, especially if the error is high, more should be deduced . . ., and 1.5 to 2.0 dioptres can well be deducted'.

Refractive errors and atropine cycloplegia

It may be of some assistance here to summarize separately the management of the different forms of refractive errors that may be disclosed under cycloplegic examination.

Myopia

In the absence of exotropia or uncompensated exophoria, a full correction of a child's myopia should normally be prescribed, as this places him in the position of an emmetrope, permitting the natural balance of the accommodation and convergence to be resumed. It should be explained to the parent, and if his age permits to the child as well, in simple language, that 'although the child may read and see near objects quite well without his glasses, the normal balance of the focusing and simultaneous converging of his eyes is disrupted without them'. The glasses will also help the child to hold his reading matter at the correct distance. On the other hand, constant wear (as opposed to use for critical vision, such as in the classroom, reading, television, cinema, etc.) need not be advised until the child's vision, without correction, has fallen to 6/12 or less. Even at this stage for vigorous play, and when he is a few years older when 'contact' sports (for example, rugby and soccer) are commenced, and for swimming, the spectacles should not be worn, while for 'hard ball' games (for example cricket and hockey) toughened or plastic lenses should be specifically recommended. Another important reason for advising constant spectacle wear in young children, even with moderately low myopia, is that it is in the best interests not only of their eyes but of their normal mental development, so that they may show a full interest in the 'world' around them, which they cannot be expected to do if they cannot see distant objects. It is of interest to note that this reason for constant wear would not apply with equal force to adults, who, in the absence of symptoms, might on occasion be willing to surrender to their blurred distance vision, as long as they had no special need to see clearly in the distance. In the young, however, with their developing eyes and visual habits, avoidance of disruption of the accommodation–convergence balance, and incorrect reading and close work distances, and restriction of mental and visual horizons, make the advantages of virtually constant wear of prime importance (Miller, 1978). Annual, or if necessary 6-monthly or even more frequent, refractive examinations should be the rule, as with the usual type of simple myopia a gradual increase of this refractive error, reaching a fairly static amount between the ages of 16 and 20 years, is to be expected.

Whereas low to moderate degrees of myopia up to 5 or 6D occurring in children (above the age of 8 or 10 years) and young adults have a good prognosis, such findings in a child under the age of 6 years must give rise to some concern in case the condition should happen to be the progressive and degenerative type of myopia. On the other hand, a number of cases of myopia found early in life are truly congenital and may be stationary.

Apart from the necessary refractive treatment of young myopic children, attention should be directed to their visual hygiene, which should include not only the use of a correct reading distance and good print, but correct position when holding books, and good lighting. The maintenance of a good all round standard of general health, with wholesome food, adequate outdoor games and exercises, all may help in keeping the 'final' minus correction as low as possible. The old idea that 'excessive close work' (many hours of reading) had a deleterious effect on the increase of the myopia has now given way to a more positive approach, where, 'the amount of work is adjusted in accordance with the general physical and mental development of the child rather than the degree of myopia' (Duke-Elder, 1978).' A robust healthy child will, as he approaches full physical maturity, tend to develop less myopia than if his health were otherwise.

It is not proposed here to enter into a discussion on 'myopia control' by such methods as the myopic child reading without spectacles (for low degrees of myopia), or using bifocals (with about a +1.50DS addition), or wearing a reduced (say by 0.50D) distance prescription, or the possible influence of contact lenses on the development of myopia in the young. All of these methods have their advocates and undoubtedly, for some patients at least, each of them have proved valuable. These facts do not, however, vitiate against the great value of the basic knowledge of the full myopic error present that a cycloplegic refraction provides. Full details of these various techniques should be studied by the student in such original publications as those of Kelly, *et al.* (1975), Oakley and Young (1975), Young (1978), Black (1978) and Stone (1976).

Hypermetropia

When one examines young patients under atropine cycloplegia and the objective findings reveal the presence of hypermetropia, it is usual to add the −1.00D to allow for the tone of the ciliary muscle. In cases of convergent squint and high esophoria, slightly less tonus allowance may be given to encourage the relaxation of an over-active ciliary muscle and lessen the tendency to excessive convergence. Mitchell (1964) suggests, however, 'even in cases in which the fullest possible correction is required, as in high esophoria or convergent squint, not less than +0.75D* should be deducted; a higher plus correction, though repressing accommodation in near vision and so lessening the tendency to converge, may defeat its object by blurring distance vision and rendering fusion more difficult'. An exception to this view, and one mentioned earlier in this chapter and also by Miller (1978), refers to very young hypermetropic convergent strabismic patients, where 'if the error is small no deduction may be made'. In the author's opinion no allowance need be made for the atropine with hypermetropic errors in the region of 1.00D or less in children with convergent strabismus up to about the age of 3–4

---

* Deducting + 0.75D is, of course, equivalent to adding 0.75D

years. The visual world of such children does not take much account of details of objects at infinity. Once the child reaches the age of about 4 years or more this attitude gradually begins to change, and Mitchell's suggestion would appear to be more applicable. The practitioner must use his judgment and treat each case individually on its merits, and with due regard to the mental and physical development of the child concerned. In all cases every endeavour should be made to see that the hypermetropic child is wearing any spectacles prescribed, before the effects of the atropine cycloplegia have worn off in about 10 days. The greatly improved visual acuity noticed by the child when the correction is worn, whilst his accommodation is still unable to assist him 'correct' his vision, is a powerful psychological incentive for him to wear his glasses and become used to them, and then continue to do so after full recovery from the atropine ointment has occurred. In the absence of any manifest or high degree of oculo-motor imbalance, after the normal $-1.00D$ allowance has been added, the proportion of the full hyper-metropic error prescribed for is arrived at by consideration of the following factors.

In general, all high-plus prescriptions are reduced somewhat when being given on the first occasion, the patient being more comfortable if allowed to follow his natural tendency to accommodate somewhat for distance, albeit only to an amount insufficient to cause symptoms. The amount to reduce the full plus spherical correction can only be based on experience, for it depends on the age (on which the available accommodation depends), the general health, the severity of symptoms and the presence of any heterophoria (esophoria, for example, necessitating more plus spherical lens than exophoria). Also, one should not disrupt too violently established accommodative-convergence relationships. This last factor applies particularly to the age-group we are discussing (that is, those under the age of 6 years) and after making the usual tonus allowance of 1.00D, in the absence of any signs of squint or moderate to high esophoria, these young patients may well have a further $-0.5D$ or $-1.00D$ added to their retinoscopy results, in view of the abundant power of their accommodation, especially if their refractive error is high. Another fact that should be taken into account is the purpose for which the spectacles are to be worn. A healthy boy aged 5 years with only 2Δ of esophoria at distance and 4Δ of esophoria at near, and a full correction of $+3.50D$ (under complete atropine cycloplegia), complaining of frontal headaches, associated only with prolonged near work, cinema and television (that is, prolonged critical vision at near and distance) might, for example, be adequately treated by being prescribed $+1.75D$ (that is, a tonus allowance of $-1.00D$ with a further reduction of $-0.75D$ for comfort), for wear only when performing the visual tasks that appeared to be causing his original symptoms. The same child, after a 6-week debilitating illness, might be made symptom-free with a fairly constant correction of $+2.25D$ for 3 months, until his health had recovered. Again, a child of about the same age where a periodic convergent strabismus, originally successfully treated with a $+2.50D$ prescription worn constantly and orthoptic exercises, had become, due to the illness, a constant manifest low esotropia, might well be prescribed a slight over-correction. This might be $+3.00D$ for constant wear for a few months, the case being frequently (every 3–4 months) reviewed refractively, and orthop-tically, as the practitioner saw fit according to the progress made.

It should be remembered that some degree of hypermetropia is physiological, especially in children below the age of 6 or 7 years, about 90% of whom are hypermetropic, and to a diminishing extent in older children, approximately 50% of whom remain so up to the age of 16 years, which is about the time of termination of the growth factor (Duke-Elder, 1978). If (1) accommodative squint, (2) appreciable esophoria, (3) subnormal vision, and/or (4) asthenopic symptoms are present, any error should be corrected. If the error is over about 3.00D the lenses should be worn constantly, and if lower they may suffice for near work only (Duke-Elder, 1969). But in the absence of (1) and (2) above, as long as sufficient positive power is given to result in normal visual acuity and overcome any asthenopic symptoms, especially with children and also young adults, with their abundance of available accommodative power, an undercorrection of the plus sphere is preferable for the following reasons.

(1) There will then be no violent disruption of the established accommodative-convergence relationship. Often the symptoms are due to excessive accommodation related to the convergence being used, and this disproportion must be corrected gradually, in stages if the refraction necessitates a high prescription, for example, a full refractive error of +4.50D may have initially to be corrected with a +2.50D or +3.00D sphere and this lens power then increased in 6 weeks to +3.50D or +4.00D, which should allay any symptoms and provide normal visual acuity.

(2) If appreciable exophoria (for example, over 5 or 6Δ) is present with hypermetropia, it may be advisable to undercorrect, in order to stimulate the accommodation and the synergic convergence, the latter lending to counteract the exophoria.

(3) Partial correction for young hypermetropes keeps their accommodation active, and makes them less dependent on their spectacles, especially when they may have to leave them off for games, etc.

(4) The long-term view should include the intention of preserving a highly developed amplitude of accommodation.

Previous prescription
This has an important bearing on any new refractive treatment. A patient whose atropine cycloplegic correction is +6.0D sphere (after tonus allowance), who has already been wearing +4.50D, but now complains of asthenopic symptoms from prolonged close work, might well be prescribed +5.25D or +5.50D, but if the +6.0D were an initial finding, in the absence of any undue esophoria +3.50D or +4.0D would probably be adequate to solve both visual and symptomatic problems. It becomes apparent from the few examples discussed that each patient, with his history, symptoms, signs, oculo-motor balances, visual needs, etc., has to be considered individually, and experience coupled with general guidelines dictates the final optical treatment and prescription, if any is considered necessary. These same principles, in general, apply to the refractive management of older children examined under milder cycloplegics (except for omitting any tonus allowance), and later still older patients not requiring these drugs at all.

Oculomotor balance
This should be recorded, whenever possible, at pre-cycloplegic and post-cycloplegic examination, both with and without the refractive findings.

Normally, hypermetropia (without cycloplegia) with high esophoria at distance calls for a maximum plus correction, and myopia with high distance exophoria usually needs a full minus correction. Under cycloplegia, with the accommodation fully relaxed, the refractionist uncovers and can prescribe these full corrections with confidence. Especially when correcting with minus sphere it is known that no overactive (or spasmodic) accommodation is deceiving the refractionist's judgment, and a possible pseudo-myopia causing him to prescribe a stronger lens power than is actually present, thus inadvertently perpetuating and exacerbating the original condition. The correct minus lens necessary to give maximum distance visual acuity can be given with certainty even when esophoria is present. Undercorrection of hypermetropia when exophoria is present is to be preferred (*see above*). Esophoria which is greater at near than at distance (convergence excess type) may well be the cause of discomfort, and excessive (latent) accommodative effort is usually to blame. In children this condition, although more frequently treated by orthoptic exercises, may (as in non-presbyopic hypermetropic adults) be treated by prescribing whatever spherical addition is necessary to render the esophoria compensated.

A near exophoria, greater than distance by up to 6, is regarded by some as a physiological exophoria, and more than this as a convergence weakness type of exophoria, but up to 15 or even 20 for near may (depending on the amount of near work undertaken and the state of the general health) be controlled without symptoms. This is understandable when it is remembered that the positive functional reserve for near may be as high as 36 or more. If symptoms do occur in this type of case (unlikely in the young, more likely in the elderly), fixation disparity techniques (Mallett, 1964, 1983) can indicate the spherical or prismatic correction necessary for the relief of symptoms. In pre-presbyopic patients, orthoptic treatment will be appropriate in many cases. It should be borne in mind that in the young (from early childhood up to 30 years or so) high exophoria at near, with orthophoria or low esophoria at distance, may be due to exhaustion caused by an excessive accommodative effort to compensate a latent hypermetropia. A cycloplegic refraction would confirm such a diagnosis.

Strabismus

Esotropia　When atropine cycloplegia is used in esotropic cases, a full plus correction, adding a −1.00D (or possibly only −0.50D) for tonus allowance in hypermetropic errors, should be prescribed with no further reduction, as this is contra-indicated in these cases where the fullest possible relaxation of the accommodation is being attempted. Further addition of plus power above that arrived at by granting the minimum tonus allowance (0.50D), even if it forced greater relaxation of the ciliary muscle, must inevitably blur the distance vision beyond an acceptable limit to a child over the age of about 4 years, and can only be considered for a near work segment in a bifocal combination.

Exotropia　Where the correction has been determined under cycloplegia the full minus lens power with maximum tonus allowance of 1.00D can be given and where necessary an excess of minus power compatible with the amplitude of accommodation and the results of the cover test using a small fixation object.

Latent and manifest error

In children refracted under cycloplegia the full latent error need only be corrected if a heterotropia or high heterophoria is present and the uncorrected latency is contributing to this (for example, if a latent hypermetropia is causing a high distance esophoria, say over 5Δ). In the absence of these two conditions, with other cases the portion of the full error to be corrected is that which will give adequate comfort and normal vision. In the case of adults, who, where necessary, would be refracted under a weaker cycloplegic, if the full manifest correction fails to relieve their asthenopic symptoms, Donders suggested correction of a further quarter of any latent error present. As the latter has become virtually fully manifest, in nearly all cases, soon after the age of 30 years, this suggestion applies mainly to those between the ages of 16 and 30 years.

Binocular balancing techniques
Although not applicable to the under 6 years age-group, which has been the main subject of discussion in this chapter dealing with cycloplegia, it may be convenient to mention here some of the simpler post-cycloplegic equalization tests that can be appreciated and interpreted by many children from the age of 7–8 years upwards, thus adding to the comfort and efficiency of any corrections prescribed for them. It might be added that, in the opinion of the author, these simpler tests usually produce quite as satisfactory results with adults as other more sophisticated and complex instrumentation and techniques he has also used with this latter group.

Only brief descriptions of these techniques will be given here, as references are quoted so that the reader may study such methods in greater detail. The reason for their inclusion is that they contribute to the 'refinement' of findings that have originally been obtained during the cycloplegic objective refraction. They are, of course, equally valid where no cycloplegic examination has been found necessary or where a post-cycloplegic examination is being carried out.

Distance corrections, to be worn constantly or occasionally, can be balanced using a mirror and septum at 3 metres, the septum so placed as to divide the patient's binocular field so that two images of selected letters, one for each eye, are seen simultaneously. Positive spherical lens power (in 0.25D steps) is added to the eye which sees more clearly, until an equality of vision for each eye is obtained, but if this balance is not obtainable, then it is generally desirable to leave the normally (habitually) dominant eye with the better acuity. This latter qualification appears to be indicated whatever method of balancing is adopted. The procedure just described is based on a technique developed by Turville about 1927, and along with some less precise methods sometimes used, for example, successive comparison, and simultaneous comparison tests, was described by Giles (1965).

Gillie (1959) devised a simple and very effective binocular balance technique he called 'The Flipper Test', which does not even require the additional use of a septum. It can be performed by using separate plus and minus 0.25D spheres, from the trial case, held in the right and left hands of the refractionist and rapidly alternated. The use of a +/−0.25D sphere in a combination holder ('flipper'), is both more convenient for the practitioner and easier for the patient to make the rapid comparisons necessary. With the patient binocularly fixating a single letter on the line immediately above that read by the eye with the poorer visual acuity, the +0.25D sphere is held in front of the right eye, and then rapidly exchanged for a −0.25D sphere—the advantage of a 'flipper' combination can be seen here. The patient is asked to state which lens (one, the +0.25DS, or two, the −0.25DS) gives the clearer vision. If the +0.25D spherical lens is preferred +0.25DS of trial case lens power is added to the correction before the right eye and the test repeated until the patient states a preference for vision with the −0.25DS held up before his eye. The procedure is repeated for the left eye, finally leaving, on re-checking each eye, a preference for vision when the −0.25DS rather than the +0.25DS is held up monocularly, whilst constantly maintaining binocular fixation. The binocular visual acuity is now considered to be 'balanced'. If the patient notices no difference in either eye, this may be due to relaxation of the accommodation and binocular +0.25DS should be put up and, if accepted given. The test then proceeds as before. The patient is in effect being asked whether it is easier to relax a quarter of a dioptre of his accommodation, or exert a quarter of a dioptre; a difference of half a dioptre is present in this contrast. It should be emphasized that this technique in practice is very accurate and very quick: it takes very much longer to describe than perform. Humphriss and Woodruff (1962) have since developed an alternative technique in which foveal vision in the eye not being refracted is suspended by fogging it with a 0.75D sphere.

*Bichromatic tests**

Davies and O'Connor (1957) were able to demonstrate that, at least as important as their use in binocular balancing, using a septum technique, the bichromatic comparison tests could be used both monocularly and binocularly virtually to eliminate the possibility of overcorrecting myopic patients for distance. If 'equality' of preference for the red and green letters or targets cannot be achieved, a definite 'green' preference indicates an excessive minus correction, whereas the patient would be far more comfortable in these circumstances left with his 'natural' preference for 'red'. After this test has been performed monocularly with,in the absence of 'equality', a 'red' preference being 'accepted' by the practitioner, it should be repeated binocularly with the same principles in mind. Most children aged from 7 or 8 years upwards are capable of co-operating with reliable answers as to whether the letters or targets are clearer (the practitioner's question should indicate that the answer must be whether the latter are 'blacker', not larger or smaller) on the red or green panel, or are equally clear, in this simple straightforward check at their post-cycloplegic examination. This test is, of course, applicable to adults as well, where cycloplegics are not usually required.

Millodot and Sivak (1973) demonstrated in controlled experiments that 'the eye is focused in the red end of the spectrum when looking in the distance and the eye is focused for radiation of decreasing wavelengths as the eye looks at objects closer to it'. These experimental observations are in accord with the clinical findings for distance corrected vision discussed above, and also with the additional clinical recordings of 'equality' or 'green' patient preferences for appropriate presbyopic corrections, included in the conclusions of the 1957 analysis of bichromatic refractive techniques.

Further uses of atropine

Atropine cycloplegia of the fixing eye of strabismic infants and children has been used in order to encourage the use of the amblyopic eye in near vision. Use of this technique, which is sometimes described as penalization, during the period of visual immaturity may induce amblyopia in the eye subjected to cycloplegia. Three such cases have been reported by von Noorden (1981). Experiments in monkeys raised with unilateral cycloplegia have demonstrated shrinkage of cells in the lateral geniculate nucleus and loss of cortical binocularity and of neurons responding to stimulation of the atropinized eye. The results of such animal experiments and the

---

* British Standard 3668:1963, 'Specification for red and green filters used in ophathalmic dichromatic tests', would appear to indicate a present day preference for the term dichromatic rather than bichromatic.

occurrence of atropine-induced amblyopia in children point to the need to exercise the greatest caution in the application of this technique.

Cyclopentolate

Cyclopentolate is the most widely used cycloplegic today. The paralysis of accommodation is not complete but it gives a depth of cycloplegia which is sufficient for the majority of cases. Sowden (1974) considers it the cycloplegic of choice when complete cycloplegia is not required. Although the recovery is not as quick as that following the use of tropicamide, the eye returns to normal much quicker than after the use of atropine. It is available in two strengths for cycloplegia — 0.5% and 1.0%.

Aged up to 12 years

Usually only one drop of the 1% solution is necessary, but it should be repeated if little effect is measurable after 15 minutes. Retinoscopic refraction may then be performed in 40–60 minutes (or sooner, if desired, when the maximal cycloplegic effect is obtained earlier than this).

Aged 12 years and above

One drop of the 0.5% solution, only repeated if within 15–20 minutes there is no significant measurable reduction in the amplitude of the accommodation. This second drop is sometimes necessary in white patients with dark hair and irides. For dark skinned adults, one drop of the 1% solution should be instilled, and the dose only repeated if the amplitude of accommodation is not falling at a satisfactory rate. Again, retinoscopy is generally carried out in 40–60 minutes, that is, the average time taken for the maximum effect of the drug to reduce the accommodation to less than 2.00D. Mitchell, Linfield and Francis (1959) have suggested that, where a deeper cycloplegia is not considered essential, a 0.125% solution, two drops of which will reduce the accommodation to approximately 1.50D (one drop to about 2.00D) in around 30 minutes, may be convenient with patients between the ages of 20 and 40 years. But it has to be considered that this maximal effect then lasts for only 10–15 minutes, which would appear to restrict the use of this concentration in general practice to fairly infrequent occasions.

Time course

One or two drops of the cyclopentolate solution instilled into the conjunctival sac produce a mydriasis commencing in a few minutes and becoming maximal in 30–60 minutes, but sometimes as rapidly as in 15 or, on rare occasions, even in 10 minutes. Cycloplegia commences almost simultaneously with mydriasis, and is also generally at its maximum between 30 and 60 minutes, with variations from an exceptional 10 minutes to 60 minutes or thereabouts. Because of the variation in the time taken to produce maximum cycloplegia, and also in view of the fact that the duration of this condition varies from 10 to 60 minutes (averaging about 40 minutes), the amplitude of accommodation should be measured every 10 minutes, after a time lag of 20 minutes following instillation, until no further fall in the accommodation is recorded (Mitchell, Linfield and Francis, 1958).

Depth of cycloplegia

As in nearly all cases the residual accommodation is 1.50D or less around 40–60 minutes after instillation (although not infrequently a second drop of the solution may be necessary to reduce the accommodation level to this), a period during this interval is the most usual time for retinoscopic refraction.

Priestley and Medine (1951) considered that cyclopentolate (then known as Compound 75 G.T.) more closely approximated their ideal criteria for a cycloplegic or mydriatic than any other drug discovered up to that time. The author is of the opinion, judging on their criteria, that this statement is still valid today.

Priestley and Medine compared the depth of cycloplegia reached after 1 hour following instillation of two drops of a 0.5% solution of cyclopentolate with the same dosage of a 5% solution of homatropine in a group of over 50 patients which included children and young adults. The cyclopentolate was instilled in the right eye and the homatropine in the left eye.

Their results showed that the residual accommodation for cyclopentolate ranged between 0.50 and 1.75D, with an average of 1.25D, whereas with homatropine this range was between 1.00 and 3.00D, with an average of 2.00D. In an endeavour to ensure that any anisocycloplegia present did not vitiate their findings, the series was later repeated using cyclopentolate in both eyes. Anisocycloplegia, a term originated by Beach (1942), who found it a phenomenon of fairly frequent occurrence, is the difference that may occur in the residual accommodation between the two eyes of the same patient to the same dose of a cycloplegic (often it amounts to about 0.5D, but exceptionally as much as 10.0D).

Rosenfield and Linfield (1986) proposed the use of what they termed 'a distance accommodation ability' measurement in which negative spherical lenses are introduced until the patient is no longer able to clearly read a line of Snellen letters as a measure of the degree of cycloplegia. They considered it an easier test to perform than apparent near point, especially on young children. It is interesting that the average minimum near and distance accommodation were not significantly different for 1% cyclopentolate as compared with 0.5%.

The residual accommodation was found again to be invariably less in these eyes than the homatropine recordings, whereas anisocycloplegia might well occur in either eye.

Stolzar (1953), in a further series, this time of 80 patients, using two drops of a 0.5% solution of the original American proprietary brand of cyclopentolate hydrochloride (Cyclogyl), found an average residual accommodation after 1 hour of 1.03D. His results (with average residual accommodation measured after correction of any distance refractive error), were as shown in Table 5.2.

Further analysis of this range of residual accommodation is also interesting (Table 5.3).

Full recovery of the accommodation, without the instillation of a miotic, usually occurred between 4 and 12 hours, but in a few cases this was delayed for 24 hours. Reading, in practice a more important consideration than full restoration of accommodation, was usually possible after 3–4 hours. Recovery from mydriasis was shown as occurring between 24 and 48 hours, in all instances without the aid of a miotic.

Table 5.2

Age-group (years)	Number of cases	Residual accommodation (D)
10–20	28	1.14
20–30	29	0.97
30–40	23	0.97

Table 5.3

Residual accommodation (D)	Percentage of cases
0.50	2.5
0.75	13.7
1.00	55.0
1.25	27.5
1.50	1.3

   Stolzar, in his investigations, presumably carried out on normal eyes, found no increase in intra-ocular pressures. He made no direct comparisons of residual accommodations against those encountered using a homatropine–hydroxyamphetamine combination, the latter formerly being one of the most popular combinations of cycloplegic and sympathomimetic drugs used by American ophthalmologists, but considered that the cycloplegic effect obtained with cyclopentolate was either equal to or more profound than that of this combination. Gettes and Leopold (1953) actually confirmed this view. Mitchell, Linfield and Francis (1958) made such a comparison with the comparable homatropine–ephedrine combination used by optometrists in Great Britain and came to much the same conclusions. They confirmed the more rapid onset and shorter duration of cyclopentolate cycloplegia. In one study, one drop of a 0.5% cyclopentolate hydrochloride solution was instilled into the eyes of 16 Caucasian students (32 eyes) (O'Connor-Davies unpublished data 1972) with an age range of 20–27 years (average 22.75 years (see Table 5.4). It was found necessary to instil a second drop of the solution with four subjects (eight eyes), in order to reduce the

Table 5.4

Range of residual accommodation (11)	Number of eyes	Percentage of total number of eyes
0.50	3	9.4
0.75	5	15.5
1.00	9	28.2
1.25	4	12.5
1.50	10	31.3
1.75	1	3.1

residual accommodation (measured with any distance refractive error corrected) to below 2.00D within 60 minutes. Three of these students (six eyes) had, as might be expected, dark brown eyes and hair (it is well established that dark complexioned people with dark irides are more resistant to cycloplegics and mydriatics), but the fourth subject was fair-haired and blue-eyed. In the whole group the findings were as follows.

Average time to reach maximum cycloplegia, 34.2 minutes

Range of time to reach maximum cycloplegia, 10–55 minutes

Average residual accommodation, 1.16D

As with all other cycloplegics, with the exception of atropine, distance fixation during retinoscopy is necessary to relax as much of the residual accommodation as possible. Measuring of the latter before and after examination may be carried out with reasonable accuracy using a +3.00D sphere monocularly with the near point rule.

Where children, under the age of 7 years, who have previously shown allergic reactions to atropine, require cycloplegic refraction, one or two drops of cyclopentolate hydrochloride eyedrops 1% may be substituted, immediately followed by very careful occlusion of the canaliculi for half a minute or so.

Medical uses

Cyclopentolate may be used in the treatment of corneal ulceration, iritis, iridocyclitis and keratitis, one or two drops of the 0.5% solution being instilled every 6–8 hours, to prevent the formation of posterior synechiae, and 'rest' the painful ciliary and sphincter pupillae muscles. For long-term treatment in these conditions, cyclopentolate does not compare favourably with the longer acting more conventional drugs such as atropine and homatropine. When breaking down lenticular adhesions, one or two drops of the 0.5% solution are instilled, followed 6 hours later by one or two drops of a 2% solution of pilocarpine nitrate; this alternating treatment is repeated daily.

Summary

The cycloplegic effect of cyclopentolate may, therefore, be summarized as giving an extensive depression of accommodation, of rapid onset and shorter duration than either atropine or homatropine, and it is, therefore, less incapacitating to the patient. In the appropriate concentration, for patients over the age of 6 years and up to the age of 42 or 43 years, where a cycloplegic refraction is considered necessary, cyclopentolate may well prove to be the drug of first choice.

Even in children under the age of 6 years, where a full refraction is called for, and where, for one reason or another, atropine cannot be used, the instillation of one or two drops of the 1% solution of cyclopentolate, although the depth of cycloplegia may not be so profound, would appear to be a suitable alternative.

Havener (1978) aptly sums up the great value of cyclopentolate when he describes its effects in the field of cycloplegia as superior to homatropine (even the 5% concentration of the latter) in its rapidity of onset, shortened duration of action, and greater intensity of effect.

As has already been mentioned, but it may not be inappropriate to reemphasize, in no instance of the use of cyclopentolate (or any other cycloplegic, with the exception of atropine) is a tonus allowance appropriate. This does not, of course, preclude adjustments being made to any prescription found under cyclopentolate cycloplegia for other reasons, some of which have been discussed in the previous chapter.

Any residual accommodation should always be measured at the time of a cycloplegic refraction (with all cycloplegics), otherwise an anisometropic prescription error may occur if an unequal cycloplegic effect between the two eyes remains undetected.

Tropicamide (Bistropamide)
(Proprietary preparation: *Mydriacyl*, USA)

Tropicamide is another rapidly acting synthetic antimuscarinic drug. It is used as a mydriatic in a 0.5% solution and a cycloplegic in a 1.0% solution.

As a mydriatic two drops of the weaker solution instilled into the conjunctival sac produce a full mydriasis in about 15 minutes, the pupil returning to normal in 8–9 hours if no miotic is used to counteract the pupillary dilatation.

To produce cycloplegia two drops of the 1% solution are instilled into the eye allowing a 5-minute interval between each drop. The full cycloplegic effect is achieved in about 30 minutes, when the retinoscopy is performed. If the latter examination has to be delayed beyond 35 minutes because of the very brief maximal effect of the cycloplegia, a further (third) drop of the 1% solution should be used. Complete recovery of the accommodation usually occurs within 6 hours, and reading is generally possible after 2–4 hours from the time of the initial instillations.

Excellent cycloplegia (with residual accommodation below 2.00D) is usually obtained, according to Gettes and Belmont (1961), following the procedures outline above, but due to the very brief duration of maximum effect the third drop is not infrequently necessitated in routine practice. In a series of 193 patients, Gettes and Belmont (1961) were only able to examine 60% of these during the interval of 20–35 minutes (when cycloplegia was maximal) and 40% had to receive the third drop. However, as Havener (1978) emphasizes, the great advantage of tropicamide is its very rapid action and very short duration of action, the patient having fully recovered from cycloplegia in 2–6 hours, and these very qualities make it also a very useful mydriatic in its weaker concentration of 0.5% (Smith, 1971).

The speed of onset allowed Harding (1970) to see more patients in his working day and the short duration of action allowed patients to return to work within 2 hours.

On the other hand, Milder (1961) did not find when using two drops of the 1% solution that it was as satisfactory a cycloplegic as the same number of drops of a 1% cyclopentolate or a 5% homatropine solution. He instilled tropicamide in one eye and cyclopentolate or homatropine in the other. In a series of 50 consecutive cases (100 eyes) he found better cycloplegia produced by the cyclopentolate in 23 out of the 25 cases and homatropine in 20 out of 25 cases in comparison to the tropicamide instilled in the second eye in each case. Thus, in only seven eyes (five with homatropine in the other eye and two with cyclopentolate in the other eye) out of the 100 eyes was tropicamide superior in its cycloplegic effect to these other drugs. In children in particular, his results indicated a poor paralysis of the ciliary muscle, in the six cases in this series up to the age of 9 years an average of 6.25D of residual accommodation was present after 30 minutes, and in 20 cases from 10 to 14 years this reading was still averaging 3.65D. Tropicamide would, therefore, appear to be a relatively inadequate cycloplegic for use with children. This is confirmed by Hiatt and Jenkins (1983) who found that tropicamide was less effective as a cycloplegic for preschool esotropia.

Other cycloplegics

Homatropine

Homatropine is a semi-synthetic alkaloid prepared from atropine; the base tropine obtained by hydrolysis of atropine is chemically combined with mandelic acid.

Homatropine Hydrobromide Eyedrops BP, the standard solution, contains up to 2% w/v homatropine hydrobromide. It is commonly used in in 1%, 2% and 5% concentrations for cycloplegia, and 0.25–0.50% strengths as a mydriatic.

It does not produce as satisfactory a cycloplegia in children. Its use for this purpose is therefore usually restricted to the over-15-years age-groups. Conventional dosage of the eyedrops is one drop of the 2% solution repeated twice at 10 minute intervals (that is, a total of three drops).

Mydriasis commences in 15 minutes and is maximal in about 30–40 minutes, with complete abolition of pupillary reflex to light and accommodation. Complete recovery of the pupil may take between 24 and 48 hours, depending on dosage. The amplitude of accommodation begins to fall in 15 minutes and is usually at its lowest between 45 and 90 minutes. Therefore, cycloplegic retinoscopic refraction should not commence until about 60 minutes after instillation, and the residual accommodation should be measured to ensure that it is below 2.00D. Refraction should be completed before 90 minutes has elapsed from the time of instillation of the drops. Accommodation may fully recover in 24 hours (12 hours when the drug is used in combination with ephedrine). Usually sufficient accommodation is available for close work with 2% homatropine hydrobromide in around 12–24 hours (this time is reduced to around 6 hours with the additional use of 5% ephedrine). The advantage of the synergist (in the optometrist's technique—ephedrine) is the quicker recovery of the ciliary muscle, with the subsequent ability to resume near work sooner. The pupil also participates in this recovery and is normal, usually, after about 24 hours. The presence of a synergist allows a smaller dosage of the principal drug and this explains the more rapid recovery. The onset of cycloplegia is also somewhat hastened, but, as in both cases (that is, with or without the ephedrine) 60 minutes may still, in some individuals, be required to reduce accommodation to less than 2.00D: this is only of academic interest.

Not infrequently the depth of cycloplegia in the under-20-years age-group is not reduced much below 2.00D, but if under this amount is recorded (the first reading being taken after half an hour and then every 10 minutes until no further fall of accommodation is noted) cycloplegic retinoscopy can usually be adequately performed, with the patient gazing at a distant target to relax the small amount of accommodation left unparalysed. No tonus allowance is made as the dependent tone of the ciliary muscle has not been affected.

Lachesine

Lachesine chloride is a synthetic antimuscarinic drug. It is a white amorphous powder, soluble 1 in 3 parts of water, with mydriatic and cycloplegic properties when instilled in solution into the eye. Lachesine is not taken internally. Lachesine Eyedrops, *BPC*, consist of a sterile solution containing up to 1% w/v of lachesine chloride with phenyl mercuric acetate or nitrate (as the antimicrobial) in purified water. These drops may be used as a substitute for those of atropine or homatropine in patients showing idiosyncrasies to these two cycloplegics.

The degree and duration of the cycloplegia is about mid-way between that produced by atropine and that by homatropine, reaching a maximum in about 1 hour, and being accompanied by a maximum mydriasis. The latter begins to subside in 5 or 6 hours. In old people, however, the response to miotics is slower and less complete after lachesine than when homatropine has been used, so lachesine's use, even in weaker concentrations for mydriatic purposes, is not recommended for patients over the age of 40 years. Mitchell (1964) does not consider it as reliable a cycloplegic as atropine or hometropine, especially in young people.

When used as a cycloplegic in the young, two drops of the 1% solution is the recommended dose, and retinoscopy is performed in about 1 hour's time when the residual accommodation has been measured and found to be at it's lowest.

Hyoscine hydrobromide (scopolamine hydrobromide)

Hyoscine is employed in general medicine for its sedative properties. Although its peripheral action resembles atropine (for example, it causes cycloplegia and mydriasis), its central action differs by producing immediate depression of the cerebral cortex, especially of the motor areas. It is used as a hypnotic in mania, alcoholism and pre-operative medication, in the last-named case usually being combined with morphine or possibly pethidine (known as meperidine in the USA). It is administered also in the treatment of motion sickness, and to depress memory of recent events. It reduces the tremors of paralysis agitans and chorea and relieves the salivation and, to a lesser extent, the muscular rigidity of post-encephalitic parkinsonism.

Peripherally its antimuscarinic (anticholinergic) action in the eye is qualitatively similar to atropine, but its action is more rapid and its effects are not as prolonged.

Hyoscine hydrobromide is instilled in eyedrops containing 0.05%, 0.25% and up to 0.5% of the drug and in a 0.25% eye ointment. Maximal cycloplegia is reached in about 40–60 minutes. Some doubt appears still to exist as to the depth and reliability of this cycloplegic in children, as compared to atropine. Sorsby *et al.* (1955) claim that a single instillation of two drops of a 0.05% solution produces as satisfactory a cycloplegia in children as is achieved by repeated instillations of atropine over a period of several days. The near maximal cycloplegia reached in about 1 hour persists for about 6 hours, with recovery for reading being reached in approximately 24 hours, and a normal ciliary muscle amplitude in 48 hours.

With stronger concentrations of this drug these recovery times will of course be extended, for example, after instillation of a 0.5% solution 3–4 days are required for half the cycloplegic effect to wear off, and complete ciliary muscle recovery takes more than a week (Marron, 1940).

This drug is more toxic than atropine, and with the eyedrops pressure over the canaliculi is mandatory. Giddiness and ataxia have been reported after its use, and because of its potency and possible unpleasant adverse reactions, which include hallucinations and psychotic disturbances in patients who have an idiosyncracy to the drug, it is not in common use by optometrists, although with the 0.05% solution the danger of toxic effects should be considerably reduced.

Adverse effects of cycloplegics

Antimuscarinic drugs are potent agents which can produce effects on several structures in the body. Atropine was a favourite of the medieval professional poisoners and is probably the most toxic compound that is used routinely as a diagnostic agent. Other cycloplegics also have the potential to produce marked side effects.

Toxic effects from topical ophthalmic use have been known for a long time (Wise, 1904). These consisted of a high temperature and central nervous system effects of hallucinations and ataxia. Daly (1959) and Harel, Frydman and Kauschansky (1985) also reported psychotic reactions to atropine eye drops. Hoefnagel (1961) reported confusion, hallucinations, ataxia and restlessness after the use of atropine. Death from the use of atropine has been reported by Heath (1950).

CNS effects represent an advanced stage of atropine poisoning. Milder effects can be seen at earlier stages of poisoning. These affect peripheral tissues, including exocrine glands such as the salivary glands and the sweat glands. Patients suffering from atropine poisoning are said to be:

blind as a Bat;
dry as a Bone;
red as a Beetroot;
mad as a Hatter.

Patients are as blind as a bat because of the effect on accommodation. They are as dry as a bone because of the inhibition of the sweat glands and salivary glands. A dry mouth is one of the earliest signs of atropine poisoning. The inhibition of sweat glands deprives the body of one of its methods of losing heat. In order to compensate for this there is a dilatation of skin blood vessels, giving the patient the appearance of being as 'red as a beetroot'. When CNS effects occur patients become as 'mad as a hatter'.

CNS effects have also been reported following the use of cyclopentolate. In the majority of cases these effects followed the administration of a higher than recommended dose or a combination with other drugs. CNS effects manifest themselves as confusion, difficulty in speaking, hallucinations and ataxia. Fortunately there have been no fatal reports following these effects of cyclopentolate, and the patient is back to normal in a matter of hours.

These effects would appear to be dose related, as Cher (1955) used two drops of 0.5% with a 10-minute interval between applications on 159 patients without producing CNS problems. Beswick (1962) used 2% cyclopentolate (not available in the UK) and noted hallucinations in a 9-year-old child. Binkhorst *et al.* (1953) found that 2% cyclopentolate elicited reactions in 4 patients out of 40.

One case has been reported in which CNS effects were seen after the use of 0.2% cyclopentolate (Carpenter, 1967) but the patient had a history of chronic dementia.

From the above, it would appear that 0.5% cyclopentolate should be used whenever possible and cyclopentolate 1% should be used sparingly.

Recently, problems in the gastro-intestinal tract following the use of cyclopentolate in premature babies have been reported (Isenberg, Abrams and Hyman, 1985). It was found that cyclopentolate 0.5% decreased gastric acid secretion while 0.25% did not. Bauer, Trepanier Trottier and Stern (1973) had earlier reported necrotizing enterocolitis following the use of cyclopentolate.

Homatropine, although less toxic than atropine, has produced problems in the past. Hoefnagel (1961) reported CNS effects such as ataxia and hallucinations in four children who had received six drops of homatropine 2% at 10-minute intervals. Such a dose must be considered excessive and it is not surprising that problems arose.

Tropicamide compared with other cycloplegics is relatively free from adverse reactions. Wahl (1965) reported unconsciousness and pallor following one drop of 0.5%. As there have been no similar reports, it would appear that the reaction is probably not drug-related.

Allergic reactions can occur to many compounds. Atropine is probably the most notorious for producing reactions but cycloplentolate has also been implicated.

It may appear that the use of cycloplegics is potentially hazardous. If the following rules are applied then this potential will be markedly reduced.

(1) Question the patient or parent about the previous use of eyedrops and any problems that may have occurred.

(2) Ask if there is a history of allergy.

(3) Check whether the patient is receiving any medication.

(4) Use the lowest concentration and the weakest drug possible.

(5) If multiple applications are necessary then they should be separated by at least 10 minutes.

(6) Only consider an atropine refraction when you feel that the parent can be trusted to administer the ointment correctly.

(7) Ensure that you are prepared for any problems that can occur. A course in first aid is a sensible precaution.

(8) If you prescribed atropine for domiciliary use, ensure that the tube is brought to the practice with the child on the day of refraction. This will enable you to verify the amount of drug used and to dispose safely of any surplus.

References

Amos, D. M. (1978) Cycloplegics for refraction. *Am. J. Optom. Physiol. Opt.*, **55**, 223–226

Bauer, R., Trepannier Trottier, M. C. and Stern, L. (1973) Systemic Cyclopentolate (Cyclogyl) toxicity in the new born infant. *Paediatr. Pharmacol. Ther.*, **82**, 501–505

Beach, S. J. (1942) Anisocycloplegia. *Am. J. Ophthal.*, **26**, 522

Beswick, J. A. (1962) Psychosis from cyclopentolate. *Am. J. of Ophthalmol.*, **53**, 879–880

Binkhorst, R. D., Weinstein, G. W., Baretz, R. M. and Clahane, A. C. (1963) Cyclopentolate toxicity in paediatric patients. *Am.J. of Ophthalmol.*, **55**, 1243–1246

Black, K. T. S. (1978) Letters to the Editor. *Optician*, **176**, 34

Carpenter, W. T. (1967) Precipitous mental deterioration following cycloplegia with 0.2% cyclopentolate. *Arch. of Ophthalmol.*, **78**, 445–447

Cher, I. (1959) Experiences with Cyclogyl. *Transact. Ophthalm. Soc. UK.*, **79**, 665–670

Daly, P. J. (1959) Psychotic reactions to atropine poisoning. *Br. Med. J.*, **2**, 608

Davies, P. H., O'Connor (1957) A critical analysis of bichromatic tests used in clinical refraction. *Br. J. Physiol. Optics*, **14**, 170–182

Duke-Elder, S. (1978) Practice of Refraction, 9th edn, Churchill Livingstone, Edinburgh and London pp. 39, 41, 51, 71, 77, 119

Gettes, B. C. and Belmont, O. (1961) Tropicamide. Comparative cycloplegic effects. *Arch. Ophthalmol.*, **66**, 336

Gettes, H. C. and Leopold, I. H. (1953) Evaluation of five new cycloplegic drugs. *Archs. Ophthalmol. N. Y.*, **49**, 24

Giles, G. H. (1965) *The Principles and Practice of Refraction and its Allied Subjects*, 2nd edn Hammond Hammond, London: pp. 155–156, 389–390

Gillie, J. Calder (1959) The flipper technique. *Optician*, **138**, 371

Harding, R. (1970) Benefits for office practice using tropicamide – A short acting mydriatic cycloplegic. *Eye, Ear Nose and Throat Monthly*, **49**, 75–76

Harel, L., Frydman, M. and Kauschansky, A. (1985) Prolonged parasympathetic paralysis and psychosis caused by atropine eye drops. *J. Paediatr. Ophthalmol. Strabis*, **22**, 38–39

Havener, W. H. (1978) *Ocular Pharmacology*, 4th edn, Mosby, St Louis pp. 253–256

Heath, W. E. (1950) Death from atropine poisoning. *Br. Med. J.*, **2**, 608

Hiatt, R. L. and Jenkin, G. (1983) Comparison of atropine and tropicamide in esotropia. *Ann. Ophthalmol.*, **15**, 341–343

Hodd, F. A. B. and Freeman H. (1955) Comparative analysis of retinoscopic and subjective refraction. *Br. J. Physiol. Optics*, **12**, 31–33

Hoefnagel D. 91961) Toxic effects of atropine and homatropine eye drops in children. *N. Engl. J. Med.*, **264**, 168–171

Humphriss, D. and Woodruff, E. W. (1962) Refraction by immediate contrast. *Br. J. Physiol. Optics.*, **19**, 15–20

Ingram, R. M. and Barr, A. (1979) Refraction of 1 year old children after cycloplegia with 1% cyclopentolate: comparison with findings after atropinisation. *Br. J. Ophthalmol.*, **63**, 348–352

Isenberg, S. J., Abrams, C. and Hyman, P. E. (1985) Effects of cyclopentolate eyedrops on gastric secretory function in pre-term infants. *Ophthalmology*, **92**, 698–700

Kelly, T. Stuart-Black, Chatfield, C. and Tustin, G. (1975) Clinical assessment of the arrest of myopia. *Br. J. Ophthal.*, **59**, 529–538

Kelly, T. Stuart-Black, (1978) Letters to the Editor. *Optician*, **176**, 34

Mallett, R. F. J. (1964) The investigation of heterophoria at near and a new fixation disparity technique. *Optician*, **148**, 547–551, 574–581

Mallett, R. F. J. (1983) A new fixation disparity test and its application. *Optician*, **186**, 11–15

Mallett, R. (1979) Personal (verbal) communication

Marron, J. (1940) Cycloplegia and mydriasis by use of atropine, scopolamine and homatropine. *Arch. Ophthalmol.*, **23**, 340

Martin-Doyle, J. L. C. (1967) *A Synopsis of Ophthalmology*, 3rd edn, p. 7, Wright, Bristol

Milder, B. (1961) Tropicamide as a cycloplegic agent. *Arch. Ophthal.*, **66**, 70

Miller, S. J. H. (1978) Parsons' diseases of the eye, 16th ed. Churchill Livingstone, Edinburgh and London pp. 86–88, 236, 499

Millodot, M. and Sivak, J. (1973) Influence of accommodation on the chromatic aberration of the eye. *Br. J. Physiol. Optics*, **28**, 169–174

Mitchell, D. W. A. (1964) *The Use of Drugs in Refraction*, 3rd edn, The British Optical Association, pp. 42–44, 56

Mitchell, D. W. A., Linfield, J. A. and Francis, J. L. (1958) A comparison of the effects of cyclopentolate with those of homatropine and ephedrine in the eye. *Optician*, **135**, 3

Oakley, K. H. and Young, L. A. (1975) Bifocal control of myopia. *Am. J. Optom. Physiol. Optics*, **52**, 758–764

Priestley, B. S. and Medine, M. M. (1951) A new mydriatic and cycloplegic drug. *Am. J. Ophthal.*, **34**, 572

Rosenfield, M. and Linfield, P. B. (1986) A comparison of the effects of cycloplegics on accommodation ability for distance vision and the apparent near point. *Ophthal. Physiol. Opt.*, **6**, 317–320

Smith, Redmond, J. H. (1965) *Clinical Glaucoma*, Cassell, London, pp.6–13

Smith, S. L. (1971) Mydriatic drugs for routine fundal inspection, *Lancet*, **2**, 837

Sorsby, A., Sheridan, M., Moore, N. and Haythorne, J. (1955) Hyoscine cycloplegia in children *Lancet*, **2**, 214

Sowden, A. S. (1974) The pre-school child: indications for cycloplegic examination. *Aust. J. Optom.*, **57**, 215–218

Stolzar, I. H. (1953) A new group of cycloplegic drugs. *Am. J. Ophthalmol.*, **36**, 110

Stone, J. (1976) The possible influences of contact lenses on myopia. *Br. J. Physiol. Optics*, **31**, 89–114

Von Noorden, G. K. (1981) Amblyopia caused by unilateral atropinisation. *Ophthalmology*, **88**, 131–133

Wahl, J. W. (1969) Systemic reactions to tropicamide. *Arch. Ophthalmol.*, **82**, 320–321

Whittington, J. H. (1958) *The Art of Clinical Refraction*. Oxford University Press, London, pp. 66–67, 232, 238–244

Wise, C. H. (1904) A case of poisoning from atropine eye drops. *Br. Med. J.*, **1**, 189

Young, J. A. (1978) Accommodation and the control of myopia. *Optician*, **176**, 7–9

Chapter 6

Mydriatics

Mydriatics are drugs which dilate the pupil to facilitate a more thorough examination of the fundus, lens periphery and vitreous. They are mostly used on elderly patients, as here the pupils are usually smaller and lens opacities and abnormal retinal conditions are not uncommon, but their use may be essential in any age-group, especially where the macula or the peripheral areas of the retina need particularly careful observations, for example, suspected macular cyst or hole, location of a penetrating foreign body, intra-ocular tumours, peripheral detachments, etc. Martin-Doyle (1967) considers the instillation of a mydriatic indispensible for an adequate examination of the macula (Table 6.1).

Ideal properties of mydriatics

(i)   Quick in onset.
(ii)   Adequate duration.
(iii)   Fast recovery after examination.
(iv)   Light reflex abolished.
(v)   No cycloplegia.
(vi)   Capable of quick reversal in an emergency.
(vii)   No rise in intraocular pressure.
(viii) No other pharmacological effect.
(ix)   No local toxic reaction.
(x)   No systemic toxic reaction.

The indications and contra-indications for mydriatic examination have been admirably summarized by Havener (1975).

Indications

The occasions where there is a special need for a thorough fundus inspection through a dilated pupil, where the latter does not already exist, include the following.

(1) Recent onset of floating opacities in the vitreous.
(2) A relatively sudden decrease in visual acuity, necessitating a careful study of the macula.

Table 6.1 Mydriatics*

Official name	Trade name	Strengths % w/v	Single dose	Mode of action	Mydriatic onset	Mydriatic duration	Reversed by	Adverse reactions	Notes
Atropine sulphate	—	1.0	Yes	Antimuscarinics	40 min	7 days	Ecothiopate or DFP	Allergic reactions and general antimuscarinics effects	Too strong for routine mydriatic use. Causes unwanted cycloplegia
Homatropine hydrobromide	—	1.0 2.0	2% only	Antimuscarinics	40 min	48 h	Physostigmine		Rarely used Cycloplegic
Cyclopentolate hydrobromide	Mydrilate	1.0 0.5 0.1	Yes except 0.1%	Antimuscarinics	30 min	24 h	Physostigmine	CNS effects	Too strong for routine examination Cycloplegic
Tropicamide	Mydriacyl	0.5 1.4	Yes	Antimuscarinics	15 min	8–9 h	Physostigmine Thymoxamine	Some CNS effects	Mydriatic of choice
Eucatropine	—	5.0 10.0	No	Antimuscarinics	30 min	6 h	?	—	Little used
Phenylephrine	—	2.5 10.0	Yes	Sympathomimetic	30 min	12–24 h	Thymoxamine	Systemic Hypertension	10% hypotensive
Cocaine	—	2.5 4.0	No	Sympathomimetic	30 min	20 h	?	Local anaesthetic	Not for use by optometrists
Hydroxy amphetamine	—	1.0 to 3.0	No	Sympathomimetic	45 min	3 h	?	—	Not for use by optometrists
Ephedrine	—	5.0	No	Sympathomimetic	30 min	12 h	—	—	Effects are variable

*All mydriatics have the ability to precipitate angle closure glaucoma in susceptible patients

(3) Unexplained loss of visual field.

(4) Unexplained ocular pain, not accompanied by raised intra-ocular tension.

(5) 'Redness' of the eye not attributable to superficial infection, allergy, or to raised intra-ocular tension.

(6) After contusion to rule out eye damage.

(7) Cloudiness of the vitreous or lens, when good mydriasis will reveal fundus detail hidden by a small pupil.

Obviously only some patients need mydriatic examination. If none of the specific ocular signs or symptoms enumerated above is present, or if the patient has a (systemic) disease not known to produce eye manifestations, a reasonable view of the optic disc and retinal vessels through the undilated pupil may be considered an adequate examination. Spontaneously large pupils are commonly found in many young people conveniently permitting a relatively thorough fundus examination. It is usually with the older age-groups, with their smaller pupils, that mydriatics are, on occasion, necessary. In his typically succinct style Havener aptly compares 'the view of a fundus through a small pupil or a dilated pupil with the view of a room as seen through a keyhole or with the door open'!

Adequate dilatation of the pupils reveals small details of great diagnostic significance, for example, diabetic micro-aneurisms, hypertensive arteriolar atte-nuation, early signs of macular degeneration, small traumatic retinal holes, peripheral retinal lesions, etc. Newell (1969) emphasizes an important clinical principle when he comments 'that there is more danger of missing significant ocular or systemic disease by failing to dilate than there is of precipitating glaucoma by dilatation'. This 'approach' is reflected in Havener's remark that 'a physician who dilates many eyes may expect to precipitate not more than one case of acute glaucoma in a lifetime'. It is to be hoped that such views expressed by eminent authorities, taken in conjunction with the precautions listed in the following contra-indications will give the optical student and practitioner a balanced attitude to the use of mydriatics in appropriate cases. It is the optometrist's moral and legal duty to refer pathological conditions (ocular or systemic) for medical attention; he will obviously be unable to do this unless he can 'see' such conditions in the first instance.

Contra-indications

Before instillation of any mydriatic (whether of the antimuscarinic or sympathomi-metic group) the optometrist must first confirm (as indicated in the previous Chapter for cycloplegia in older patients) that no contra-indications to the dilatation of the pupil(s) are present. Contra-indications will include the following.

(1) The known presence of glaucoma, ascertained by questioning the patient and inspection of the eyes for signs of 'therapeutic miosis' (patient on 'drops' with very small pupils) or previous glaucoma surgery.

(2) Evidence of elevated intraocular tension, derived from visual field and/or tonometric investigations.

(3) The presence of an abnormally shallow anterior chamber, which is almost invariably associated with a narrow anterior angle, such an eye being predisposed to acute glaucoma (which is the only type of glaucoma that can be precipitated by a mydriatic) occurring solely in such structurally designed eyes. The central depth of

the anterior chamber in the normal adult eye is about 3 mm. Assessing this depth by oblique illumination using a small source of light held close to the temporal limbus and observing the shadow cast by the lens displacing the iris forwards towards the cornea on the opposite nasal side of the iris and use of the slit-lamp also provides a good indication of this and the state of the angle.

The current ready availability of slip-lamp microscopes in optometric practices should encourage an excellent alternative technique, using this instrument to ascertain that the angle of the anterior chamber is a wide open one, and not the narrow or extremely narrow angle of the eye predisposed to primary angle-closure glaucoma. Originally, Van Herick, Shaffer and Schwartz (1969), and subsequently Polse (1975) and Stone (1979), described a technique for estimation of the width of the anterior chamber angle which should contribute appreciably to establishing the safety or otherwise of the diagnostic use of mydriatics (or miotics) (Figure 6.1).

The technique consists of observing with the microscope (using low magnification (6x or 10x) and the microscope/light-beam angle set at approximately 60 degrees) an optical section of the angle in the immediate vicinity of the limbus. Temporal and nasal observations are made employing the narrowest light beam, with the patient fixating the microscope positioned directly in front of him.

The ratio of aqueous interval to corneal thickness is carefully assessed: 1:1 (or more) corresponds to Grade 4 (with reference to Shaffer's gonioscopic classification); 1:2 to Grade 3; 1:4 to Grade 2; and less than 1:4 to Grade 1.

Grade 2 is a narrow angle capable of closure, and Grade 1, an extremely narrow angle, is likely to do so. Both these grades are contra-indications for the diagnostic use of mydriatics (or miotics).

It must be stated, however, that gonioscopy is the sole definitive test of the latter. In established glaucoma, where the pupil is to be dilated, it is the practice of ophthalmologists (the only consultants competent to dilate in these circumstances) to perform a prior gonioscopy for this assessment.

Not only full mydriasis, in such predisposed eyes, will result in an increased intra-ocular tension by mechanical blockage of the angle by the iris, but a state of semi-dilatation of the pupil may initiate this rise by producing pupillary block. This may occur in these eyes, with their shallow anterior chambers and anteriorly placed lens, the iris being more closely opposed to the lens capsule over a much wider area than in the normal depth chamber where the pupillary iris margins lightly touch the anterior lens surface. The passage of aqueous between the posterior and anterior chambers is then hindered and, with the semi-dilated pupil, a physiological iris bombé results. The peripheral iris bulges forward to come in contact with the posterior corneal surface, thus impeding the drainage of the aqueous via the filtration channels of the angle.

Where any of these three contra-indications exist (that is, known glaucoma, raised intra-ocular tension or abnormally shallow anterior chamber and angle), no mydriatic should be instilled and the patient must be referred to his doctor with a full report.

Mode of action

Because of the presence of the two opponent muscles, the pupil sphincter and dilator muscles, there are two different modes of action of mydriatics.

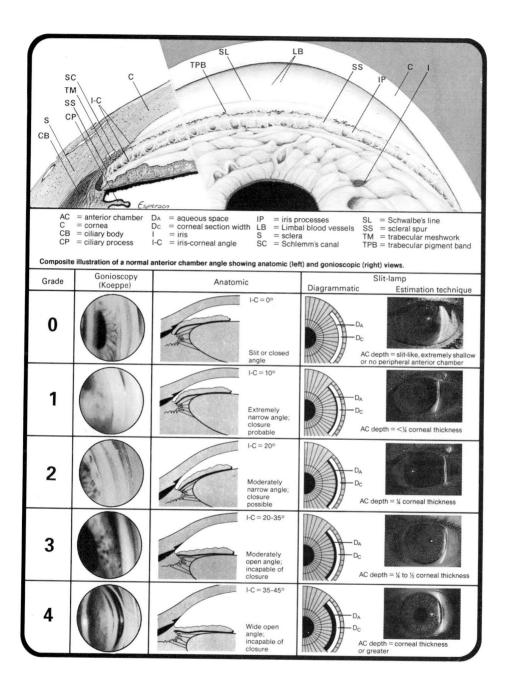

Composite illustration of a normal anterior chamber angle showing anatomic (left) and gonioscopic (right) views.

Figure 6.1 Van Herrick's Test (courtesy of Allergan Pharmaceuticals)

The dilator pupillae muscle is innervated by the sympathetic nervous system and sympathomimetic drugs will cause a contraction of the dilator muscle causing mydriasis. The parasympathetic system is largely unaffected by such drugs and thus the pupillary light reflex remains active. Sympathomimetic drugs also have little effect on accommodation.

On the other hand, the sphincter pupillae muscle, which is innervated by the parasympathetic system, can be paralysed by the same class of drugs which cause cycloplegia, the antimuscarinic agents. With this type of drug the pupillary light reflex is reduced or abolished.

Antimuscarinic mydriatics

By using weak concentrations of 'strong drugs' (for example, homatropine) or 'weak drugs' (for example, tropicamide) of the antimuscarinic group, mydriasis can be produced with a much less profound cycloplegia, with the latter's attendant incapacitating effect on near vision thereby considerably reduced, as the sphincter pupillae is more susceptible than the ciliary muscle to these substances.

Tropicamide

Tropicamide is the antimuscarinic mydriatic of choice today. Normally available as 0.5% and 1.0% strengths, it is the weaker of the two that is used most often for mydriasis. Davidson (1976) states that the mydriatic effect is greater than the cycloplegic effect and that this propensity for mydriasis is of clinical value. The 1% strength is used for cycloplegia. Tropicamide is quick in onset and short in duration, and the depth of mydriasis is adequate for most examinations since the pupil light reflex is depressed. Pollack, Hunt and Polse (1981) investigated the dose/response relationships of tropicamide's mydriasis and cycloplegia under two levels of illumination. They found that the mydriatic effect was independent of dose (range 0.25–1.0%) and level of illumination, whilst the cycloplegic effect was greater for the stronger concentrations.

This confirms that 0.5% should be used for mydriasis and 1% for cycloplegia. Pollack *et al.* used patients with a range of eye colours but did not collate the findings for different degrees of pigmentation. Hence it is possible that the strength may need to be varied with the level of pigmentation. The mydriasis caused by tropicamide can be reversed if necessary with weak solutions of physostigmine.

Other antimuscarinic mydriatics

All cycloplegics can be used as mydriatics but the effect is usually too long lasting. The following have been used in the past.

Cyclopentolate
The mydriatic concentration of cyclopentolate is 0.1% (compared with 0.5% and 1.0% for cycloplegia). Mydriasis commences in about 10 minutes and is maximal in about 30. The effect may last up to 24 hours (Davison, 1970). It produces similar mydriasis but more cycloplegia than homatropine (Table 6.2). Cyclopentolate is sometimes used pre-operatively to produce maximal mydriasis.

Table 6.2

Average pupil diameter before instillation (mm)	Average pupil diameter after 0.1% cyclopentolate hydrochloride solution (mm)	Average pupil diameter after 0.5% homatropine hydrobromide solution (mm)	Average reduction in accommodation after 0.1% cyclopentolate solution (D)	Average reduction in accommodation after 0.5% homatropine solution (D)
R.E 4.3	7.7		7.60	
L.E 4.3		7.5		4.50

Homatropine

At one time, homatropine was the principal mydriatic and was often used in mixtures such as homatropine and cocaine or homatropine and ephedrine. The mydriatic effect commences in 10–20 minutes and is maximal in 30–40 minutes. At 30 minutes both light and accommodative reflexes are absent and the examination may be carried out. Recovery takes the same time as cyclopentolate if a miotic is not used, but may be as prolonged as 3 days (Davidson, 1970). It can be employed as 0.25% or 0.5%. As would be expected, the higher strength produces a slightly larger pupil but a much more marked effect on the ciliary muscle in reducing accommodation (Table 6.3).

Table 6.3

Average pupil diameter before instillation (mm)	Average pupil diameter after 0.5% homatropine hydrobromide solution (mm)	Average pupil diameter after 0.25% homatropine hydrobromide solution (mm)	Average reduction in accommodation after 0.5% homatropine solution (D)	Average reduction in accommodation after 0.25% homatropine solution (D)
R.E 4.2	7.4		4.60	
L.E 4.2		7.1		3.20

Eucatropine

Instillation of a drop of a 5% or 10% solution produces a dilatation of the pupil which commences in 10–20 minutes and is complete in approximately 30 minutes: the pupil is then inactive to light. Recovery without a miotic usually occurs in between 2 and 6 hours or more depending on the concentration used. Unlike the other atropine-like examples given above, eucatropine has little, if any, effect on the accommodation, and there is little danger of an increase in intra-ocular pressure.

Sympathomimetic mydriatics

Phenylephrine

This is the only sympathomimetic mydriatic in regular use and the only one available in single use units. Phenylephrine is used in a variety of strengths but 2.5% and 10.0% are the ones most often used. Mydriasis commences in about 10 minutes and is maximal in 30 minutes. The mydriasis lasts for several hours. Phenylephrine has been compared with ephedrine, which it has replaced as the most commonly used mydriatic (Table 6.4).

Table 6.4

Average pupil diameter before instillation (mm)	Average pupil diameter after ephedrine hydrochloride 5% solution (mm)	Average pupil diameter after phenylephrine hydrochloride 10% solution (mm)	Average reduction in accommoda- tion after ephedrine 5% solution (D)	Average reduction in accommoda- tion after phenylephrine hydrochloride 10% solution (D)
R.E 4.3	7.2		0.45	
L. E 4.3		7.3		0.76

Phenylephrine is an alpha-agonist and as well as producing mydriasis, it causes vasoconstriction of the conjunctiva. In low concentrations (0.125%) it is used as a vasoconstrictor in some over-the-counter eye brightening drops.

There is little doubt that sympathomimetic amines produce less effect on accommodation than antimuscarinics, and some authors (Kanski, 1969) suggest that phenylephrine produces mydriasis without any cycloplegic effect at all. On the other hand, larger decreases in near point accommodation than can be attributed to the increase in the size of the pupil have been reported (Garner *et al.*, 1983).

Phenylephrine, like all sympathomimetics, is less effective in highly pigmented patients and will allow the light reflex to remain.

The average apparent fall of accommodation in this small series (14 subjects) would appear to be insignificant, and although this reduction might well be explained by the increased pupillary size, despite the pupillary reflex to accommodation-convergence still being present, Biggs, Alpern and Bennett (1959) found the mydriasis lasted long after the accommodation had returned to normal. This discussion appears to the author to be merely academic with little reference to consulting room practice as such small reductions of accommodation are involved. It might be mentioned here that the small numbers involved in all the author's tabulated series in this chapter are only intended to give students an idea of the average kind of results to be expected when they are working in general ophthalmic practice. The number of subjects, their age range, irides and skin pigmentations, etc., were not varied enough to give these results statistical significance. It should be clearly understood that the responses using the same drug vary considerably from patient to patient, and sometimes even between the two eyes of the same individual. However, even with these averaged recordings under discussion, by allowing a ±2 mm variation in final pupillary diameter 40 minutes after instillation of a specific mydriatic, the resultant range will include nearly all patients and embrace those individuals who show maximal or minimal response to a particular mydriatic.

When mydriasis is necessary with pupils that are obviously going to be difficult to dilate, as in those cases discussed previously, one of the more powerful antimuscarinic mydriatics should be the drug of choice without hesitation. It is a waste of the patient's and practitioner's time to attempt to dilate such pupils with one of the weaker sympathomimetic drugs; for example, Barbee and Smith (1957) concluded that phenylephrine is a relatively ineffective mydriatic when used on Negro patients. They found that only the antimuscarinic drugs, and these in cycloplegic concentrations, were really adequate in these patients, and even then cyclopentolate 1% produced only a 1.5 mm mean increase in pupillary diameter, compared to the approximate 3.0 mm increase obtained with atropine 1%, hyoscine 0.2%, and homatropine 4%. Phenylephrine 10% actually proved slightly more effective than the cyclopentolate, giving an average 1.75 mm increased pupil width. As Havener (1978) remarks, the eyes of Negroes are only dilated with great difficulty, especially when using phenylephrine, cyclopentolate or hydroxyamphetamine as the mydriatic.

Priestley and Medine (1951) have also carried out a comparative study of the mydriatic responses, to various drugs, of white and coloured subjects. They found that after 20 minutes the speed of mydriasis with cyclopentolate 0.5% was surpassed by homatropine (2%) and phenylephrine (neosynephrine) 10%, and at the end of 60 minutes the latter ranked first. Nevertheless, after this time the cyclopentolate drops did produce an average 7.0 mm pupil in the Negro subjects compared to 7.5 mm in the white subjects.

The recently introduced 2.5% strength of phenylephrine has led to some discussion as to its effectiveness relative to the 10% strength. Although Duffin, Pettit and Straatsma (1983) found a greater effect from 10% phenylephrine than from the 2.5%, it must be pointed out that they were using a viscolized 10% solution against an aqueous 2.5% and this difference in vehicles could have had an influence on the mydriatic action. The disparity in mydriasis was greater for darkly pigmented eyes as opposed to those with lightly coloured eyes. Neuhaus and Hepler (1980) found similar mydriatic effects with 2.5% and 10% phenylephrine and recommend 2.5% for routine dilatation.

Cocaine

This alkaloid, derived from the leaves of the *Erythroxylum coca*, is a colourless, crystalline substance, the official salt being the hydrochloride; maximum therapeutic dose 15 mg. Solubility of the alkaloid is 1 in 300 in water, and 1 in 10 in castor oil; solubility of the salt is 2 in 1 in water. Cocaine is a powerful local anaesthetic, blocking nerve conduction on topical application to sensory nerve endings, for example, those in the corneal epithelium. The hydrochloride salt is usually ordered in 2–4% w/v concentration in an aqueous eyedrop solution, Cocaine Eyedrops, *BPC*, and is also present in a 2% w/v concentration in combination with homatropine hydrobromide 2% w/v in Cocaine and Homatropine Eyedrops, *BPC*. Because of the difficulties of ensuring sterility, the oily eyedrops of the alkaloid (where castor oil was the vehicle) have been omitted from the current *Codex*.

Lamellae 0.65 mg, also no longer official, may now be obtained only to special (medical) order, that is, they have to be specifically prepared.

Mydriatic effect

The mydriatic effect of cocaine commences in 5–20 minutes, reaching a maximum in about 30 minutes. Dilatation of the pupil may last as long as 20 hours, though more usually the duration is around 6 hours. It is a sympathomimetic drug, whose mechanism of action is interference with the normal fate of noradrenaline. Specifically, cocaine prevents noradrenaline, either already in the circulation, or released by stimulation of sympathetic nerves, from being taken up by a transport mechanism in the nerve membrane into storage sites in the adrenergic nerve endings. This results in an increased amount of noradrenaline being left available for activation of the adrenergic receptors, and this increases the magnitude and prolongs the duration of activity of this neuro-transmitter.

Instillation of cocaine into the conjunctival sac does not cause cycloplegia, and although a mydriasis occurs the pupil is not immobile to light. Accommodation–convergence reflexes will still cause a pupillary constriction, indicating that the parasympathetic is not affected, and on excitation the sphincter pupillae overcomes the stimulated dilatator pupillae. Cocaine's mydriatic effect may be described as the result of the indirect action of a sympathomimetic drug.

Constriction of the blood vessels accompanies the mydriasis when this drug is applied to the eye, the noradrenaline in the blood stream initiating an alpha-receptor response in the smooth muscle coat of the vessels and causing blanching of the conjunctival membrane and sclera.

Anaesthetic and analgesic effects

Its anaesthetic and analgesic effects develop in 5–10 minutes when suitable concentrations are applied to mucous membranes, including the conjunctiva of the eye, and persist for 20–30 minutes. Corneal sensitivity is lost in about half a minute, but usually four drops of a 2% solution, instilled at 3-minute intervals, are used in ophthalmic surgery to produce complete analgesia of the cornea. This method does not leave the iris fully analgesic, infiltration with procaine (or a suitable substitute) being employed to effect this. Adrenaline need not be added to the drops to prolong their effect (as is necessary with other local anaesthetics), as cocaine is itself a vasoconstrictor. It should never be applied in unnecessarily high concentration as, being readily absorbed from mucous membranes (including the conjunctival), in addition to risks following absorption, it may produce lasting local damage. This includes oedema and desquamation of the corneal epithelium, with possible ulceration. Cocaine has been largely replaced as a local anaesthetic, because of these tendencies, by other synthetic local anaesthetic agents. The aqueous drops of the salt are generally used, but oily (in a castor oil solution) drops of the alkaloid are an alternative, although no longer included in the *BPC* or *BP*. Cocaine and its salts are controlled by the Misuse of Drugs Act 1971 and its Regulations 1973, and are also Prescription Only Medicines (that is, they are CD, POM), so that the eyedrops may not be obtained for practice purposes by an optometrist, and remain available only on a medical prescription. Injected intravenously, cocaine is a very dangerous drug of dependence. It causes exhilaration and a sense of well-being, due to stimulation of the cerebral cortex, but this may be followed, after large doses, by restlessness, tremors and hallucinations, and some people with idiosyncracy may collapse and die even after quite small doses.

An individual physically dependent on the drug suffers from sleeplessness, loss of memory and mental deterioration.

Cocaine is not given orally, being largely hydrolysed in the gastro-intestinal tract and thus having little effect if given by this route. It has been used in medicine, with morphine, for patients suffering from terminal malignant disease, to reduce post-morphine depression, but now its medical use is almost entirely confined to the application of solutions for surface anaesthesia to cornea, nose and throat.

Hydroxyamphetamine hydrobromide (*Paredrine*, USA)

This is a white crystalline powder, soluble 1 in 1 in water; it is a sympathomimetic agent with direct and indirect effects on adrenergic alpha- and beta-receptors. It may be given in a single dose of up to 60 mg by mouth, 20 mg by intramuscular injection and 10 mg by intravenous injection.

In general medicine its main use is in nasal sprays as a decongestant, by intramuscular or intravenous injection to maintain blood pressure in spinal anaesthesia, and for its direct stimulatory effect on the heart in the treatment and prevention of bradycardia due to excessive carotid sinus irritability. When used as a mydriatic in 1–3% eyedrops full mydriasis occurs in about 30–45 minutes and lasts 2–3 hours. It has been used for cycloplegic refraction in conjunction with one drop of 4% homatropine hydrobromide or one drop of 1% atropine sulphate. Eyedrops of this drug (usual strength 1%) are included in the *USNF* (Martindale, 1977). It is CD, POM.

Gambill, Ogle and Kearns (1967) in a comparative study of the mydriatic effects of homatropine hydrobromide, phenylephrine hydrochloride, tropicamide and hydroxyamphetamine hydrobromide, considered the first two of these agents produced comparable mydriasis, tropicamide induced the most rapid and greatest pupillary dilatation, and hydroxyamphetamine hydrobromide was the least effective.

Ephedrine hydrochloride

Ephedrine is a colourless crystalline alkaloid obtained from species of Ephedra, or prepared synthetically. Both the alkaloid, and the official hydrochloride salt, which may occur as a colourless crystalline substance or as white crystalline powder and has a maximum therapeutic dose of 60 mg, are soluble in water (1 in 36, and 1 in 4, respectively).

Ephedrine is a sympathomimetic amine which resembles adrenaline and amphetamine in its action, but systemically its central stimulatory actions are less pronounced than those of amphetamine and methamphetamine, which have superseded it for this purpose. This drug is now used clinically, mainly for its peripheral effects. When given by mouth in therapeutic doses, ephedrine constricts the peripheral vessels, thus raising the blood pressure, it relaxes the bronchioles, decreases the tone and peristaltic movements of the intestine, but contracts the uterus and the sphincter of the bladder, whilst at the same time relaxing the detrusor muscle of the latter. It stimulates the respiratory centre as well as the cerebrum and dilates the pupils. These effects explain its employment, sometimes by intramuscular or subcutaneous injection, as its action is delayed and only fully established after about an hour when given by mouth, to combat a fall in blood pressure: to treat allergic conditions, such as hay fever, urticaria and serum sickness; to prevent attacks of bronchial spasm (in milder cases of acute asthma), and to control nocturnal enuresis in children. When given orally its effects last about 4 hours. To relieve the symptoms accompanying painful swelling and catarrh of mucous membranes, which it does when applied locally to the latter, it constricts blood vessels causing blanching and reduces the secretions of the area so treated. Finally, it is used in eyedrops as a mydriatic in a 5% w/v concentration.

According to Innes and Nickerson (1975) it has a direct stimulatory effect on both alpha- and beta-receptors, but also owes part of its peripheral action to release of noradrenaline (an indirect action) from sympathetic nerve endings. Both Bowman and Rand (1980) consider the ephedrines (there are four isomers, the most active being the one included in the pharmacopoeia) have largely an indirect action. They describe the action of indirectly acting sympathomimetic amines as displacing noradrenaline from the storage sites in the adrenergic neurones; in the process these compounds themselves have the affinity to attach themselves to these sites.

Vale and Cox (1978) consider the ratio of direct to indirect activity of ephedrine is approximately 20–80%, respectively.

Mydriatic effect
Instilled into the conjunctival sac one drop of a 4 or 5% solution of ephedrine hydrochloride initiates a mydriasis in 10–15 minutes which is maximal in about 30 minutes, and without the aid of a miotic the effect lasts for several hours. Although some authorities do not agree, Mitchell (1964) considers that a slight reduction of the accommodation is present in nearly every case varying from 0.25D to 2.00D or even more. The author has not infrequently encountered this phenomenon, which does not seem to be easily explicable whilst accepting the established fact that innervation of the ciliary muscle is via the parasympathetic system, and pupillary constriction to light and the accommodation–convergence reflexes are not abolished by ephedrine. Mydriasis is not as maximal as with the antimuscarinic mydriatics, and ephedrine eyedrops are often ineffective in the presence of highly pigmented irides, dark-skinned and even dark-haired people, diabetics, and in patients over the age of 60 years. The pupils in all such individuals are usually more difficult to dilate with any mydriatic. In the older group arteriosclerosis may exist and be present in the radial vessels of the iris, these vessels resisting the pull of the comparatively weak dilatator pupillae as long as the more powerful sphincter pupillae remains active. In all such cases, where mydriasis to sympathomimetic drugs is unsatisfactory, resort should be made to the more certain effects of the antimuscarinic class. Usually, however, especially in younger patients, sympathomimetic mydriatics prove quite effective, cause little or no reduction in the accommodation and, when requested or especially required, but essentially in the near-presbyopic and presbyopic age-group, a miotic following their use is very effective. The pupillary dilatation produced by sympathomimetic mydriatics is quite satisfactorily counteracted by weaker miotics such as 1% pilocarpine hydrochloride (or nitrate)

Mitchell (1964) has suggested in these difficult arteriosclerotic cases to employ a synergistic combination of 0.25% homatropine hydrobromide with 4.0% ephedrine hydrochloride, but if such a procedure is adopted physostigmine 0.25% must then be considered the miotic of choice, as homatropine now has additionally to be counteracted.

Ephedrine hydrochloride eyedrops may be employed in the differential diagnosis of pathological and non-pathological anisocoria. If reaction to light and accommodation are equal, in speed and degree, the constrictor apparatus (the sphincter pupillae) is normal in both eyes. Again, if dilatation of the pupils, in speed and degree, to ephedrine is equal, the dilatator apparatus (the dilatator pupillae) in both eyes is normal, and if both these conditions can be so demonstrated any inequality of pupillary size has been shown to be an idiosyncrasy and not a pathological entity.

It should be mentioned that the instillation of ephedrine eyedrops also causes a noticeable widening of the palpebral aperture. This is due to the drug's stimulatory effect on the sympathetic nerve supply to the smooth muscle (Müllers) that aids in opening the upper and lower lids. In addition, after a transitory hyperaemia due to the irritation (stinging) caused by the drops, there will be a blanching of the conjunctiva as vasoconstriction of its blood vessels supervenes.

Antimuscarinic or sympathomimetic

In his selection of a mydriatic, the optometrist will no doubt invoke some personal preference. In the majority of practices, the probable choice will be between phenylephrine and tropicamide.

Tropicamide is the more effective mydriatic, especially if photography is contemplated, as the pupillary light reflex will be abolished. However Mordi, Tucker and Charman (1986), when comparing 0.1% cyclopentolate and 10% phenylephrine as mydriatics, concluded that neither were ideal since both caused a loss of accommodation signified by a recession of near point and a slowing of the accommodation response.

Tropicamide has the ability to cause a rise in intraocular pressure in eyes with a deep anterior chamber as opposed to phenylephrine, which causes a fall (like all sympathomimetics). However, the rise in IOP is likely to be small and transient and not likely to cause a problem.

Phenylephrine can have effects on blood pressure (see below) and is contra-indicated in patients with cardiovascular problems and patients taking certain drugs.

In summary, it would appear that tropicamide 0.5% is the first choice as a mydriatic, but special conditions require special considerations. Huber, Smith and Smith (1985) found that diabetic patients responded poorly to tropicamide and recommended a combination of this agent with phenylephrine to give adequate mydriasis with a minimum of accommodative paralysis. Chang, McCann and Hitchcock (1985) found that phenylephrine produced better sector pupil dilatation than tropicamide. Sector pupil dilatation in which the pupil becomes oval or pear-shaped is recommended for dilating eyes with narrow filtration angles because it reduces the risk of acute angle closure glaucoma.

Mixed mydriatics

When the mydriasis produced by one or other of the two types of mydriatic will not produce sufficient depth of mydriasis, mixtures of an antimuscarinic and a sympathomimetic may be employed. The following mixtures are some of the ones that have been employed:

homatropine and cocaine
homatropine and ephedrine
tropicamide and phenylephrine
cyclopentolate and phenylephrine

The strengths of the compounds in the mixtures can be varied according to the degree of mydriasis required. Apt and Hendrick (1980) investigated the mydriatic effect of three combinations:

cyclopentolate 0.5% and phenylephrine 2.5%
tropicamide 0.5% and phenylephrine 2.5%
tropicamide 1.0% and phenylephrine 2.5%

and found no significant difference between any of the mixtures. They recorded dilations of around 7 mm within 60 minutes, which must be approaching maximal effect. The light reflex was abolished. Unfortunately, they did not report on the duration of effect.

Mydriatics for Horner's syndrome

Sympathetic denervation of the iris dilator muscle will lead to a slightly miosed pupil. The iris will be supersensitive to sympathomimetic amines but subsensitive to parasympathomimetics such as pilocarpine or carbachol. Colasanti, Chui and Trotter (1978) demonstrated these phenomena in rabbits. As a differential diagnostic test, a weak sympathomimetic mydriatic may be used. Adrenaline 0.1% or phenylephrine 0.125% is instilled, and if the muscle is sympathetically dener-vated, it will be hypersensitive to the mydriatic and dilate. Normally innervated irides will not respond. As a further test, indirectly acting sympathomimetics will have no effect.

Adverse effects of mydriatics

With any topically applied, ophthalmic drug there is a possibility of producing an undesirable effect, either on the eye or on the body as a whole. Mydriatics have the ability to do both.

The use of a mydriatic causes pupil dilatation which in turn introduces the possibility of angle block. The danger will be dependent on the degree of dilatation, not on the mydriatic employed. The probability of inducing an attack of closed angle glaucoma is remote (figures vary from 0.06% to 0.09% of the population: (Lowe, 1967; Hollows and Graham, 1966) and it can be made even more remote by careful prior examination of the patient and detailed history taking. Keller (1975) concludes that providing proper precautions are taken, the risk of precipitating angle closure is virtually nil. Prevention is better than cure and the time to find out that the patient has a shallow anterior chamber depth is before the mydriatic is instilled, not after.

Obviously, it is important that the optometrist is aware of the signs and symptoms of such an attack, which can occur not only from the injudicious use of a mydriatic, but also spontaneously. An optometrist may expect to see an attack of closed angle glaucoma about once in 40 years.

The classical symptoms of closed angle glaucoma are well known but are worth repeating here. The patient experiences intense pain which may be severe enough to induce vomiting. The conjunctival blood vessels are dilated, giving an appearance to the inexpert eye of conjunctivitis. The cornea loses transparency slightly because the high intraocular pressure causes it to imbibe water and swell. The patient may report this as seeing haloes around lights. Through the hazy cornea the pupil can be seen, often mid-dilated (Chandler, 1952) and probably non-circular. The pupil will not constrict to light, accommodation or to the action of miotics. The intraocular pressure, whether measured with a tonometer or assessed digitally, is very high. The situation is an emergency one, but not requiring panic measures. Providing the intraocular pressure is reduced over the ensuing period, there should be no long lasting damage.

Angle closure glaucoma is not the only adverse reaction which can be induced by the use of mydriatics and the optometrist should be especially alert to other problems. The other side effects of antimuscarinics have been dealt with under cycloplegics (Chapter 5), but as it is usual to use lower concentrations, they should be less likely to occur.

Other local toxic effects from topical sympathomimetic drugs include a toxic epithelial desquamation of the cornea similar to that seen with local anaesthetics (Havener, 1978).

Liberation of iris pigment into the anterior chamber has been reported by Aggarwal and Beveridge (1971) following the use of 10% phenylephrine. The pigment appeared as aqueous floaters within 45 minutes of the drug being instilled, causing an aqueous flare which could be confused with anterior uveitis. There were apparently no symptoms.

Sympathomimetic mydriatics, like any other topically applied drug, can produce systemic effects and the cardiovascular system is the one most sensitive to their effects. The problem with sympathomimetics is exacerbated by the high concentration of active agent that is used relative to the normal systemic dose. Topically administered drugs may gain access to the vascular system either by direct absorption through the conjunctival blood vessels or via the naso-lacrimal system to the alimentary tract. Absorption can be very quick, with maximum levels being reached in 10–20 minutes after instillation (Kumar *et al.*, 1985).

There are several predisposing risk factors which will increase the possibility of severe systemic reaction (Hopkins and Lyle, 1977). These are:

(1) Prior use of a local anaesthetic.
(2) Conjunctival disruption and/or bleeding.
(3) Patients with high blood pressure, heart disease or thyrotoxicosis.
(4) Multiple applications.
(5) Concomitant medication.

Fraunfelder and Scafidi (1978) reviewed 33 cases of adverse reactions following the topical ocular use of 10% phenylephrine. There were no cases following 2.5% phenylephrine. Fifteen patients suffered myocardial infarcts which could not be definitely attributed to the use of phenylephrine, but seven patients showed significant increases in systemic blood pressure. They recommend the use of 2.5% phenylephrine in infants and the elderly. Accordingly, the use of sympathomimetic mydriatics in patients with cardiac disease, hypertension, aneurysms, advanced arteriosclerosis and patients receiving monoamine oxidase inhibitors or tricyclic antidepressants should be avoided.

Apparently healthy patients may also be at risk, a case of coronary artery spasm having been reported in a healthy 28-year-old patient (Alder, McElwain and Martin, 1981).

When used properly, the incidence of a blood pressure rise from the use of phenylephrine should be low. Epstein and Murphy (1981) found that only 2 patients out of 62 responded with a change in blood pressure of more than 20 mm Hg to the use of phenylephrine 10% with cyclopentolate 1%. Brown, Brown and Spaeth (1980) failed to find significant changes in patient who had received 10% phenylephrine.

References

Aggarwal, J. C. and Beveridge, B. (1971) Liberation of iris pigment in the anterior chamber after instillation of 10% phenylephrine hydrochloride solution. *Br. J. Ophthalmol.*, **55**, 544–545

Alder, A. G., McElwain, G. E. and Martin, J. H. (1981) Coronary artery spasm induced by phenylephrine eyedrops. *Arch. Int. Med.*, **141**, 1384–1385

Apt, I. and Henrick, A. (1980) Pupillary dilatation with single eyedrop mydriatic combinations. *Am. J. Ophthalmol.*, **89**, 553–559

Barbee, R. F. and Smith, W. O. (1957) A comparative study of mydriatic and cycloplegic agents. *Am. J. Ophthal.*, **44**, 617

Biggs, R. A., Alpern, M. and Bassal, D. K. (1959). The effect of sympathomimetic drugs upon the amplitude of accommodation. *Am. J. Ophthal.*, **48**, 169

Brown, M. M., Brown, G. C. and Spaeth, G. (1980) Lack of side effects from topically administered 10% phenylephrine eyedrops. *Arch. Ophthalmol.*, **98**, 487–489

Chandler, P. (1952) Narrow angle glaucoma. *Arch. Ophthalmol.*, **47**, 695–716

Chang, F. W., McCann, T. A., and Hitchcock, J. R. (1985) Sector pupil dilatation with phenylephrine and tropicamide. *Am. J. Optom. Physiol. Optics*, **62**, 482–486

Colasanti, B. K., Chui, P. and Trotter, R. R. (1978) Adrenergic and cholinergic drug effects on rabbit eyes after sympathetic denervation. *Eur. J. Pharmacol.*, **47**, 311–318

Davidson, S. I. (1976) Mydriatic and cycloplegic drugs. *Transact. Ophthalmol. soc. UK*, **96**, 327–329

Duffin, R. M., Pettit, T. H. and Straatsma, B. R. (1983) 2.5% vs 10% phenylephrine in maintaining mydriasis during cataract surgery. *Arch. Ophthalmol.*, **101**, 1903–1906

Epstein, D. L. and Murphy, E. (1981) Effects of combined 1% cyclopentolate – phenylephrine eye drops on systemic blood pressure of glaucoma patients. *Ann. Ophthalmol.*, **13**, 735–736

Fraunfelder, F. T. and Scafidi, A. F. (1978) Possible adverse effects from topical ocular 10% phenylephrine. *Am. J. Ophthalmol.*, **85**, 447–453

Gambill, H. D., Ogle, K. N. and Kearns, T. P. (1967) Mydriatic effects of four drugs determined with a pupilograph. *Arch Ophthal., NY.*, **77**, 740

Garner, L. F., Brown, B., Baker, R., and Colgan, M. (1983) The effect of phenylephrine hydrochloride on the resting point of accommodation. *Invest. Ophthalmol. Vis. Sci.*, **24**, 363–395

Havener, W. H. (1975) *Synopsis of Ophthalmology*, 4th ed, Mosby, St Louis, pp. 307, 491–494

Havener, W. H. (1978) *Ocular Pharmacology*, 4th ed, Mosby, St Louis, pp. 233, 237

Hollows, F. C. and Graham, P. A. (1966) Intraocular pressure, glaucoma and glaucoma suspects in a defined population. *Br. J. Ophthalmol.*, **50**, 570–586

Hopkins, G. A. and Lyle, W. M. (1977) Potential systemic side effects of six common ophthalmic drugs. *J. Am. Optom. Assoc.*, **48**, 1241–1245

Huber, M. J. E., Smith, S. A. and Smith, S. E. (1985) Mydriatic drugs for diabetic patients. *Br. J. Ophthalmol.*, **69**, 425–427

Innes, I. R. and Nickerson, M. (1975). In Goodman and Gilman's. *The Pharmacological Basis of Therapeutics*, 5th ed, Macmillan, New York. pp. 500, 503

Kanski, J. J. (1969) Mydriatics. *Br. J. Ophthalmol.*, **53**, 428–429

Keller, J. T. (1975) The risk of angle closure from the use of mydriatics. *J. Am. Optom. Assoc.*, **46**, 19–21

Kumar, V., Schoenwald, R. D., Chien, D. S., Packer, A. J. and Choi, W. W. (1985) Systemic absorption and cardiovascular effects of phenylephrine eyedrops. *Am. J. Ophthalmol.*, **99**, 180–184

Lowe, R. F. (1967) Primary angle closure glaucoma, a review of provocative tests. *Br. J. Ophthalmol.*, **51**, 727–732

Martindale. (1977) *Extra Pharmacopoeia*, 27th ed, The Pharmaceutical Press, London (1) pp. 14, 193, 227, 987–990, 227; (2) p.14; (3) pp. 987–990; (4) p. 193

Martin-Doyle, J. L. C. (1967) *A Synopsis of Ophthalmology*, 3rd ed, Bristol, p. 8

Mitchell, D. W. A. (1964) *The Use of Drugs in Refraction*, 3rd edn, The British Optical Association, London

Mordi, J., Tucker, J. and Charman, W. N. (1986) Effects of 0.1% cyclopentolate or 10% phenylephrine on pupil diameter and accommodation. *Optom. Physiol. Optics.*, **6**, 221–227

Neuhaus, R. W. and Hepler, R. S. (1980) Mydriatic effect of phenylephrine 10% (aq) vs phenylephrine 2.5% (aq). *Ann. Ophthalmol.*, **12**, 1159–1160

Mordi, J., Tucker, J. and Charman, W. N. (1986) Effect of phenylephrine 10% (aq) vs phenylephrine 2.5% (aq). *Ann. Ophthalmol.*, **12**, 1159–1160

Newell, E. (1969) *Ophthalmology, Principles and Concepts*, 2nd ed, St Louis, p. 140

Pollack, S. L., Hunt, J. S. and Polse, K. A. (1981) Dose-response effects of tropicamide HCl. *Am. J. Optom. Physiol. Optics*, **58**, 361–366.

Polse, K. A. (1975) Technique for estimating the angle of the anterior chamber using the slit lamp. *Optom. Weekly*, **66** (22), 524

Priestley, H. S. and Medine, M. M. (1951) A new mydriatic and cycloplegic drug. *Am. J. Ophthal.*, **34**, 572

Stone, J. (1979) The slit lamp biomicroscope in ophthalmic practice. *Ophthal. Optician*, **19**(12), 439

Vale, J. and Cox, B. (1978) *Drugs and the Eye*, Butterworths, London, p. 41

Van Herick, W., Shaffer, K. N. and Schwartz, A. (1969) Estimation of width of the anterior chamber: incidence and significance of the narrow angle. *Am. J. Ophthal.*, **68**(4), 626

Chapter 7

Miotics

Miotics are drugs which constrict the pupil. In the hands of the optometrist they are used to reverse the mydriasis produced by drugs such as phenylephrine and tropicamide, but may also be used in the emergency treatment of closed angle glaucoma (Table 7.1).

In medicine their principal use is in the treatment of primary open angle glaucoma. As the ideal properties for a glaucoma treatment vary greatly from those of an anti-mydriatic miotic, this chapter will only deal with the latter. Anti-glaucoma treatments will be dealt with in Chapter 17.

Ideal properties

(i) Quick in onset.
(ii) A length of action appropriate to the mydriatic previously employed.
(iii) An effect on the ciliary muscle which leaves the patient without cycloplegia or cyclospasm.
(iv) An effect on the iris which allows a normal pupil light reflex.
(v) No other pharmacological effect.
(vi) No local toxic reaction.
(vii) No systemic toxic reaction.

From the above it can be seen that there will be no perfect miotic. Much will depend on the appropriate selection of a miotic to follow the mydriatic.

Indications for use

At one time it was routine to instil a miotic after mydriatic examination in all patients over the age of 40. Nowadays, with the use of short-acting mydriatics such as tropicamide, the necessity for their routine use must be questioned and the advantages of the miotic must be carefully weighed against its disadvantages.

Miotics have also been used in the treatment of accommodative esotropia. Hiatt (1983) found that miotics were no better than, and often not as good as, glasses in correcting the deviation and enhancing binocularity and therefore they are little used for this purpose today.

Table 7.1 Miotics

Official name	Trade name	Strengths % w/v	Single dose	Mode of action	Mydriatic onset	Mydriatic duration	Recommended after	Adverse reactions	Notes
Pilocarpine	Isoptocarpine Sno Pilo	1.0 2.0 4.0	Yes	Parasympathomimetic	10 min	6 h	—	Ciliary spasm	
Carbachol	Isopto-carbachol	3.0	No	Parasympathomimetic	?	?	—	Ciliary spasm	Poorly absorbed
Acetylcholine	Miochol	1.0	Yes	Parasympathomimetic	?	?	Cataract operations	—	Used intra-ocularly during surgery
Bethanechol	—	1.0	No	Parasympathomimetic	?	?	—	Ciliary spasm	Rarely used
Methacholine	—	5.0 10.0	No	Parasympathomimetic	?	?	—	—	—
Physostigmine, eserine	—	0.25 to 1.0	No	Anticholinesterase	10 min	12 h	Tropicamide & cyclopentolate	Ciliary spasm	—
Thymoxamine	—	0.5	Yes	L Blocking agent	30 min	5 h	Sympathomimetic	—	—

Advantages

The use of a miotic:

(1) Reduces the danger of angle closure. It nevertheless introduces the danger of pupil block and, as previously indicated, all patients should have their angles assessed before a mydriatic is instilled.
(2) Avoids photophobia, especially on a bright, sunny day.
(3) Speeds the return of accommodation.
(4) Lowers the intraocular pressure. This should not be too elevated if the anterior chamber is sufficiently deep and some mydriatics, e.g. phenylephrine, actually cause a fall.

Disadvantages

(1) The small pupil can lead to dimness of vision. This can be a problem at twilight, especially if the patient is proposing to drive a car.
(2) A spasm of accommodation may be caused, leading to pseudomyopia.

Mode of action

Mydriatics can cause mydriasis either by paralysing the sphincter (antimuscarinics) or by stimulating the dilator (sympathomimetics). Conversely, miotics may cause their effect by either inhibiting the dilator (alpha-blocking agents) or by stimulating the sphincter (parasympathomimetics or anticholinesterases).

Miotics acting on the pupil sphincter muscle

The sphincter muscle is stimulated to contract by the action of acetylcholine on muscarinic receptors, so drugs can act by mimicking the action of acetylcholine on the muscarinic receptor (parasympathomimetic) or by preventing the breakdown of acetylcholine by the cholinesterase present at the cholinergic neuro-effector junctions (anticholinesterases).

Miotics acting on the pupil dilator muscle

As the sympathetic innervation to the dilator muscle is stimulatory (motor), it is logical that alpha-receptors predominate. The effect of noradrenaline on this muscle can be blocked by an alpha-blocking agent. There are many alpha-blocking agents available for use in general medicine. They are used in the treatment of hypertension and peripheral vasospastic conditions, but only thymoxamine is available as an eyedrop.

Parasympathomimetic miotics

Parasympathomimetic miotics can be grouped into choline esters, which are derivatives of acetylcholine, and cholinomimetic alkaloids which include pilocarpine, arecoline and muscarine. By far the most commonly used parasympathomimetic miotic is pilocarpine.

Pilocarpine

Obtained from the leaves of *Pilocarpus microphyllus* (jaborandi plant) and other species of Pilocarpus, it is a colourless, syrupy, liquid alkaloid which is soluble in water. The hydrochloride salt, which is freely soluble in less than one part of water, is now preferred to the nitrate (previously used) in the preparation of the eyedrops, because it is compatible with a wider range of antimicrobial preservatives.

Mechanism of action

Pilocarpine is a direct acting parasympathomimetic agent (compare with the indirect acting physostigmine). Like all such agents (including also such synthetic choline esters as carbachol and bethanecol) its primary action is the stimulation (or inhibition) of autonomic effector cells in a similar manner to that accomplished by the acetylcholine released by stimulation of post-ganglionic parasympathetic nerves, that is, it acts primarily at muscarinic receptors of autonomic effector cells. Koelle (1975) also states that, in addition it has some *nicotinic* ganglionic effects, but part of this secondary ganglionic action involves stimulation of muscarinic receptors which are now known also to be present in varying proportions on autonomic ganglion cells. The nicotinic actions of parasympathomimetic drugs refer to their initial stimulation, and in higher dosage to subsequent blockade (as with nicotine) of autonomic ganglion cells and neuromuscular junctions. All the actions of pilocarpine and other parasympathomimetic drugs (as well as ACh) can be blocked by atropine, through competitive occupation of the cholinoceptive sites on autonomic effector cells, and on the secondary muscarinic receptors of autonomic ganglion cells.

Bowman and Rand (1980) consider the nicotinic action to be very weak. In this nicotinic action it resembles the endogeneous mediator acetylcholine, but it does not, like the latter, stimulate the motor end-plates of skeletal muscle in normal doses. Its effects systemically are also similar to its fellow cholinomimetic alkaloid muscarine; it slows the heart and pulse, increases peristalsis, constricts the bronchioles, increases the secretions of the salivary, lacrimal, gastric, pancreatic and intestinal glands, and also the mucous glands of the respiratory tract. Pilocarpine causes marked sweating, due to the drug's direct stimulatory action on the sweat glands and vasodilatation of blood vessels in the skin, this latter effect producing flushing in man. Langley, as long ago as 1875, described pilocarpine's peripheral dilator actions. Large doses of pilocarpine at first stimulate then depress the CNS. It will have been noted that physostigmine, taken orally, produces all these effects, but in this case they are caused by this anticholinesterase prolonging the activity of acetylcholine and not, as with pilocarpine, by the direct excitatory (or inhibitory) action of the alkaloid itself on the cholinoceptive receptor sites.

Ophthalmic preparations

Applied locally to the eye as a 0.5–5% solution (the 1% strength is the most commonly used by practitioners), pilocarpine hydrochloride (or nitrate) causes a miosis which, after commencing in about 10 minutes, is maximal within half an hour and gradually decreases over a period of 6 hours with the 1% solution (Lowenstein, 1956). While the spasm of the ciliary muscle may last for up to 2 hours, unlike that following physostigmine once this spasm has worn off it does not return if near work is commenced.

Whilst pilocarpine 1% adequately reconstricts the mydriasis produced by sympathomimetic agents it appears unnecessary to use the more powerful but also more uncomfortable physostigmine, although the latter appears necessary to satisfactorily reverse the mydriasis following antimuscarinic eyedrops. This is a view which coincides with that of Anastasi, Ogle and Kearns (1968), who found that pilocarpine 1% counteracted the effects of phenylephrine and hydroxyamphetamine (another sympathomimetic mydriatic) in concentrations usually used in ophthalmology within 30 minutes, but after mydriasis with anti-parasympathomimetic agents, such as tropicamide and homatropine, pilocarpine did not cause effective miosis.

Table 7.2 illustrates the general effectiveness of one drop of a 1% solution of pilocarpine hydrochloride within 30 minutes, subsequent to a dilatation for 40 minutes of the right pupils of 14 students (aged between 20 and 27 years—average age 24 years) with 5% ephedrine hydrochloride, and the left pupils of the same group with 10% phenylephrine hydrochloride.

Table 7.2

Average pupil diameter before instillation of any drug (mm)	Average pupil diameter after instillation of ephedrine 5 % solution (mm)	Average pupil diameter after instillation of phenylephrine 10 % solution (mm)	Average pupil diameter of instillation of pilocarpine 1 % solution (mm)	Average pupil diameter after instillation of pilocarpine 1 % solution (mm)
R.E 4.3	7.2		5.5	
L.E 4.3		7.2		5.8

As with physostigmine, it is ineffective in the presence of atropine, the latter successfully competing for the effector cell receptor, but not resulting in the excitation of these as does pilocarpine.

The miotic effect of pilocarpine in various patients produces rather marked individual differences in the latent period before miosis, in the rate, the degree, and the duration of contraction and the time factor for redilatation (Lowenstein and Loewenfeld, 1953). Strength for strength it is only about half as powerful a drug as physostigmine, and thus a 1% solution does not produce the extreme degree of miosis that the anticholinesterase agent does in this concentration. Neither is the spasm of accommodation nearly as marked or as painful as when physostigmine is used.

After pilocarpine has diffused out of the eye, the pupil on recovery remains slightly more dilated than normal, because of a diminished response of the sphincter pupillae to normal reflex stimulation after the direct action of the pilocarpine. The lack of recurring accommodative spasm on attempting close work, together with the absence of pain and discomfort, are advantages of pilocarpine over physostigmine, but the latter is a more reliable miotic in counteracting the dilatation of the pupil caused by the antimuscarinic mydriatics, as the effects of these may outlast those of the pilocarpine, in which case the pupils will re-dilate.

In addition to the effect of the drug on the ciliary and sphincter pupillae muscles, pilocarpine increases the flow of blood through the vasculature of the anterior uvea (Alm and Bill, 1973).

Carbachol (*Doryl; Carcholin*)

Carbachol, maximum therapeutic dose 0.5 mg by subcutaneous injection or 4 mg orally, occurs as very hygroscopic colourless crystals or a white crystalline powder. It is used in general medicine to produce motility of the gut in post-operative paralytic ileus, and contraction of the bladder in non-obstructive conditions of urinary retention. Carbachol, a quaternary ammonium parasympathomimetic drug (direct action), has muscarinic and nicotinic properties and is not rapidly inactivated by cholinesterase. It may be used as a miotic in 0.75–3% solution in the treatment of glaucoma, and is a useful alternative to pilocarpine, and to other miotics where resistance or intolerance has developed. In such cases, generally the 0.75% solution will be more effective than 2% pilocarpine (Havener, 1978). However, it was not considered a suitable agent in the treatment of accommodative esotropia because of its irregular onset and short duration of action.

The *BPC*, 1973, eyedrops contain up to 3% of carbachol but, as an alternative miotic for pilocarpine allergic patients, the optometrist should find a 0.5% strength adequate to reverse sympathomimetic mydriatics. As the only prepacked proprietary ophthalmic solution (*Isopto Carbachol*) is 3%, extemporaneous preparation of a 0.5% eyedrops by the pharmacist is required. As it is poorly absorbed through the cornea the drops include a wetting agent such as benzalkonium chloride, which also performs the additional role of acting as a bactericide. It is a derivative of, but more stable than, acetylcholine.

Acetylcholine chloride + mannitol (*Miochol*)

Synthetically manufactured acetylcholine chloride has a maximum therapeutic dose of 200 mg subcutaneously or intramuscularly; a white very hygroscopic crystalline powder, very soluble in water, it is a powerful parasympathomimetic agent, but when injected its action is very transient as it is so rapidly hydrolysed by cholinesterase. It has, of course, the same action as endogenous acetylcholine, but has been largely replaced in medicine by the more stable synthetic parasympathomimetics discussed above. However, a freshly prepared 1% solution incorporating 5% mannitol, a white crystalline powder, soluble 1 in 6 in water, acting as an osmotic agent in the combination, intensifies the effect of the acetylcholine. This preparation is used in intra-ocular surgery after cataract extraction to constrict the pupil in seconds. A solution of acetylcholine instilled into an intact eye will not cause miosis as this substance would be hydrolysed by acetylcholinesterase long before it could reach an effective concentration in the anterior chamber aqueous.

Bethanecol chloride (*Urecholine; Mecothane*)

Bethanecol chloride, maximum therapeutic dose 5 mg subcutaneously, 30 mg orally, occurs as white hygroscopic crystals or a crystalline powder, soluble 1 in 1 in water. It has the same uses in general medicine as carbachol. A quaternary ammonium parasympathomimetic agent that is not inactivated by cholinesterase (Martindale, 1977), it has a muscarinic, but unlike carbachol no nicotinic, action (Koelle, 1975). Bethanecol is used in a 1% solution as a miotic and like carbachol also needs a wetting agent to help it penetrate the cornea.

It may be used as an alternative to pilocarpine but as there are no official or proprietary ophthalmic preparations available, eyedrops have to be extemporaneously prepared by the pharmacist if required.

Methacholine chloride

Methacholine chloride, maximum therapeutic dose 25 mg by subcutaneous injection, occurs as deliquescent colourless or white crystals or a white crystalline powder, soluble in less than one part of water. It has the muscarinic action of acetylcholine but is more stable, and is used in general medicine to terminate attacks of atrial paroxysmal tachycardia when simpler methods have failed. Of the two synthetic parasympathomimetic drugs, carbachol and methacholine, although they possess in general the same muscarinic actions as acetylcholine (slowing of the heart, increased peristalsis, dilatation of peripheral blood vessels and increased salivary, sweat and bronchial secretion) there is some selectivity on particular structures; for example, carbachol is relatively more effective on the gastro-intestinal tract and bladder, whilst methacholine is relatively more effective on the cardiovascular system. Normal pupils require a 10–20% solution to produce miosis, and this drug has also been used in these strengths for the treatment of simple glaucoma, but other miotics are now generally preferred. In eyedrops form it is a Pharmacy Medicine (P) and therefore available for use by optometrists.

Contra-indications and precautions are similar to those appertaining to pilocarpine. Methacholine is hydrolysed by acetylcholinesterase, but even alone in an adequate concentration it is successful in producing a marked miosis (and spasm of accommodation and lid twitching) by its direct action, as it has some resistance to this enzyme.

Anticholinesterases

Anticholinesterase agents can be divided into reversible and irreversible agents depending in their duration of action. Anticholinesterases are taken up by cholinesterase in the same way as acetylcholine. There then follows a series of reactions in which the acetylcholine or anticholinesterase is broken down and the enzyme regenerated. The difference is that the reactions for acetylcholine are very fast while for anticholinesterase they are very slow. If the anticholinesterase is an irreversible one the regenerating reactions are thought to take place at such a slow rate that they do not effectively take place and the body manufactures new enzyme.

Reversible anticholinesterases

The principal agents in this group are physostigmine (eserine) and neostigmine.

Physostigmine (eserine)

Physostigmine is an alkaloid obtained from the seeds of *Physostigma venenosum* (Calabar beans) and may also be prepared synthetically.

Properties

Large, colourless crystals, sparingly soluble in water (1 in 75), but the official salt, the sulphate, is deliquescent and has a solubility in less than 1 part of water, and the salicylate (which stings rather less when used in the eyedrops) is soluble 1 in 90 parts water. Because of the greater solubility of the sulphate and its compatibiilty with a wider range of preservatives, it is now preferred to the salicylate for the preparation of eyedrops. No doses are stated for physostigmine sulphate or salicylate in the *BP* 1980, as today this drug is used mainly as a miotic.

Although Physostigmine Eyedrops, *BP* contain up to 1% w/v of the sulphate (the BNF instructs a strength of 0.25% to be dispensed unless otherwise stated by the prescriber), the salicylate eyedrops are not now available prepacked by pharmaceutical manufacturers in the United Kingdom, but, of course, may be prepared extemporaneously, if necessary, by the pharmacist. Solutions of physostigmine salts, like the alkaloid itself, on exposure to light and air become pink, especially the sulphate, due to oxidation. This results in the formation of rubreserine, which is more irritating to the eye than eserine, even though the miotic effect is maintained. Physostigmine Eyedrops, *BP*, contain 0.2% w/v sulphur dioxide equivalent (an antoxidant) to retard formation of this degradation product. Rogers and Smith (1973) have brought this problem into perspective by their investigations into the stability of physostigmine eyedrops. They found that the 0.25%, 0.5% and 1% eyedrops, prepared in accordance with the *PBC*, 1973 formula (pH 3.6–3.8), and sterilized by heating or filtration, retained more than 99% of their activity after storage at 25°C for 1 year. A faint pink colour appeared after sterilization by heat, and was also present in all samples after storage for this time. It would appear from these researches that filtration may be the method of choice to obtain colourless eyedrops from the date of manufacture. On the other hand, despite a faint pink colouration, as long as the date of manufacture is within a year, and the interval after first opening the container not more than a month, it would appear to be in order to use these drops.

Mechanism of action

Physostigmine is an anticholinesterase (anti-AChE) drug. The role of this enzyme in terminating the action of the transmitter acetylcholine, liberated by cholinergic nerve impulses at junctions with their effector organs, and at synaptic sites, has already been discussed in Chapter 2. Thus the acetylcholine is allowed to accumulate at sites of cholinergic transmission, and as the action of the acetylcholinesterase on the acetylcholine is being inhibited, the effect will be similar to continuous stimulation of these cholinergic fibres. Physostigmine is an excellent example of this class of drug, but because the chemical complex of drug and acetylcholinesterase is only temporary and finally dissociates, its effects are limited to about 12 hours or so, and it is termed a reversible anticholinesterase. This is in contrast to the effects of very much more potent organophosphate compounds, which also act in this manner, but for very prolonged periods (from days to weeks); these are called irreversible anticholinesterase drugs, for example, dyflos (*see* later). The latter are extremely toxic compounds and are never used by optometrists. The irreversible anticholinesterases form extremely stable complexes with the enzyme (acetylcholinesterase), whilst in the case of the physostigmine-enzyme complex slow hydrolysis eventually results in regeneration of the cholinesterase.

Physostigmine, when topically applied to the eye, therefore, permits a prolonged stimulation by acetylcholine of the ciliary and sphincter pupillae muscles resulting in spasms of accommodation and miosis, respectively. Conjunctival hyperaemia also occurs due to the peripheral vasodilatory effects of this miotic.

In the body the cholinergic fibres of the parasympathetic system slow the heart and pulse rate, and increase peristalsis, salivary, bronchial and gastric secretions and dilate peripheral blood vessels. Taken orally, physostigmine therefore enhances these cholinergic effects. It is not surprising that this drug in toxic doses causes slow pulse, vomiting, diarrhoea, intestinal colic and flushing.

Ophthalmic preparations

The main use of physostigmine today is as a miotic and it is seldom given internally. Ophthalmic aqueous solutions of 0.25%, 0.5% and 1% (or even 2% in an acute attack of glaucoma), of either the official sulphate, or salicylate, and the alkaloid itself in similar strengths in a castor oil vehicle (although the latter are no longer official), are the usual forms in which it is administered.

Strength for strength physostigmine is about twice as active as pilocarpine, that other most useful miotic. On instillation of eyedrops of this anticholinesterase drug constriction of the pupil commences in between 5 and 10 minutes and miosis is maximal in about 30 minutes. The effects last up to about 12 hours or more with a 0.5% solution, and somewhat less with the 0.25% solution more generally used by optometrists.

Physostigmine ointment 0.5% (the *BPC* 1963 eye ointment was 0.125%) causes an intense miosis continuing for 12–36 hours (Havener, 1978).

The 1% eyedrops of this drug should not be used by the optometrist even in the emergency produced by a sudden attack of acute glaucoma. Because of the pain and discomfort this concentration causes, this strength is unsuitable for constricting the dilated pupil of the normal eye after mydriatic examination. The marked pupillary contraction resulting from instillation of a 1% solution, the pupil diameter being less than 2 mm, persists for more than 12 hours, and its normal size may not be regained for a few days. Eyedrops of this concentration of the drug should be reserved for the medical treatment of the later stages of simple glaucoma, when weaker strengths and weaker miotics (for example, pilocarpine) no longer control the rise in tension.

The 0.25–0.5% solutions of physostigmine, particularly the former, are the more usual concentrations of this miotic, and the 0.25% proves to be quite adequate in constricting the pupil in about half an hour, following the dilatation produced by the mydriatic concentrations of such antimuscarinic eyedrops as cyclopentolate hydrochloride 0.1%, homatropine hydrobromide 0.25–0.5%, eucatropine 2–5%, and tropicamide 0.5%.

Table 7.3 illustrates the type of response that may be expected after 30 minutes when employing physostigmine 0.25% as a miotic, following a 40-minute dilatation of the pupils (the right and left eyes of 20 students—40 eyes—age range from 20 to 26 years, average 23.4 years) with cyclopentolate hydrochloride 0.1% (in the right eyes) and homatropine hydrobromide 0.5% (in the left eyes).

The majority of subjects reported some mild to moderate accommodative spasm and some lid twitching in both eyes after instillation of the miotic. Physostigmine 0.25% appeared to produce very adequate constrictions of the pupil in overcoming both cyclopentolate 0.1% and homatropine 0.5% mydriasis in the chosen time interval.

Table 7.3

Average pupil diameter before instillation of any drug (mm)	*Average pupil diameter after instillation of cyclopentolate 0.1 % solution (mm)*	*Average pupil diameter after instillation of homatropine 0.5 % solution (mm)*	*Average pupil diameter after instillation of physostigmine 0.25 % solution (mm)*	*Average pupil diameter after instillation of physostigmine 0.25 % solution (mm)*
R.E 4.2	7.4		3.7	
L.E 4.2		7.5		3.5

Comparison of 0.25% physostigmine (Table 7.3) and 2% pilocarpine (Table 7.4)
At a further clinical class with the same 20 students the identical procedures (using 0.1% cyclopentolate in their right eyes, and 0.5% homatropine in their left eyes, and allowing a period of 40 minutes for the mydriatic effects to occur) were followed. Then instead of instilling a drop of 0.25% solution of physostigmine sulphate as the miotic into each eye, one drop of a 2% solution of pilocarpine hydrochloride was substituted, and the results are recorded in Table 7.4.

From this series it would appear that an adequate average constriction of the pupil was obtained with 2% pilocarpine in 30 minutes in the eyes the pupils of

Table 7.4

Average pupil diameter before instillation of any drug (mm)	*Average pupil diameter after instillation of cyclopentolate 0.1 % solution (mm)*	*Average pupil diameter after instillation of homatropine 0.5 % solution (mm)*	*Average pupil diameter after instillation of pilocarpine 2 % solution (mm)*	*Average pupil diameter after instillation of pilocarpine 2 % solution (mm)*
R.E 4.3	7.5		6.9	
L.E 4.3		7.4		4.9

which had previously been dilated with 0.5% homatropine, but that, in this interval of time, 2% pilocarpine was an inadequate miotic to counteract the mydriasis produced by 0.1% cyclopentolate.

Irreversible anticholinesterases

There are many agents in this group which are chemically related to the organo-phosphorus compounds. They were originally developed as nerve gases and insecticides but some have found medical uses, e.g. Di-isopropylfluorophosphonate (*Dyflos*) and ecothiopate.

Dyflos (DFP) or di-isopropylfluorophosphonate (Isofluorophate, USP)

This is an irreversible anticholinesterase drug used in 0.05–0.1% concentration, in arachis oil, as it is unstable (spontaneous hydrolysis occurring) in aqueous solution. It has a very rapid onset of action, 5–10 minutes, and very prolonged miotic effect, lasting 2–4 weeks; the ciliary muscle spasm, which may cause macropsia, continuing from 3 to 7 days (Havener, 1978). This miotic can also be used by ophthalmologists to overcome the mydriasis caused by atropine. It is used mainly in the treatment of aphakic glaucoma. The adverse reactions that occur with this drug including blurring of vision, severe pain and frontal headache, and treatment with dyflos carries a high risk of cataract formation (Martindale, 1977). Systemic toxic effects, which may occur even after inhalation of the vapour (another reason for the use of the oil preparation) are prolonged and similar to those caused by ecothiopate (*see* below). It is a POM.

Organophosphorous substances are used as insecticides in agricultural and horticultural activities and their use is not without risk when protective measures are inadequate.

Insecticide solutions in contact with the eyes of workers in these occupations will, of course, produce the adverse reactions described under dyflos, with the accompanying extreme miosis and ciliary spasm, and ophthalmic practitioners with patients employed in the agricultural or horticultural industries may be confronted with such cases on occasion.

Ecothiopate iodide (Ecothiophate iodide *USP*) (*Phospholine Iodide*)

Ecothiopate iodide is a further irreversible, organophosphorous, anticholinesterase miotic, used in 0.06–0.25% solution mainly in the treatment of open-angle glaucoma. It considerably improves the facility of outflow in these glaucomatous eyes (Drance and Carr, 1960), but is not without some adverse effects (as for other long-acting anticholinesterase drugs, for example, dyflos). These include such systemic toxic effects in some patients (frequency of dosage is an important factor here) as diarrhoea, nausea, abdominal cramps and general weakness and fatigue (Humphreys and Holmes, 1963), and locally iris cysts. It is also used on occasion in the treatment of accommodative esotropia in children. The iris cysts (which also occur with prolonged dyflos therapy) fortunately disappear when the miotics are discontinued, or may usually be prevented from forming by the simultaneous use of phenylephrine (2.5–10%) which does not impair the therapeutic effect of the ecothiopate (Abraham, 1964).

Ecothiopate eyedrops must be freshly prepared by the pharmacist in a diluent supplied by the manufacturers, the drops only remaining stable if the solution is kept refrigerated.

Ecothiopate iodide is a POM and like the other irreversible anticholinesterase miotics, not available for use by optometrists.

Alpha-blocking agents

The principal agent in this group is thymoxamine, which is purely an alpha-blocker, having little beta-blocking activity. Many other alpha-blockers have been isolated, e.g. tolazoline, phentolamine and ergotoxine, but only thymoxamine is used ophthalmically. It causes miosis by relaxing the pupil dilator muscle. Its main indication is the reversal of mydriasis caused by sympathomimetic agents, but it would appear to have some activity in overcoming the mydriasis caused by tropicamide. It can be used intraocularly (Grehn, Fleig and Schwarzmuller, 1986). It produces no endothelial damage when used in very dilute concentration (e.g. 0.02%), and is potentially useful in cataract surgery and penetrating keratoplasty.

In addition to its miotic action, thymoxamine paralyses the smooth muscle of the upper lid, causing a slight ptosis. For this effect it has been used in the treatment of exophthalmos. These effects are most notable in patients with thyroid problems. There would appear to be little effect on normal patients (Dixon, Anderson and Hatt, 1979). Its effects last for about 5 hours.

There would appear to be little effect on ciliary muscle or on intraocular pressure in eyes with deep anterior chambers. The latter is surprising as phenylephrine, which it antagonizes, lowers intracocular pressure and thus a small rise would have been expected, but the mydriatic and ocular hypotensive effects of sympathomimetics have separate time-courses and probably involve different receptors. Conversely, in closed angle glaucoma, thymoxamine does, for several reasons, appear to have a role in reducing pressure (Halasa and Rutkowski, 1973). Firstly, it is thought that during such attacks the sphincter becomes less effective than the dilator and the latter muscle dominates. Secondly, a relaxed sphincter reduces the possibility of pupil block and Halasa and Rutckowski (1973) explain this by the use of a mathematical model. In pupil block, forces trying to pull the iris back towards the anterior lens capsule should be avoided. If both muscles are relaxed there are no posterior vector forces. Thirdly, it may have an overall synergistic effect with other miotics.

Because thymoxamine reduces the pressure in closed angle but not open angle, it can form the basis of a useful differential test.

It is effective in concentrations between 0.01% and 1.3% (Lee *et al.*, 1983) but is only available in single use containers as a 0.5% solution.

Choice of miotic

The choice of miotic will to a large extent be determined by the mydriatic used. As far as the optometrist is concerned there is a choice of three agents: pilocarpine, physostigmine and thymoxamine.

Other miotics are available, e.g. neostigmine, but these three are very representative of their groups.

If an antimuscarinic has been used then an anticholinesterase is recommended, because pilocarpine is insufficiently active to cause a reversal. Pilocarpine or thymoxamine can be used after a sympathomimetic. In other words, there is a possibility of using either a physiological or a pharmacological antagonist. A physiological antagonist works on different receptors to produce an opposite effect, e.g. pilocarpine after phenylephrine, whilst a pharmacological antagonist works on the same receptor to produce the antagonism, e.g. thymoxamine after phenylephrine.

Saheb *et al.* (1982) compared the use of thymoxamine with pilocarpine in the reversal of phenylephrine-induced mydriasis. Pilocarpine was quicker in onset and produced a deeper miosis. Thymoxamine took twice as long (20 minutes) to return the pupil to its normal size, but was significantly longer in action than was pilocarpine, having a half-life of 12 hours compared with 5 hours for pilocarpine. The maximum effect has been separately reported to occur at 60 minutes after instillation (Lee *et al.*, 1983).

The problems of using a parasympathomimetic after a sympathomimetic are twofold:

(1) Both muscles are under spasm, pulling in opposite directions.
(2) There is a spasm of accommodation because of the much greater effect of the parasympathomimetic on the ciliary muscle, compared with the sympathomimetic.

The effect of the two muscles contracting concurrently makes the iris fairly rigid, with the consequences that the lens bulges forward and the rim of the iris meets the anterior lens capsule, reducing the depth of the anterior chamber (Wilkie, Drance and Schulzer, 1969). The situation impedes the flow of aqueous from the posterior chamber to the anterior chamber, resulting in a pressure differential across the iris, which causes it to bulge forward (iris bombé). If the anterior chamber is shallow, there is a possibility of angle closure developing (Garin, 1966). Since the miotic was instilled as a precaution against the risk of angle closure glaucoma being induced by the use of a mydriatic, such an occurrence would be unfortunate to say the least.

Since pilocarpine is not recommended after an antimuscarinic because of lack of efficacy and is contra-indicated after parasympathomimetics because of pupil block, the question must be asked, "What use is pilocarpine ?" It represents a compromise between using a miotic and not using a miotic, i.e. use a less effective one, but in reality its use cannot be justified on pharmacological grounds. It is nevertheless, useful for the emergency treatment of glaucoma.

Miotics strong enough to overcome the action of atropine ecothiopate or dyflos are not available for use by optometrists.

Mixed miotics

Just as it has been the practice in the past to use mixed mydriatics containing agents with different modes of action in order to produce synergy, mixtures of miotics have also been employed. Whereas mixed mydriatics always contain an agent acting on the pupil dilator muscle and an agent acting on the pupil sphincter muscle, mixed miotics have tended to contain a parasympathomimetic and an anticholinesterase, e.g. pilocarpine and physostigmine, both of which are active on the sphincter. Their use has been based on empiricism rather than pharmacological evidence.

It would appear to be more logical to mix, for example, thymoxamine and pilocarpine or physostigmine in order to reverse a mixed mydriatic. Because thymoxamine has not been generally available in ophthalmic form until recently, there is little experience with such a mixture.

Miotics for Adie's pupil

Adie's pupil is the parasympathomimetic counterpart of Horner's syndrome. In the differential diagnosis of anisocoria, a weak solution of a directly acting miotic may be used, e.g. 0.125% pilocarpine or 2.5% methacholine (normal miotic strength—20%). Because the sphincter muscle is parasympathetically denervated it is supersensitive to acetylcholine and other parasympathomimetrics. Because there is no natural release of acetylcholine, anticholinesterases will have no effect.

Bourzon, Pilley and Thompson (1978) compared 2.5% methacholine and 0.125% pilocarpine in the diagnosis of Adie's pupil. They found methacholine effective in 64% of patients, while pilocarpine was effective in 80%, so that the latter can be considered to be the better drug for this differential test.

Adverse reactions to miotics

In the main, the most serious side-effects from miotics arise from their chronic use in glaucoma or from possible overdosage during acute glaucoma treatment rather than the single application used to reverse mydriatics.

However, miotics can cause transient effects which may trouble some patients and may therefore discourage the optometrist from using them.

Thymoxamine is irritant on instillation, as are some other miotics. Miotics whose principal action is on the sphincter pupillae may also cause a spasm of accommodation even in some apparently presbyopic patients.

Abramson, Franzen and Coleman (1973) demonstrated an axial thickening of the lens and a decrease in anterior chamber depth in patients between 60 and 80 years of age. Even when this effect has apparently worn off, it may return when close work is attempted. If the miotic is much stronger than the mydriatic, then the patient will have smaller than normal pupils. This dimness of vision can be a problem, especially if combined with a pseudomyopia from the spasm of accommodation.

The blood vessels of the conjunctiva will dilate in response to parasympathomimetic agents and conjunctival injection may result. Additionally, some patients may be allergic to pilocarpine, but this is unlikely to develop after one instillation.

Anticholinesterases can have nicotinic as well as muscarinic effects and these will be manifested as lid twitching. Anticholinesterases have been implicated in cataract formation (Pietsch *et al.*, 1972).

The parasympathetic nervous system supplies many of the visceral structures and theoretically these may be affected by topically administered agents. In particular, one could expect effects on the respiratory system, cardiovascular system and the gastro-intestinal system.

Drugs which stimulate muscarinic receptors will cause bronchoconstriction and may cause respiratory embarassment to asthmatic patients, but this is a theoretical possibility rather than an actual danger. Bradycardia (slowing of the heart) and vasodilation similarly do not appear to be a problem. Anticholinesterase can reduce the level of plasma cholinesterase, leading to diarrhoea and adverse interaction with certain muscle relaxants used in surgery, but this is only from chronic use. Few systemic effects should therefore result from the post-mydriatic use of miotic.

However, gastro-intestinal symptoms such as diarrhoea and vomiting and respiratory problems have been reported following large doses of topical pilocarpine (Epstein and Kaufman, 1965).

References

Abraham, S. V. (1964) The use of an ecothiopate-phenylephrine formulation (Ecophenyline – B3) in the treatment of convergent strabismus and amblyopia with special emphasis on iris cysts. *J. Paedriatr. Ophthalm.*, **1**, 68

Abramson, D. H., Franzen, L. A. and Coleman, D. J. (1973) Pilocarpine in the presbyope. *Arch. Ophthalmol.*, **89**, 100–102

Alm, A. and Bill, A. (1973) The effects of pilocarpine and neostigmine on the blood flow through the anterior uvea of the monkey. A study with radioactively labelled microspheres. *Exp. Eye Res.*, **15**, 31–36

Anastasi, I. M., Ogle, K. N. and Kearns, I.P. (1968) Effects of pilocarpine in contracting mydriasis. *Archs. Opthal., NY.*, **79**, 710–715

Bourzon, P., Pilley, S. F. J. and Thompson, H. S. (1978) Cholinergic supersensitivity of the iris sphincter in Adie's tonic pupil. *Am. J. Ophthalmol.*, **85**, 373–377

Bowman, W. C. and Rand, M. J. (1980) *Textbook of Pharmacology*, 2nd ed. Blackwell, Oxford and London.Dixon, R. S., Anderson, R. L. and Hatt, M. V. (1979) The use of thymoxamine in eyelid retraction. *Arch. Ophthalmol.*, **97**, 2147–2150

Drance, S. M. and Carr, F. (1960) Effects of phospholine iodide (217MI) on intraocular pressure in man. *Am. J. Ophthalmol.*, **49**, 470

Epstein, E. and Kaufman, I. (1965) Systemic pilocarpine toxicity from overdosage. *Am. J. Ophthalmol.*, **59**, 109–110

Garin, G. (1966) Angle closure glaucoma induced by miotics. *Am. J. Ophthalmol.*, **62**, 1063–1067

Grehn, F., Fleig, T. and Schwarzmuller, A. (1986) Thymoxamine: a miotic for intraocular use. *Graefe's Arch. Clin. Exp. Ophthalmol.*, **224**, 174–178

Halasa, A. H. and Rutkowski, P. C. (1973) Thymoxamine therapy for angle closure glaucoma. *Arch. Ophthalmol.*, **90**, 177–180

Havener, W. H. (1978) Ocular pharmacology, 4th edn, Mosby, St Louis, pp. 289, 298–299

Hiatt, R. L. (1983) Medical management of accommodative esotropia. *J. Pediatr. Ophthalmol. Strabis.*, **20**, 199–207

Humphreys, J. A. and Holmes, J. H. (1963) Systemic effects produced by ecothiopate iodide in the treatment of glaucoma. *Arch. Ophthalmol.*, **69**, 737

Koelle, G. B. (1975) In Goodman and Gilman's Pharmacological basis of therapeutics, 5th edn, New York, p. 473.

Lee, D. A., Rimele, T. J., Brubaker, R. F., Negatki, S. and Vanhoutte, P. M. (1983) Effect of thymoxamine on the human pupil. *Exp. Eye Res.*, **36**, 655–662

Lowenstein, O. (1956) The Argyll Robertson pupillary syndrome. *Am. J. Ophthal.*, **42**, 105

Lowenstein, O. and Loewenfeld, I. I. (1953) Effect of physostigmine and pilocarpine on iris sphincter of normal man. *Arch. Ophthalmol.*, **50**, 311

Martindale, (1977) *Extra pharmacopoeia*, 27th edn, The Pharmaceutical Press, London

Pietsch, R. L., Bobo, C. B., Finklea, J. F. and Valloton, W. W. (1972) Lens opacities and organophosphorus cholinesterase-inhibiting agents. *Am. J. Ophthalmol.*, **73**, 236–242

Roger, A. R. and Smith, G. (1973) Stability of physostigmine eye-drops. *Pharm. J.*, **211**, 353

Saheb, N. E., Lorenzetti, D., East, D., and Salpter-Carllon, S. (1982) Thymoxamine versus pilocarpine in the reversal of phenylephrine-induced mydriasis. *Can. J. Ophthalmol.*, **17**, 266–267

Wilkie, J., Drance, S. M. and Schulzer, M. (1969) The effects of miotics on anterior chamber depth. *Am. J. Ophthalmol.*, **68**, 78–83

Chapter 8

Local anaesthetics

Local anaesthetics are chemical agents that reversibly block the transmission of nerve impulses along sensory fibres. They will also block motor nerves but in higher concentrations than are normally obtained by topical instillation. Different sensations are lost according to the size of axons serving them. Pain, which is carried by the smallest fibres, is lost first, followed by touch and temperature sensitivity. Pressure, which is carried by the largest nerve fibres, is lost last, if at all (Table 8.1).

Not all local anaesthetics are suitable for topical ophthalmic use. This is because of the poor absorption characteristics of some agents, e.g. procaine, an excellent injectable anaesthetic which because of the highly polar nature of the compound has poor lipid solubility and therefore crosses mucous membranes very slowly.

Ideal properties

Topical anaesthetics should:

(1) Be quick in onset of action.
(2) Be effective for a reasonable duration of time. (It should allow the practitioner time to carry out the procedure and then reverse completely, returning to the patient the protection of the sensitive eye.)
(3) Not affect the pupil, accommodation or intraocular pressure.
(4) Not antagonize or enhance the effects of other drugs, e.g. mydriatics, cycloplegics, antimicrobials etc.
(5) Be comfortable to the patient on initial application.
(6) Not interfere with the healing process.
(7) Be non-toxic, both locally and systemically.

Indications for use

The surface of the eye is very sensitive and there are several techniques which require contact with the cornea. These are facilitated by the prior use of a topical anaesthetic.

Table 8.1 Local anaesthetics*

Official Name	Trade Name	Strengths % w/v	Single dose	Onset of anaesthesia	Duration of anaesthesia
Amethocaine (tetracaine)	—	0.5 1.0	Yes	1 min	20 min
Benoxinate (oxybupro-caine)	Novesine	0.4	Yes	1 min	15 min
Proxymeta-caine (proparacaine)	Ophthai-ne	0.5	No	1 min	15 min
Lignocaine	—	2.0 to 4.0	Yes (mixed with fluor-escein)	1 min	30 min

*All local anaesthetics will depress epithelial oxygen uptake to some extent. Repeated instillation will lead to desquamation to corneal epithelium and eventually loss of vision.

They include:

(1) *Foreign body removal.* The blepharospasm which normally accompanies a superficial foreign body makes examination of the eye very difficult, so a drop of local anaesthetic will make location and removal of the offending object very much easier.
(2) *Tonometry.* Unless a non-contact tonometer is used or tonometry is carried out on the sclera, topical anaesthesia is essential for the assessment of intraocular pressure.
(3) *Contact lens fitting.* Some procedures may be more easily carried out if a topical anaesthetic is instilled initially.
(4) *Certain diagnostic procedures.* Some practitioners prefer to use a topical anaesthetic prior to a Schirmer test of lacrimal function. It is argued that this gives a truer assessment of the basal tear secretion rather than the enhanced flow which will result if the strip is placed in the sensitive unanaesthetized eye.

Topical anaesthesia is also sometimes used prior to the instillation of rose bengal stain, but this may give a slightly false picture if the anaesthetic interferes with the integrity of the corneal epithelium.

Advantages

(1) Certain procedures would be impossible without a topical anaesthetic. For example, most simple portable tonometers which can be used for domiciliary visits all require a local anaesthetic.
(2) Use of a local anaesthetic makes procedures more comfortable for the patient.
(3) They correspondingly make procedures easier for the practitioner.

Disadvantages

(1) While the surface of the eye is insensitive, it is susceptible to damage from superficial foreign bodies.
(2) Some topical anaesthetics cause initial stinging.
(3) The effects of other drugs may be enhanced. This is probably due to a reduction in tear flow rather than an increase in corneal permeability.
(4) Topical anaesthetics can delay the healing processes.

Mode of action

Information passes along nerve fibres via 'electrical impulses' or action potentials. When the nerve is at rest, the interior has a negative charge. An action potential is generated by the influx of sodium ions into the interior of the nerve, causing it to have a positive charge (depolarization). The nerve fibre is returned to its resting potential (negative state) by the efflux of potassium ions (repolarization). The action potential is then generated along the axon by successive depolarizations and repolarizations of adjacent regions, the exact mechanism of action at the cellular level having been the subject of much study. Schoen and Candida (1979) found that the chloride permeability of corneal cells was reduced by the application of local anaesthetics.

Choice of topical anaesthetic

Cocaine is, of course, the original local anaesthetic against which the newer synthetic agents are assessed. It is now better known for its abuse rather than its use as a local anaesthetic. It has many undesirable properties in addition to its local anaesthetic action. It has a sympathomimetic action which leads to mydriasis on topical application. It has deleterious effects on the corneal epithelium, leading to desquamation and an increased penetration of other substances across the cornea. This is a property which is peculiar to cocaine and not to local anaesthetics in general. Cocaine is also a CNS stimulant which leads to euphoria and addiction.

Cocaine is controlled by both the Misuse of Drugs Act and The Medicines Act under which it is available only on prescription (Prescription Only Medicine). It is not legally available to optometrists for use in their practice.

There is, nevertheless, an extensive range of topical anaesthetics which are available to optometrists for professional use, i.e. amethocaine, proxymetacaine, benoxinate and lignocaine. All are available in commercial preparations but proxymetacaine is not manufactured in single dose units.

The property in which respect the agents vary most is the initial stinging on instillation. In descending order of comfort, the agents can be listed thus:

Proxymetacaine—most comfortable
Benoxinate
Lignocaine
Amethocaine—least comfortable

Whichever local anaesthetic is selected, the concentration chosen should be as low as possible. Polse, Keener and Jauregui (1978) plotted the dose-response curves of benoxinate and proxymetacaine. They found benoxinate at concentrations as low as 0.1% and proxymetacaine at 0.125% produced a maximal increase in threshold to touch. Although the concentrations currently employed (0.4% and 0.5%, respectively) are definitely supramaximal with respect to the depth of anaesthesia, the recovery time was found to be proportional to the concentration used. At the lowest concentration the duration of effect was sufficient to carry out normal optometric procedures, so at the normally used concentrations it was plainly excessive.

Draeger, Langenbucher and Bannert (1984) similarly found a prolongation of effect when 0.5% was used compared with 0.1%. The vehicle and preservative had little effect on the performance of the local anaesthetic.

Proxymetacaine hydrochloride (Proparacaine Hydrochloride, USP) (*Ophthaine: Alcaine*, Canada, USA: *Ophthetic*, Australia, Canada, South Africa, USA)

Proxymetacaine is a white or almost white crystalline powder soluble 1 in 30 of water. A synthetic topical anaesthetic, it has a greater potency than amethocaine, but there is little clinical difference. The instillation of one drop of 0.5% solution of proxymetacaine produces anaesthesia lasting about 15 minutes. In ophthalmology deep anaesthesia, as required for cataract extraction, may be obtained by instilling one drop every 5–10 minutes until 5–7 drops have been administered (Martindale, 1977).

Time of onset of anaesthesia is very similar, 6–20 seconds (average 12.9 seconds), to that with amethocaine, 9–26 seconds (average 14.7 seconds) (Boozan and Cohen, 1953).

In this series, using 0.5% solutions of three local anaesthetics, amethocaine, proxymetacaine (proparacaine), and benoxinate, Linn and Vey (1955) found essentially similar duration and intensity of anaesthesia among all three.

Instillation of proxymetacaine is, on the other hand, considerably more comfortable than the use of amethocaine; it causes much less stinging and squeezing of the eyes and is often painless (Boozan and Cohen, 1953).

The eyedrops should be stored protected from light and when opened kept at a temperature of between 2 and 10°C. Sensitivity reactions are rare and Havener (1978) describes the only case he observed in several years, occurring in a patient where the drug had been used for repeated tonometries. The allergic reaction manifested itself as marked epithelial stippling and slight stromal oedema, with considerable conjunctival hyperaemia and slight puffiness of the lids: pain and profuse lacrimation were severe for some hours. Sensitivity of patients to proxymetacaine is not experienced when amethocaine is used, and vice versa (Havener, 1978).

Proxymetacaine is a POM.

Oxybuprocaine hydrochloride (benoxinate hydrochloride) (*Novesine*, Australia, South Africa; *Dorsacaine*, USA)

Oxybuprocaine is a synthetic local anaesthetic which occurs as white crystals or a white crystalline powder and is very soluble in water. It is used in a 0.4% solution and has clinical characteristics essentially similar to proxymetacaine, both drugs causing less irritation and stinging than amethocaine (Emmerich, Carter and Berens, 1955). As both cocaine and amethocaine cause more or less punctate epithelial staining, which may be confusing during applanation tonometry, this procedure is performed with more accuracy with oxybruprocaine or proxymetacaine than with amethocaine (Havener, 1978). One drop instilled into the conjunctival sac anaesthetizes the surface sufficiently to allow tonometry to be performed in 60 seconds. Three drops instilled over an interval of about 4 to 5 minutes will produce sufficient surface anaesthesia, after a further 5 minute interval, for an ophthalmologist to remove a foreign body embedded in the corneal epithelium, or for incision of a Meibomian cyst through the conjunctiva (Martindale, 1977). The sensitivity of the cornea after three drops is normal again in about 1 hour, whereas after one drop (for example, as used for removing a superficial non-embedded corneal foreign body, or tonometry) the effective anaesthesia lasts 10–15 minutes. This topical anaesthetic has an additional advantage in that it possesses bactericidal properties.

'In a series of more than 1000 patients anaesthetized with benoxinate, no toxic effects were encountered, either locally or systemically.' (Havener, 1978).

Lignocaine hydrochloride (Lidocaine Hydrochloride, *Eur. P., USP*) (*Xylocaine*)

Lignocaine occurs as a white crystalline powder soluble in less than 1 part of water. Unlike the other three topical anaesthetics (amethocaine hydrochloride, proxymetacaine hydrochloride and oxybuprocaine hydrochloride) which are all of the ester type, lignocaine hydrochloride is a local anaesthetic of the amide type. A 2–4% (the latter strength is available as a proprietary preparation) will anaesthetize the cornea. It is an alternative agent in individuals sensitive to ester type local anaesthetics (Ritchie and Cohen, 1975). As a topical eyedrops preparation it is a POM. It is also used in ophthalmology for infiltration analgesia (*see* below).

Amethocaine hydrochloride (Tetracaine Hydrochloride *Eur. P., USP*) (*Anethaine, Decicain,* Australia: *Pontocaine,* Canada, USA)

Amethocaine hydrochloride, a white crystalline powder soluble in 1 in 7.5 water, is one of the most popular topical anaesthetics and is used in 0.25–1% solutions. Solutions stronger than 1% should be avoided as they may damage the cornea. On instillation an initial burning sensation is often complained of, but this passes off in about half a minute or less, by which time the anaesthetic effects are well advanced. Employed in these concentrations amethocaine does not normally cause desquamation of corneal epithelial cells. The peculiar numb sensation persists for 10–20 minutes, depending on the concentration of the drops, but the patient must be warned (and this applies with other topical anaesthetics) not to rub his eyes during this time (and especially during the initial stinging), as the corneal epithelium can unwittingly be damaged in the process. Within a minute or two of instillation of one drop of 0.5% solution of this drug a tonometry can be carried out painlessly. The instruction to the patient gently to close his eyes immediately on instillation of these (or any eyedrops) will definitely reduce the amount of stinging experienced. Tears should be patted away from the closed eyes with a fresh paper tissue or cotton wool, by the practitioner.

Removal of a non-embedded foreign body should generally not necessitate more than one drop of a 0.5% solution, although more applications will be required for taking eye impressions.

Topical anaesthetics, including amethocaine, should not be prescribed even in very dilute concentrations for home use in an attempt to tide a prospective contact lens patient over the more difficult initial stages of wear. Repeated instillations of even very weak concentrations of these drugs, will intensify those tiny superficial corneal epithelial lesions commonly seen with the slit-lamp microscope after use of these eyedrops. Healing of corneal abrasions is significantly retarded by local anaesthetics, and even removal of a foreign body should be performed, if this is possible without blepharospasm and severe discomfort to the patient, without their use. Epithelial regeneration, both mitosis and cellular migration, have been shown to be affected by their employment (Gundersen and Liebman, 1944), which should, therefore, be avoided unless absolutely necessary, and even then only the weakest concentration that will adequately suit the specific situation should be instilled.

Sensitivity to amethocaine is extremely uncommon and only likely to occur after repeated use of the drug (unlikely in optometric practice). The lids become red, swollen, then irritated and itching, and this lasts for some days (Havener, 1978).

Amethocaine is relatively stable in solution, but it is affected by light; it should therefore be stored in an amber bottle or dark cupboard as after long periods it hydrolyses in solution.

Adverse reactions to local anaesthetics

As with all topically applied drugs there is a possibility of both local and systemic adverse effects. With their action of modifying trans-membrane ionic flow it is inevitable that local effects will be produced on the cells with which it comes in contact. Before they can reach the nerve fibres they must first cross corneal epithelial cells. Sturrock and Nunn (1979) examined the cytotoxic effects of three local anaesthetics, procaine, lignocaine, and bupivacaine, and they found an inhibition of cell growth and cell survival of cultured cells. Oxygen flux was investigated by Augsberger and Hill (1973), who found that while cocaine depressed the uptake of oxygen by corneal epithelial cells, benoxinate, even in multiple applications, did not.

Local anaesthetics in ointment form produced morphological changes in the corneal epithelium, cocaine being the most toxic. Benoxinate and proxymetacaine caused a decrease in microvilli and microplicae. Repeated administration caused changes to the plasma membrane and cytoplasm (Brewitt, Bonatz and Honegger, 1980). Gundersen and Liebman (1942) tested several local anaesthetics, including cocaine and amethocaine, on the healing of wounds in the guinea pig cornea. All anaesthetics tested caused a delay in wound healing and a similar result was obtained when lignocaine was tested on the healing of skin wounds in rats (Morris and Tracey, 1977).

It is well known that cocaine is subject to abuse for its CNS effects. The other local anaesthetics are subject to abuse for their ability to remove temporarily the feeling of discomfort from the surface of the eye. The people who abuse them, more often than not, are those who should know better, i.e. medical personnel who have access to these agents. Burns and Gipson (1978) warned that paramedical personnel may abuse topical anaesthetics. The irritation which may persist after a foreign body has been removed can lead someone to instil a local anaesthetic repeatedly. Exposure keratitis is an example of another condition which may lead to the misguided supply of a topical anaesthetic for domiciliary use.

It is recognized that topical anaesthetics can be used incorrectly and that is why they are restricted to use by optometrists in their practice and may not be supplied to patients for use at home under any circumstances. As they are POM drugs, they are not available to the general public.

Unfortunately, this is not the case in all countries of the world. Penna and Tabbara (1986) reported keratopathy following the use of benoxinate which was bought over the counter in Saudi Arabia. Two patients had had exposure keratitis and one a foreign body and they developed disciform keratitis and stromal infiltration. The final best corrected acuity was 6/30 in most eyes, with one eye being reduced to counting fingers at 5 feet.

They had all received bottles of benoxinate from a pharmacy and had used the drops continuously. The legislation which covers the use of drugs may be irksome and time consuming, but if it can avoid cases like these then it is worthwhile.

Three similar cases were reported in Holland by Henkes and Waubke (1978), these patients having developed a physical dependence on the drops because of the intense pain in the insensitive cornea. The local anaesthetics in these cases were supplied by an ophthalmologist. Vision was reduced to counting fingers in one eye and keratoplasty was required.

Jallet *et al.* (1980) described a case where a solution containing only 0.05% benoxinate, used for the treatment of arc eye, led to abuse and keratopathy. This solution, which contains an antiseptic in addition to the local anaesthetic, is available in France without prescription. A dramatic illustration of the problem of local anaesthetics abuse was a patient whose left eye had to be removed due to the corneal ulcer perforation and panophthalmitis which developed in the course of her use of local anaesthetic eye drops with hard contact lenses (D'Haenes, 1984).

Much has been made of the interaction of local anaesthetics with sulphonamides. The theoretical antagonism is based on the fact that some local anaesthetics are derivatives of PABA (para-amino benzoic acid). Sulphonamides exert their effect by competing with PABA, which bacteria require in order to synthesize folic acid. Folic acid is necessary for the production of new DNA and cell multiplication. It is suggested that the local anaesthetic will increase the local level of PABA and compete with the sulphonamide, thus reducing its antimicrobial effect. It must be pointed out that the amount of PABA will be small compared with the levels of sulphonamide usually encountered. Additionally, there will be a time delay between using the local anaesthetic and applying the sulphonamide. Any antagonism is likely to have little clinical significance.

Systemic effects are minimal providing that small volumes are used. Fainting or syncope is known to occur sometimes, but it is not certain to what extent this is related to the drug being used.

References

Augberger, A. R. and Hill, R. M. (1973) Topical anesthesia and corneal function. *Ophthal. Opt.*, 12–18

Boozan, C. W. and Cohen, I. J. (1953) Ophthaine. *Am. J. Ophthalmol.*, **36**, 1619

Brewitt, M., Bonatz, E. and Honegger, J. (1980) Morphological changes of the corneal epithelium after application of topical anaesthetic ointment. *Ophthalmologica*, **180**, 198–206

Burns, R. P. and Gipson, I. (1978) Toxic effects of local anesthetics, *JAMA.*, **240**, 347

D'Haenes, J. D. (1984) Le cas clinique. Complications corneenes par instillations de collyres anesthetiques sur des lentilles de contact. *Contactologica.*, **6**, 142–143

Draeger, J., Langenbucher, H. and Bannert, C. (1984) Efficacy of topical anaesthetics. *Ophthal. Res.*, **16**, 135–138

Emmerich, R., Carter, G. T. and Berens, C. (1955) An experimental clinical evaluation of Dorsacaine hydrochloride (Benoxinate, Novesine). *Am. J. Ophthalmol.*, **40**, 481

Gundersen, T. and Liebman, S. D. (1944). Effects of local anaesthetics on regeneration of corneal epithelium. *Arch. Ophthalmol.*, **31**, 29–33

Havener, W. H. (1978) *Ocular pharmacology*, 4th edn, Mosby, St Louis, p.73

Henkes, H. E. and Waubke, T. N. (1978) Keratitis from the abuse of local anaesthetics. *Br. J. Ophthalmol.*, **62**, 62–65

Jallet, G., Cleires, S., Girard, E., and Bechetoille, A. (1980) Keratopathie toxique grave a l'oxybupro-caine d'appasition particulierment rapid. *Bull. Soc. Ophthalmol.*, *France*, **80**, 385–387

Lin, J. G. and Vey, E. K. (1959) Topical anaesthesia in ophthalmology. *Am. J. Ophthal.*, **40**, 697

Martindale, W. (1977) *Extra pharmacopoeia*, 27th edn, The Pharmaceutical Press, London, p. 871

Morris, M. and Tracey, J., (1977) Lignocaine: its effects on wound healing. *Br. J. Surg.*, **64**, 902–903

Penna, E. P. and Tabbara, K. F. (1986) Oxybuprocaine keratopathy: a preventable disease. *Br. J. Ophthalmol.*, **70**, 202–204

Polse, K. A., Keener, R. J. and Jauregui, M. J. (1978) Dose-response effects of corneal anaesthetics. *Am. J. Optom. Physiol. Opt.*, **55**, 8–14

Ritchie, J. M. and Cohen, D. J. (1975) In Goodman Gilman's *The pharmacological basis of therapeutics*, 5th edn, Macmillan, New York, p.389

Schoen, H. F. and Candida, O. A. (1975) Effects of tertiary amine local anaesthetics on ion transport in the isolated bullfrog cornea. *Exp. Eye Res.*, **28**, 199–209

Sturrock, J. E. and Nunn, J. F. (1979) Cytotoxic effects of procaine, lignocaine, and bupivacaine. *Br. J. Anaesthesiol.*, **51**, 273–281

Further Reading

Burns, R. P., Forster, R. K., Laibson, P. and Gipson, I. K. (1977) Chronic toxicity of local anaesthetics on the cornea. In *Symposium on Ocular Therapy* **10**, pp. 31–44 (Leopold, I. H. and Burns, R. P.) John Wiley & Sons Inc., New York

Chapter 9

Stains

Staining agents are amongst the most useful diagnostic agents, providing information fairly rapidly without producing a pharmacological effect; their usefulness lies in their differential staining characteristics. Important clinical information is provided both by the presence and the absence of staining demonstrated by the use of these agents. (Table 9.1).

Many dyes and substances have been investigated in the past for their staining properties. Foster (1980) lists 34 chemical substances which have been used for vital staining of the eye, including such marvellous names as Magadala Red, Safranin, Brilliant Black and Victorian Blue. His bibliography contains a reference to the use of fluorescein by M. Straub in 1888, which indicates how long ago the principle of vital staining of the eye was established. Today only two stains are in regular use, fluorescein sodium and rose bengal.

Table 9.1 Stains

Official Name	Trade name	Strengths % w/v	Single dose	Uses	Adverse reactions
Fluorescein sodium	Fluorets	1.0 – 2.0	Yes — also paper strips	Tonometry, corneal abrasions, contact lens fitting	Supports growth of *Pseudomonas aeruginosa*
Rose bengal	—	1.0	Yes	Stains, dead cells, Diagnosis of dry eye	Irritant on application to dry eyes
Alcian blue	—	1.0	No	Stains mucus	Persistant staining of corneal epithelium
Trypan blue	—	1.0	No	Stains mucus and dead cells	—
Tetrazolium and iodo-nitro-tetrazolium	—	?	No	Stains degenerate but not dead cells	—
Bromothymol blue	—	?	No	pH indicator	—
Methylene blue	—	?	No		

Ideal properties

(1) They should be water soluble, because vehicles other than water will be toxic and/or interfere with staining patterns.
(2) Stains should selectively stain certain cells or structures in the eye.
(3) They should not stain skin, clothes, contact lenses or any instrument which is likely to come in contact with the eye when the stain is present.
(4) The effect should be reversible, either as a result of tear flow or by use of an irrigating solution.
(5) There should be no interference with vision.
(6) There should be no other pharmacological effect.
(7) They should be non-irritant to the surface of the eye.
(8) They should be non-toxic, especially as one is looking for pathological changes.
(9) They should be compatible with other stains and any other compound with which they are likely to be used.

Norn (1972a) has laid down an extensive scheme for the testing of dyes for vital staining of the cornea and conjunctiva. In particular, he was concerned how any new stain would fit in with characteristics of existing dyes.

Fluorescein sodium

Fluorescein is an orange-red dye which fluoresces in high dilution. As well as being used as a topical stain, it can also be used as an injection for fluorescein angiography. Fluorescein does not actually stain tissues, it merely colours the tear film. The normal corneal epithelium is impermeable to the tear film and substances dissolved in it, because the lipid membranes at the surface of the eye are an effective barrier against polar, water-soluble substances. If this barrier is breached, then the tear film can gain access to deeper layers. There is a pH difference between the surface and the deeper tissues and this causes a green colour in the area of desquamation. The factors which affect the fluorescence of fluorescein have been extensively reviewed. The pH of the solution not only influences the absorption spectrum (like any other pH indicator) but also determines the intensity of the fluorescence, which is highest at pH 8, and thus the area of defect is shown up. After gaining access, the fluorescein will diffuse sideways, giving a slightly false picture. Defects in the epithelium, whether caused by trauma or disease (e.g. dendritic ulcer), are disclosed by the stain.

Optimum conditions for observation of fluorescein

For dilute concentrations of fluorescein in aqueous solution, light with a wavelength between 485 and 500 nm is absorbed maximally. This absorbed energy excites the fluorescein molecules and the emitted light is in a lower energy state and of longer wavelength. The fluorescent light appears green, having its highest intensity at a wavelength between 525 and 530 nm.

In order to observe the fluorescein pattern of the fit of a hard lens, contact lens practitioners have commonly used a Burton type lamp which is generally fitted with a pair of 4 W 'Blacklight Blue' miniature tubular fluorescent lamps. Wavelengths produced by such a source range from approximately 305 to 410 nm, with maximal emission at 350 nm. Some hard contact lens materials have been formulated to absorb within the UV-A band of long-wave radiation which ranges from 315 to 400 nm. Since a Burton type lamp is unsuitable for evaluation of the fluorescein pattern of such lenses, it is possible to use instead the blue filter on a slit-lamp microscope as a source, since its maximum transmission is likely to be in the region of 390–410 nm. Alternatively, a Wratten filter such as a No.45A, could be placed either in the illumination system of the slit-lamp or in front of the white fluorescent bulbs fitted in some Burton type lamps. The use of a blue filter which limits illumination to wavelengths maximally absorbed by fluorescein eliminates veiling glare caused by extraneous wavelengths.

It is established practice to mount a dark yellow filter on the camera lens in order to achieve adequate contrast in the photography of contact lens fluorescein patterns (Abrams and Bailey, 1961). Lee, Courtney and Thorson (1980) have reported that similar incorporation of a barrier filter such as yellow Wratten No.15 in the observation system of a slit-lamp microscope can significantly facilitate the detection of fluorescein staining of the cornea.

Indications for use

(1) Detection of defects in the corneal epithelium.
(2) Contact lens fitting.
(3) Applanation tonometry.
(4) Determination of naso-lacrimal duct patency.
(5) Assessment of tear break up time.
(6) Tear flow assessment.

Corneal defects (Colour Plate IV)

Fluorescein should be used routinely after foreign body removal to detect any damage caused by the offending object while it is present. If a small foreign body has penetrated the eye, a corresponding green rivulet may be seen issuing from the entry hole.

Although fluorescein will also demonstrate corneal ulcers, it may be better to use rose bengal, which is more selective.

Epithelial erosions due to trichiasis will be shown up, but fluorescein is of little help in the diagnosis of keratoconjunctivitis sicca or other forms of conjunctivitis, e.g. infective, allergic or chemical in origin.

Contact lens fitting (Colour Plate V)

In the fitting of hard contact lenses, the dye is an aid in studying the areas where the lens is clearing (green fluorescence) or touching (purplish-blue) the cornea in the case of corneal lenses. With scleral lenses the same observations apply to the optic area but a green colouration, or the absence of it will show where there is clearance or contact, respectively, of the scleral portion of the lens in relation to the sclera. Textbooks on contact lens practice deal with the interpretation of these observations in the appropriate detail.

Fluorescein sodium should not be used to study the fit of soft contact lenses, as it stains them following absorption into the polymer. A high molecular weight fluorescein derivative has been developed in an attempt to overcome this disadvantage, e.g. Fluorexon (Refojo, Miller and Fiore, 1972). The use of this dye is limited, as although it will not enter pHEMA (polyhydroxyethylmethacrylate) it stains most other lenses, and even a 4% solution is not as fluorescent as 0.5% fluorescein (Ruben, 1978).

Applanation tonometry (Figure 9.1)
In applanation tonometry, a legitimate procedure for optometric practice, the visibility of the fluorescein, observed under cobalt-blue filter light, again assumes practical significance. The margin of the applanated area is delineated by a solution of the dye; the 'touch' area (purplish-black) has a diameter of 3.06 mm on the cornea. The concentration of the fluorescein is very important in this technique and it should not be too low (as occurs with excessive tearing), when the examiner's visibility of it is impaired, or too high. The best results are often obtained when using benoxinate hydrochloride 0.1% as the local anaesthetic, as recommended by Goldmann. A 2% solution of fluorescein is far too strong for this procedure. Grant (1963) suggests a 0.25% concentration and, with experience, just the right amount may be obtained by employing sterile fluorescein paper strips.

Because Goldmann-type applanation tonometers involve contact with the eye, a topical anaesthetic has to be administered with the fluorescein. Unfortunately local anaesthetics are salts of weak bases and strong acids. Sodium fluorescein is a salt of strong base and weak acid. Mixtures of the two types of compound are thus inherently unstable. A stabilized mixture of lignocaine (4%) with fluorescein (0.25%) is available in single use units. If benoxinate is the preferred anaesthetic, it should be instilled separately or used to moisten the fluorescein strip.

For a full description of the technique of accurate applanation measurements of intra-ocular pressure the reader is referred to the appropriate literature issued with the instrument, and such papers as those of Grant (1963), Moses (1960) and Spaeth (1978). Considerable practice and experience are necessary before reliable results are routinely obtained, and field examinations should always be conducted, whenever possible, in conjunction with Schiötz or applanation tonometry.

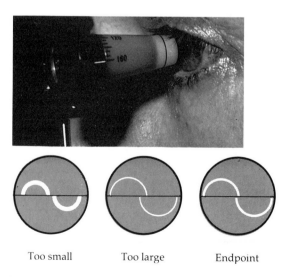

Too small   Too large   Endpoint

Figure 9.3 Applanation tonometry with Goldmann tonometer

Lacrimal patency
To demonstrate the patency of the lacrimal drainage system in patients complaining of frequent and troublesome epiphora, a drop or two of 2% fluorescein sodium eyedrops (P) may be used. Alternatively, the saline moistened fluorescein strip may be used to convey sufficient amount of the dye to the conjunctiva. Then a few drops of saline solution are also instilled into the conjunctival sac to increase the volume of liquid present, and the patient is asked to blow his nose in a white tissue. Yellow staining of the tissue proves patency of the lacrimal drainage of this particular eye, and the procedure is repeated for the other. Absence of staining of the tissue does not necessarily indicate obstruction to the passage of tears down the lacrimal passageway until observation has shown that the lacrimal punctum is in correct apposition to the globe of the eye.

Assessment of tear break up time
Since fluorescein colours the tear film, it can be used to assess the tear break up time (TBUT), which is the interval after blinking for discontinuities to appear in the precorneal tear film. After a blink, the tear film is formed anew and if the tears are coloured with fluorescein, a uniform fluorescent layer will be seen. After some time (usually much greater than the interblink period), convection currents disrupt the normal trilaminar layer, the surface active effect of the mucin is diluted and holes appear in the film. TBUT can be lengthened by the application of viscous drops. It is very much reduced in tear deficiency syndromes such as keratoconjunctivitis sicca, and Foster (1980) considers TBUTs of less than 10 seconds to be pathognomic of dry eye.

    If the tear film breaks up immediately, the eyes are open and breaks appear repeatedly in the same place, there is probably some pathological process at these sites. A short tear break up time can co-exist with a normal Schirmer tear test if the eye is mucin deficient.

Tear flow assessment
The half-life of drops in the conjunctival sac is very low. It will depend on the patency of the nasolacrimal duct and the rate of tear production. The rate at which fluorescein disappears from the conjunctival sac can be taken as a measure of the tear flow. Barendsen, Oosterhuis and van Haeringen (1979) used fluorescein to estimate the minimum permissible interval between the application of drugs. Predictably, they found that fluorescein concentration in the tear film decreased quicker in younger patients and thus viscous solutions were cleared at a slower rate than aqueous ones.

Contamination

Contamination of fluorescein eyedrops is a particularly serious risk, even greater than that encountered with the majority of other eyedrops. As these individual drops are liable to become infected with bacteria and at the same time are being used frequently on damaged tissue which is so prone to infection, very great care must be taken in their use. *Pseudomonas aeruginosa* is an especially dangerous pathological micro-organism by which fluorescein eyedrops are inclined to become invaded. Phenylmercuric acetate or nitrate in 0.002% strength is the best bactericide for preserving these particular eyedrops, and this is effective against Pseudo-

monas given adequate contact time. However, the safest method of their employment is sterile single-dose units or sterile fluorescein-impregnated paper strips,
both of which are readily available and to be highly recommended.

Rose bengal (Colour Plate VI)

Rose bengal is a brownish-red powder which is soluble in water and is normally
used as a 1% solution. Although not yet approved for sale in the UK, rose bengal
strips have been prepared (Scott, 1979). This substance is a derivative of fluorescein but has markedly different staining characteristics, crossing the cell
membranes of dead cells but not living ones. Mucus threads will also be stained.
Some practitioners prefer to examine the eye after rose bengal staining with a green
light.

Rose bengal also differs from fluorescein in its usage. While there is probably no
optometric practice which is without ophthalmic fluorescein in some form, rose
bengal is comparatively little used. This is most likely due to (a) the initial irritation
to the surface of the eye (especially, unfortunately, patients with dry eyes) and (b)
unfamiliarity with the results of staining. It is useful in the following conditions.

(1) Dendritic keratitis.
(2) Keratoconjunctivitis sicca.
(3) Keratitis neuroparalytica.
(4) Exophthalmos.
(5) Pressure areas due to contact lens wear.

Dendritic keratitis
Rose bengal will stain the areas of the dendritic ulcer. It is restricted to the
processes of the ulcer and does not diffuse to surrounding areas.

Keratoconjunctivitis sicca
The parts which are stained are the exposed triangular areas in the interpalpebral
conjunctiva. Such staining constitutes a better diagnostic indication of dry eye than
the Schirmer tear test.

Keratitis neuroparalytica
Extensive staining can occur in the same regions as in KCS.

Exophthalmos
If this is great enough to deny the eye of the normal protection of the lids, drying
will occur which will lead to changes in the exposed area.

Pressure areas due to contact lens wear
Contact lens practitioners may use rose bengal during their initial assessment of
patients for contact lens tolerance. It is equally useful in follow-up visits where
stains may be found on the cornea or bulbar or palpebral conjunctiva and although
not serious, provide an indication that modification of the lens may be necessary.

Mixtures of fluorescein and rose bengal

A mixed stain containing 1% fluorescein sodium and 1% rose bengal has been investigated by Norn (1964b, 1967), who concluded that it was better than the individual stains alone. He examined normal patients, patients with diseases of the cornea, conjunctiva and lacrimal passages and contact lens wearers. For the latter, he concluded that these vital stain are suitable for assessing damage in relation to the wearing of contact lenses. He attributed a punctate red crescent on the lower bulbar conjunctiva but considered that modification was only indicated in the presence of symptoms.

Triple staining with the above mixtures plus alcian blue has also been examined (Norn, 1964a). The three dyes stain different structures—fluorescein stains epithelial lesions, rose bengal stains degenerate cells and alcian blue, mucus.

Other stains

The following stains are seldom used but nevertheless are of interest.

Alcian blue

Alcian blue is a complex copper-containing compound which is used in 1% solution and is specific for staining mucus. It is used to counterstain rose bengal which, in addition to staining dead cells, also stains mucus (Norn, 1972b). If a break in the integrity of the epithelium exists, the exposed deeper layers may be stained a pale blue-green colour which will persist for several months (Norn, 1964b).

Trypan blue

Trypan Blue stains mucus and dead cells which have undergone structural changes (Norn, 1972b).

Tetrazolium and iodonitrotetrazolium

These compounds have been used for the vital staining of tumours and assessing corneal grafts (Norn, 1972b). They are by nature pro-stains because the compounds are reduced inside cells to a red dye formazan. The colour takes about 4 minutes to develop.

Tetrazolium stains degenerate cells, not dead cells. Living healthy cells are not stained because of the impermeability of the cell membrane and dead cells are not stained because the enzymes needed to reduce the dye to formazan are not present. It is a useful dye in the differential diagnosis of chronic simple conjunctivitis.

Bromothymol blue

This is a narrow range pH indicator which changes colour around pH 7 and it stains degenerate and dead cells and mucus. It is used to assess the damage caused by chemical agents such as lime.

Methylene blue

Dwyer Joyce (1967) reported on methylene blue, a bacterial stain which will also vitally stain nerve tissue. Like rose bengal it will outline an area of ulceration in herpetic keratitis. Hitchen (1971) refers to its ability to 'artistically' stain corneal ulcers when combined with fluorescein, the ulcer appearing as a dark blue area with a green halo.

References

Abrams, B. S. and Bailey, N. J. (1961) Black light photography. *J. Am. Optom. Assoc.*, **32**, 647–648

Barendsen, H., Oosterhuis, J. A. and van Haeringen, N. J. (1979) Concentration of fluorescein in tear fluid after instillation as eye drops. *Ophthal. Res.*, **11**, 73–82

Dwyer-Joyces, P. (1967) Corneal vital staining. *Irish J. Med. Sci.*, **6**,359–367

Foster, J. (1980) The spectrum of topical dyeagnosis. *Suid-Akrikaanse Argief vir Oftalmologie*, **7**, 23–31

Grant, W. M. (1963) Fluorescein for applanation tonometry. *Am. J. Ophthalmol.*, **55**, 1252

Hitchen, B. (1971) Corneal staining. *Ophthalmic Optician*, **11**, 23

Lee, J., Courtney, R. and Thorson, J. C. (1980) Contact lens application of Kodak Wratten filter systems for enhanced detection of fluorescein staining. *Contact Lens J.*, **9**, 33–34

Moses, R. A. (1960) Fluorescein in applanation tonometry. *Am. J. Ophthalmol.*, **53**, 1149

Norn, M. S. (1964a) Fluorescein vital staining of the cornea and conjunctiva. *Acta Ophthalmol.*, **42**, 1038–1048

Norn, M. S. (1964a) Vital staining in practise. *Acta Ophthalmol.*, **42**, 1046–1053

Norn, M. S. (1967) Vital staining of the cornea and conjunctiva. *Am. J. Ophthalmol.*, **64**, 1078–1080

Norn, M. S. (1972a) Method of testing dyes for vital staining of cornea and conjunctiva. *Acta. Ophthalmol.*, **56**, 809–814

Norn, M. S. (1972b) Vital staining of the cornea and conjunctiva. *Acta. Ophthalmol.*, Supplement 113

Refojo, M. F., Miller, D. and Fiore, A. S. (1972) A new fluorescent stain for soft hydrophilic lens fitting. *Arch. Ophthalmol.*, **87**, 275

Ruben, M. (1978) *Soft Contact Lens Clinical and Applied Technology*, Bailliere Tindall, London, p. 175

Spaeth, G. L. (1978) In *Clinical Ophthalmology* (ed. T. D. Duane), Harper and Row, Maryland, pp. 26–29

Chapter 10

Anti-infective agents

Certain procedures such as contact lens fitting or tonometry can result in disruption of the corneal epithelium. Foreign bodies may also cause a loss of integrity of the corneal epithelium. Because of the risk of infection under these circumstances, it is common practice to instill an antimicrobial as a prophylactic against this eventuality (Table 10.1). It is difficult to prove that such a prophylactic agent is effective in preventing infection, as it would be unethical to withhold it from patients in order to see whether infections occurred.

Prevention of infection extends not only to the use of antimicrobial agents but also to attention to hygiene precautions in practice (Chapter 3). For example, suitable preparation of tonometer heads and contact lenses can do much to reduce the task of the antimicrobial agent. Such procedures do not necessarily negate the use of the antimicrobial. Instead, they ensure that it will be more effective by reducing the viable count of bacteria.

The conjunctival sac is often sterile but on many occasions it will be infected by a wide spectrum of bacteria. Of course, organisms such as *Staphylococcus aureus* or *epidermis* and Streptococci are common residents but there is no guarantee as to

Table 10.1 Antimicrobials

Official Name	Trade name	Strengths % w/v	Forms available	Single dose	Adverse reactions
Sulphacetamide	Albucid	10.0 20.0 eyedrops	Eye drop	Yes (10% drops only)	Transient irritation
		2.5 – 10.0	Eye ointment		
Dibromoprop -amidine isethionate	Brolene	0.15	Eye ointment	No	—
Propamidine	Brolene	0.1	Eye drops	No	—
Framycetin	Framygen, soframycin	0.5 0.5	Eye ointment Eye ointment	No No	— —

which organisms will necessarily be present. Some may be opportunistic pathogens and a break in corneal integrity will allow them access to the deeper layers of the epithelium, where they will find an environment conducive to growth and multiplication.

The half-life of a drop in the conjunctival sac is very short and protection is afforded for a short time, but providing the total viable count in the sac is reduced, the prophylactic agent will have done its job. If an infection has gained hold then one drop will not be sufficient. In fact, the normal dose regime of 3 or 4 times a day will not be very effective either and it is perhaps fortunate that many cases of bacterial conjunctivitis are self resolving.

Ideal properties for anti-infective agents

Prophylactic antimicrobial agents should have the following ideal properties.

(1) They should have as wide a spectrum as possible. As it is not known which organism, if any, may be present, it is important to cover as many species of bacteria as possible. Notwithstanding, it would be wrong to use indiscriminately such agents as gentamicin (not available to the optometrist in any case), which is effective against *Pseudomonas* spp. This type of agent should be withheld until it is really needed, otherwise resistant strains will develop. The emergence of 'super-bugs' which are resistant to several antibiotics is mainly due to the uncontrolled use of these compounds in some countries.
(2) They should be as long-lasting as possible. The dwell time in the conjunctival sac is very short but any agent that becomes absorbed into the layers of the cornea should remain effective for some time.
(3) They should not interfere with wound healing.
(4) They should be presented sterile, preferably in single use units.
(5) They should be non-irritant.
(6) They should be non-toxic.

The following agents are available for use by optometrists:

sulphacetamide;
mafenide;
dibromopropamidine and propamidine;
framycetin.

Sulphacetamide sodium (*Albucid; Acetopt, Optamide*, Australia; *Bleph*, Australia, Canada, South Africa; *Cetamide, Optiole-S, Sodium Sulamyd*, Canada; *Op-Sulfa, Sebizon, Sulf—10/30*, USA)

Sulphacetamide sodium occurs as white or yellow-white crystals or a microcrystalline powder soluble 1 in 1.5 of water. It is used chiefly for local application in infections and injuries of the conjunctiva (for example acute conjunctivitis) and in prophylaxis (as by ophthalmic opticians). To prevent ocular infections developing after injuries and burns a 10% solution may be applied every 2 hours or a 30% solution twice a day. Alternatively, an eye ointment containing 6% of the drug in a greasy basis is available.

These are the official *BPC* eyedrops and *BP* eye ointment concentrations, respectively, but the eyedrops are also available in 20% and 30% (*Albucid*) and eye ointments in 2.5% (greasy basis) and 10% water-miscible basis (*Albucid*). Stronger solutions than 5% cause burning and stinging, therefore this effect is present with all strengths of the eyedrops mentioned, but is particularly marked with the hypertonic 30%. The brief discomfort is, however, usually tolerated without serious complaint.

The sulphonamide drugs have a bacteriostatic (rather than a bactericidal) action by virtue of their ability to prevent bacterial utilization of *p*-aminobenzoic acid (PABA) (Havener, 1978). PABA is required by sulphonamide-sensitive bacteria which use PABA to synthesize the vitamin folic acid. The latter is needed by micro-organisms for normal reproduction and metabolism. The basic structure of PABA is very similar to the sulphonamides which act as competitive antagonists or antimetabolites, substituting for the PABA in the transformation. Preformed folic acid is ingested by man so the sulphonamides do not interfere with its availability to human cells, or bacteria that utilize the preformed vitamin.

The growth of most Gram-positive micro-organisms and a variety of Gram-negative organisms, including some strains of Pseudomonas, is inhibited by sulphonamides. Sulphacetamide sodium in 10–30% solution and 6% ointment is effective, by local application, against surface ocular infection from such organisms in a manner which still compares favourably with many of the newer antibiotics. Generally, however, the antibiotics have replaced the sulphonamides as first choice in the treatment of major infections (Havener, 1978).

Sulphacetamide, although possessing a relatively 'weak' bactericidal action compared to some of the other sulphonamides, is suitable for topical application to the eye because of its acceptable pH and its solubility in aqueous solution. A 30% solution has a pH of 7.4% whilst solutions of other sulphonamides are highly alkaline. The drug penetrates into the ocular tissues and fluids in high concentrations, and its solubility in water is approximately 90 times that of sulphadimidine.

Eyedrops and eye ointments of sulphacetamide sodium are classed as POM.

As these eyedrops are affected by light and oxygen if in multi-dose containers, they are stored in dark amber bottles and contain an antoxidant (sodium metabisulphite) and the preservative phenylmercuric acetate or nitrate. As this solution is affected by heat, sterilization of the eyedrops is by (bacterial) filtration or, commercially, the single-dose units by gamma irradiation.

Combinations of sulphacetamide sodium with other antiseptics are obtainable, for example, the following proprietary preparations.

Ocusol eyedrops, containing 5% sulphacetamide sodium and 0.1% zinc sulphate as the active constituents, are POM.

Vasosulf eyedrops containing sulphacetamide sodium 15% with sodium thiosulphate 0.2%, methyl parabenzoate 0.02%, propyl parabenzoate 0.005%, in a neutral isotonic eyedrop solution (adjusted to pH 7.3–7.5) are POM.

Mafenide proprionate (*p*-aminomethylbenzenesulphonamide proprionate; alpha-amino-*p*-toluene sulphonamide proprionate) (*Sulfomyl*)

Mafenide proprionate is a colourless crystalline substance readily soluble in water. It has properties and uses similar to sulphacetamide sodium but bacteriological tests suggest it may be superior in its action against *Staphylococcus aureus, Staphylococcus albus, Streptococcus viridans, Haemophilus influenzae, Diplococcus pneumoniae* and *Pseudomonas aeruginosa* (Bain, 1954; Fraser, 1956; Perkins, 1957). Being less irritant to the conjunctiva is an additional advantage possessed by mafenide proprionate.

Although with *Sulfomyl* eyedrops no instances of allergy or irritation have been reported, these drops, or other topical ophthalmic sulphonamide preparations, should not be used in patients known to be sensitive to other sulphonamides.

Dibromopropamidine isethionate (*Brolene*)

This is a white or almost white crystalline powder soluble 1 in 2 of water. It is a member of the aromatic diamidine group of compounds which possess antibacterial and antifungal properties and is active against pyogenic cocci, *Staphylococcus aureus* as well as inhibiting certain Gram-negative bacilli, including *Escherichia coli, Proteus vulgaris*, and some strains of *Pseudomonas aeruginosa*. Dibromopropamidine's antibacterial action is not inhibited by pus or blood (Martindale, 1977). This antiseptic is effective even when instilled immediately following the use of amethocaine.

Dibromopropamidine isethionate is available as a proprietary preparation. (*Brolene* eye ointment) in a 0.15% concentration which is used for the treatment of conjunctivitis, blepharitis and other ocular infections, as well as for prophylactic ophthalmic purposes.

Propamidine isethionate

Propamidine isethionate is a white or nearly white granular powder soluble 1 in 5 of water, another member of the aromatic diamidine group of compounds. It also has antibacterial and antifungal properties. It is active against *Staphylococcus aureus, Streptococcus pyogenes* and certain other streptococci and Clostridia, but not against *Pseudomonas aeruginosa, Proteus vulgaris* or *Escherichia coli*: its antibacterial action is not inhibited by tissue fluids, serum or pus (Martindale, 1977).

Propamidine isethionate is available as a proprietary preparation (*Brolene* eyedrops) in a 0.1% concentration, which is used in the treatment (which should not exceed a week) of conjunctivitis (particularly that due to Morax-Axenfield and pyogenic cocci), as well as for prophylactic purposes.

The rare possibility of sensitization reaction to *Brolene* preparations is an indication for immediate discontinuation of their use.

Framycetin

Framycetin is the only antibiotic available for use by optometrists in the UK and is produced by certain strains of *Streptomyces fradiae* or *decaris*. Framycetin is an isomer of neomycin which is used extensively as a topical antibiotic in general medicine.

Neomycin is a mixture of three substances—neomycin A, neomycin B and neomycin C. In fact, neomycin A is an inactive break-down product of the other two and is normally present at a concentration of 10–15%.

Framycetin is otherwise known as neomycin B and preparations of framycetin contain not more than 3% neomycin C and not more than 1% neomycin A.

It has a broad spectrum of activity against Gram positive and Gram negative bacteria. It is effective against a greater range of bacteria than penicillin or streptomycin, e.g. *Proteus vulgaris, Escherichia coli, Haemophilus influenzae* and *Klebsiella* spp.

Like all antibiotics, resistance can develop with continued indiscriminate use, but this tends to develop more slowly than to other antibiotics. Of course, there will be cross-resistance between neomycin and framycetin and other aminoglycoside antibiotics.

Neomycin and framycetin are poorly absorbed from the alimentary tract. For this reason neomycin can be used to suppress normal intestinal bacteria prior to alimentary surgery. It is well absorbed from injection but produces toxic reactions, especially to the kidneys and ears. Framycetin will have similar toxicity. Because of the poor systemic absorption and the toxicity, neomycin and framycetin are principally used for topical application. Framycetin is used on gauze dressings, in skin creams, nebulizers and eye preparations.

Adverse reactions

The manner in which an optometrist will normally use an anti-infective agent will lead to few adverse effects. Single topical applications of drugs which have been chosen for their high therapeutic index are unlikely to produce toxic reactions. Hypersensitivity reactions can occur and when taking a patient's history, questions should be asked about past untoward drug reactions.

References

Bain, W. E. S. (1954) Mafenide in ophthalmology. *Practitioner*, **1/2**, 682

Fraser, I. T. (1956) Treatment of ophthalmia neonatorum with sulphonamidobenzylamine propionate. *Practitioner*, **177**, 71

Havener, W. H. (1978) *Ocular Pharmacology*, 4th edn. Mosby, St Louis, pp. 172–194

Martindale, W. (1977) *Extra Pharmacopoeia*, The Pharmaceutical Press, London, p. 517

Perkins, E. S. (1957) Antiobiotics and chemotherapy in treatment of diseases of the eye. *Practitioner*, **178**, 572

Chapter 11

Miscellaneous agents

Agents used in the treatment of inflammation

The optometrist is not responsible for treating inflammation which occurs as a response to infections, allergy or chemical stimulation. These conditions need an examination of the cause in order to remove it before treating the symptoms.

However, there are situations in which an anti-inflammatory agent may be appropriate and the optometrist has access to a variety of agents which will alleviate the symptoms of inflammation. These include vasoconstrictors, antihistamines and nonsteroidal anti-inflammatory agents.

Vasoconstrictors

In the development of some allergic responses, histamine is released, causing vasodilation. It can be reversed by the use of antihistamine working on the histamine receptor, but is best treated with a physiological antagonist—a sympathomimetic.

Blood vessels are innervated by sympathetic nerves and adrenergic receptors that produce vasoconstriction are alpha-receptors. Some blood vessels also have beta-vasodilator receptors but these are not normally found in mucous membranes.

Alpha-receptors also mediate contraction of the pupil dilator muscle and some mydriatics can be used as vasoconstrictors. The concentrations employed to produce the latter effect are very much lower than mydriatic or ocular hypotensive (anti-glaucoma) concentrations. Some sympathomimetics are used just as vasoconstrictors.

Sympathomimetics used as vasoconstrictors include adrenaline, phenylephrine, naphazoline, xylometazoline and tetrahydrozoline.

Adrenaline acid tartrate
Adrenaline acid tartrate is a white, greyish-white or light brownish-grey crystalline powder soluble 1 in 3 of water. It has the pharmacological actions of adrenaline (*see* Chapter 8), and is, in the *BP* a 1 in 1000 Adrenaline Solution, the most popular conjunctival decongestant used by ophthalmic opticians. As has already been mentioned, repeated instillations of this solution over a short period will result in a reactive hyperaemia, so on any particular occasion only 1 or 2 drops of it should be used. The solution, if in a multi-dose container, should be stored in well filled bottles, protected from light in amber bottles in a dark cupboard, and kept in a cool

place. The official solution contains preservatives (chlorbutol and chlorocresol), an antoxidant (sodium metabisulphite), sodium chloride and 0.18% w/v adrenaline acid tartrate, which is the equivalent of 1 in 1000 adrenaline. For ophthalmic purposes the solution should be sterile, and at this concentration, in the normal eye, it should have no mydriatic effect, the decongestion being obtained by a sympathomimetic vasoconstrictor action. This effect, obtained by a 0.09% adrenaline acid tartrate, has been combined with the mild antiseptic and astringent effect of 0.25% zinc sulphate in an official (*BP*) eyedrops (P).

Phenylephrine hydrochloride
This is a white crystalline powder soluble 1 in 2 of water. Its main use as a direct acting sympathomimetic mydriatic when used in a 10% solution has already been discussed in Chapter 6. Although not as popular as a vasoconstrictor with optometrists as adrenaline 1 in 1000, employed in 0.125% eyedrops (P) it may be used quite satisfactorily for this purpose to whiten the eye. Numerous proprietary eye lotions designed to produce just this effect include it in this strength. Even in this very weak concentration it may cause some mild dilatation of the pupil in some patients (Weiss and Shaffer, 1962), and to preclude the risk of precipitating an attack of acute glaucoma in those predisposed (this has occurred on rare occasions) its employment as a local decongestant should be eschewed in patients aged over 40 years.

Naphazoline hydrochloride (Albalon, Australia, Canada; Vasocon, Canada, USA) or Naphazoline nitrate
Naphazoline hydrochloride and naphazoline nitrate are white or almost white crystalline powders soluble 1 in 6 and 1 in 36 water, respectively. These are potent sympathomimetic vasoconstrictors with a direct alpha-adrenergic receptor stimulatory action, and may be used as topical decongestants in 0.05% or 0.1% eyedrops. Frequent application of these solutions will produce a reactive hyperaemia. Instillation should not be repeated in less than 4–6 hours to avoid this rebound congestion.

Naphazoline eyedrops cause slight mydriasis and are contra-indicated in patients with actual or suspected closed-angle glaucoma.

Although not administered systemically, topical application of naphazoline has resulted in systemic absorption, and it is readily absorbed from the gastro-intestinal tract (Martindale, 1977).

Xylometazoline hydrochloride (Otrovine)
This is a further sympathomimetic agent with marked alpha-adrenergic receptor stimulatory action. It may be used in eyedrops as a conjunctival decongestant in 0.05% concentration, and is available in this strength combined with the antihistaminic, antazoline sulphate (0.5%) (a white or almost white crystalline powder soluble 1 in 5 of water) in a proprietary eyedrops preparation (*Otravine-Antistin*) (P).

Tetrahydrozoline hydrochloride (USP) (Visine, Australia, Canada, South Africa, USA)
Tetrahydrozoline is a sympathomimetic vasoconstrictor with pronounced alpha-adrenergic activity. Ophthalmic decongestant eyedrops normally contain 0.05% w/v. As it is readily absorbed from the gastro-intestinal tract the usual precautions

must be observed, particularly with reference to contra-indication for topical ophthalmic sympathomimetic agents (*see* adrenaline, naphazoline, etc.). Tetra-hydrozoline is not available as a proprietary preparation in the United Kingdom but is in common use in such preparations in the USA.

Precautions. The sympathomimetic conjunctival decongestants must not be used on patients receiving monamine oxidase inhibitors (or within 10 days of their discontinuation) since severe hypertensive crisis may result, or on patients with hypertension or hyperthyroidism or children below the age of 2 years.

Antihistamines

The alternative method of antagonizing the action of histamine is by using a pharmacological antagonist—an antihistamine. Histamine receptors have been divided into two types, H1 and H2. The former are involved in the well known triple response to histamine. When histamine is injected a local vasodilation occurs, which is due to a direct effect of histamine on the blood vessels and is manifested as a bright red spot. Changes in the permeability of the blood vessels cause a loss of plasma protein into the extracellular space. This leads to an area of oedema, causing a bump which becomes red because of reflex vasodilation, with stimulation of pain and itch fibres.

H1 receptors are found on the surface of the eye as well as other mucous membranes, e.g. nasal cavities. They are blocked by antihistamines such as antazoline.

H2 receptors mediate gastric acid secretion and are blocked by drugs, such as cimetidine, which are used for the treatment of gastric ulcers. H2 receptors have been found on the surface of the eye. These receptors are thought to be involved in the dilatation of episcleral, conjunctival and perilimbal blood vessels (Havener, 1983).

H1 antagonists such as antazoline (*Antistine*) have been used in combination with sympathomimetic vasoconstrictors, since this is more effective than each component on its own. By utilizing two forms of antagonism (pharmacological and physiological), an additive effect is produced. The usual symptoms of histamine mediated allergy are lacrimation, redness, itching, pain and photophobia. Antazoline would appear to relieve the itching, while naphazoline (a vasoconstrictor) will be more effective on the blood vessels and in reducing the redness.

Many antihistamine agents also have antimuscarinic activity. Some agents are able to antagonize both histamine and acetylcholine equally. Topical application can reduce tear flow by this atropine-like effect. It is a reported side-effect of systemic use of antihistamines that contact lens tolerance may be reduced.

Non-steroidal anti-inflammatory drugs (NSAIDs)

As their name suggests, these compounds were developed as an alternative to steroids in the treatment of inflammatory disease. Steroids were hailed as wonder drugs when they were first introduced into medicine. Certainly they are very effective and reduce many of the symptoms of inflammation. Unfortunately, they produce many side-effects, e.g. cataracts and raised intraocular pressure. Alternative agents were therefore developed which it was hoped would have equal anti-inflammatory effects for much fewer adverse reactions.

One of the mechanisms (Figure 11.1) involved in the inflammatory response is the conversion of fatty acids to prostaglandin. In the eye prostaglandins produce an atropine resistant miosis. Before prostaglandins were discovered, the name irin was given to a theoretical substance which was released during mechanical manipulation of the iris.

Prostaglandins increase the permeability of the ciliary epithelium, allowing larger amounts of protein to pass into the aqueous humour which gives rise to aqueous flare and an increase in intraocular pressure. This rise is followed by a fall some 2 hours later. Prostaglandins have been implicated in corneal neovascularization.

There are many inhibitors of prostaglandin formation. The oldest, best known and cheapest is aspirin (acetylsalicylic acid). It has been tested for the prevention of cystoid macular oedema following cataract extraction.

The first of the new generation of NSAIDs was indomethacin, a compound which has been tested in topical formulation for cystoid macular oedoma.

There are now many such agents available today, although because of adverse reactions, almost as many would seem to have been withdrawn. Several have been tested for ophthalmic use but only one is currently available in an ophthalmic form—oxyphenbutazone. This compound has recently been withdrawn from systemic use.

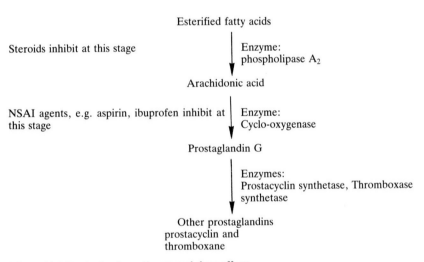

Figure 11.1 Prostaglandin pathways and drug effects

Oxyphenbutazone eye ointment (Tandaril Eye Ointment) (POM)
Oxyphenbutazone is a white crystalline powder almost insoluble in water. It is a derivative of phenylbutazone, with similar anti-inflammatory, analgesic, and antipyretic effects. It is given in general medicine, usually by mouth, for the treatment of rheumatic and allied disorders. Oxyphenbutazone may be used in a 10% concentration in a greasy eye ointment base for nonpurulent inflammatory anterior segment eye conditions. Where other conjunctival decongestants are contra-indicated, a single application of this ointment provides a useful alternative

for the ophthalmic optical practitioner. The *BNF* (1976–78) describes this preparation as 'an effective anti-inflammatory agent free from the attendant changes associated with topical steroid therapy'.

Irrigating and emollient drops

These agents have no active principal as such. In fact, the vehicle is the only component and carries out the functions of this type of product. They are used for the following purposes:

(1) Washing out excess stain in order to get a clear picture.
(2) Removal of foreign bodies.
(3) Dilution of chemical splashes in the eye.
(4) Protection of the eye during impression taking.
(5) As an emollient after trauma.

Normal saline

Normal saline (0.9% w/v sodium chloride Ph.Eur.) is isotonic with blood plasma and approximately isotonic with tears. Isotonicity is related to osmotic pressure, which is a property like boiling and freezing points, being dependent on the number of ions or molecules in solution, rather than the weight.

At one time it was thought that all solutions which came in contact with the eye should be isotonic, but it has since been shown that the eye can tolerate solutions with a range of osmotic pressures.

Rather than refer to absolute osmotic pressure, it is the practice to specify sodium chloride equivalents. The eye is able to withstand solutions with sodium chloride equivalents of between 0.5 and 2.0% (Riegelman, Vaughan and Okumoto, 1955).

Normal saline is available in many forms, for many uses. Although the contents will be the same, the packaging and the label will have a great influence on the legal category assigned in the UK.

Normal saline is available as:

(1) Single use units of 0.5 ml. These are eyedrops and are classed as Pharmacy Medicines. In these small volumes, saline can be used to moisten fluorescein strips or to wash out excess stain and can also be used as a rewetting drop for soft contact lenses.
(2) Multidose saline eyedrops. These will contain a preservative such as benzalkonium chrloride and will be packed in 10 ml dropper bottles. They will be used for the same purpose as single use eyedrops and are similarly classed as Pharmacy Medicines.
(3) Large volume eye lotions. Eye lotions are packed in volumes of 500 ml. They are used for irrigation of chemical splashes when running water is not available. They are classed as eye lotions and are General Sales List Medicines.
(4) There are a variety of saline preparations which are intended for contact lens care; these will be dealt with in Chapter 12.

Oily drops

Oily drops such as castor oil or liquid paraffin have been used as emollients (soothing lubricants) after foreign body removal, to assist in the removal of oily foreign bodies or as a protective after the removal of foreign body.

Liquid paraffin (parolein eyedrops) is one oil that has been used. Castor oil is an alternative, which has the advantage that it is available in single use eye drops.

Artificial tears

There is a wide range of artificial tears available which contain a variety of viscosity agents and preservatives. Some like Sno tears (Smith & Nephew) and Liquifilm (Allergan) contain polyvinyl alcohol, which is a surface active agent as well as increasing viscosity, whilst others contain cellulose derivatives, such as the Isopto range (Alcon) and hypromellose BPC.

Most artificial tears are isotonic but Hypotears (Coopervision) has a sodium chloride equivalent of 0.6%. They have a viscosity range from 2 cps (similar to that of water) to well in excess of 20 cps.

The principal use of artificial tears is to relieve the symptoms of dry eye but the treatment of this condition is the responsibility of medical practitioners. Artificial tears are Pharmacy Medicines and may be supplied by optometrists in an emergency only.

Artificial tears may be employed as an in-use comfort drop for contact lens wearers but caution should be exercised because of the preservative contained in them. It is important that notice is taken of the concentration as well as the type of preservative present.

Most artificial tears contain 0.01% benzalkonium chloride which at this concentration will destabilize the tear film and shorten the tear break up time (Holly, 1978; Hollis and Lemp, 1977). Some formulations (e.g. Sno tears) contain only 0.004% of this preservative, which does not interfere with tear film stability (Holly, 1978). Chlorbutol and thiomersal are used in other artificial lens formulations.

References

Havener, W. H. (1983) *Ocular Pharmacology*, 5th edn. Mosby, St. Louis

Hollis, F. J. and Lemp, M. A. (1977) Tear physiology and dry eyes. *Survey of Ophthalmology*, **22**, 69–87

Holly, F. J. (1978) The preocular tear film. *Contact Lens*, 52–55

Martindale, W. (1977) *Extra Pharmacopoeia*, 27th edn. The Pharmaceutical Press, London, p.23

Riegelman, S., Vaughan, D. G. and Okumoto, M. (1955) Compounding ophthalmic solutions. *J. Am. Pharm. Assoc.*, **16**, 742

Weiss, D. J. and Shaffer, R. N. (1962) Mydriatic effects of one-eighth percent phenylephrine. *Arch. Ophthalmol.*, **68**, 727

Chapter 12

Contact lens solutions

The development of contact lens solutions has, of course, followed that of contact lens materials. In addition, the appreciation of newer dangers such as the AIDS virus and acanthamoebae may impose further requirements in performance. Certainly, the wearing of lenses can lead to changes in the bacterial flora of the conjunctival sac with a reduction in the number of *Staphylococcus epidermidis* and an increase in the population of Gram negative rods (Hovding, 1981), both of which are non-pathogens. Infections with pathogenic organisms occur during contact lens wear, resulting in corneal ulcers; Weissman *et al.* (1984) examined 18 patients wearing extended wear soft contact lenses and found that *Pseudomonas aeruginosa* was the most common pathogen isolated from ulcers.

The solution can react with the lens at its surface, causing changes in wettability or, in the case of a soft lens, in the bulk of the lens by altering the water content, thus changing the shape or other lens parameters.

Originally, solutions were developed commercially to aid the wearing of hard PMMA lenses and with the development of soft lenses, a whole new formulation problem was posed to the pharmaceutical industry. Later on it had to cope with the special demands of the new gas permeable hard materials. Solutions perform many functions but the underlying reasons for using solutions are as follows:

(1) To facilitate the insertion, wearing and removal of the lens.
(2) To maintain the optical and physical properties of the contact lens.
(3) To reduce the adverse effects of contact lens wear.
(4) To reduce as far as possible the danger of infection.

All solutions (irrespective of use) should have the following ideal properties:

(1) They should be sterile.
(2) They should not harm or discolour (Wardlow and Sarver, 1986) the lens.
(3) They should not be toxic to the eye.
(4) Their mode of use should encourage patient compliance.

Solutions for both hard and soft contact lenses fall into one of the following categories:

(1) Disinfecting and Soaking Solutions
(2) Daily Cleaning Agents
(3) Wetting Solutions
(4) Comfort Drops
(5) Protein Remover Tablets

167

Disinfecting and soaking solutions

Suitable formulated disinfecting and soaking solutions act as a storage medium for all types of contact lens while they are not being worn.

Even an extended wear contact lens must spend some time outside the eye. Even if it were possible to insert a contact lens which was clean and sterile, it would, in all probability, come out contaminated and infected. If a lens is stored dry, it would lose water and the secretions adhering to it would harden and become difficult to remove. The amount of water loss would depend on the original level of hydration of the lens. The hard PMMA lens has a small water content, but soft lenses can contain up to 80% water.

The level of bacterial contamination would not be reduced by dry storage, as the organic contaminants would support the growth of micro-organisms.

Storage of the lens in solution is the universally accepted practice today. After removal and cleaning the lens is placed in a storage case containing one of the three types of solution.

(a) A stable disinfecting solution containing one of the preservatives mentioned in Chapter 3 (Figure 12.1).

(b) A transient disinfecting solution containing an antimicrobial agent which is inherently unstable and which is broken down by neutralizer to leave the lens in a sterile solution containing no active ingredient (Figure 12.2).

(c) A saline soaking solution in which the lens is heated. (Soft lenses only) (Figure 12.3).

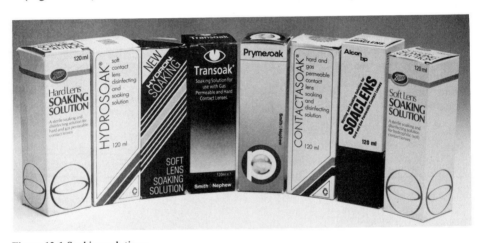

Figure 12.1 Soaking solutions

Other techniques of contact lens disinfection have been tried, such as ultrasonics or microwaves from a cooker (Rohrer *et al.* 1986).

Whatever the system used, it should have effects not only on the normal challenge bacteria, i.e. *Staph. aureus, Pseud. aeruginosa* and *Escherichia coli*, but also on bacteria such as *Serratia marcescens* (Ahearn, Penley and Wilson, 1984, Parment *et al.* 1986), *Haemophilus influenzae* (Armstrong, Cohen and McCarthy, 1984) and other organisms such as fungi (Churner and Cunningham 1983; Brooks, Lazarus and Weiner 1984) and acanthamoebae. Fungi in particular are a problem,

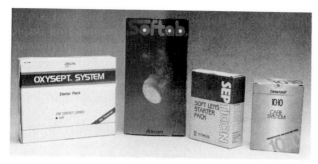

Figure 12.2 Transient solutions

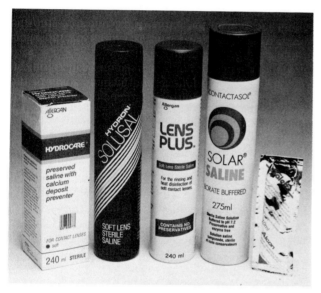

Figure 12.3 Saline solutions

as the organism can actually penetrate hydrophilic contact lenses (Bernstein, 1973; Filppi, Pfister and Hill, 1973).

Stable disinfecting solutions

These will contain one or more preservatives. Lenses can be placed in the solution and taken out at any time but to ensure that the lens is properly disinfected it should be left for a number of hours. This is a disadvantage compared with heat or oxidative methods, which are much quicker (Kreis, 1972). The efficacy of this type of solution will be affected by several factors: the level of contamination; the freshness of the solution; the volume of the solution in the lens case; and temperature.

The use of a daily cleaner will do much to reduce the bacterial contamination before the lens is placed in a soaking solution. Good hygiene practices such as hand washing before the lens is handled will reduce the work of the soaking solution.

Soaking solutions will need changing regularly, as although the solution in the case may appear to be the same as when it was poured from the bottle, it will have lost some of its effectiveness. In over half of the 217 cases reported by Barry and Ruben (1978) who exhibited contact lens related problems, bacteria were isolated from the storage case. Some of the preservatives will have been taken up by contamination and dead bacteria. Contaminants will also provide a protection for bacteria from the antimicrobial agent. The reports of eye infections in contact lens wearers often result from contaminated lens storage cases. It is necessary to have a case that is compatible with the solution and with the lens, which must be completely immersed.

Disinfecting and soaking solutions designed for PMMA and gas permeable hard lenses contain a variety of preservatives, including chlorhexidine, benzalkonium chloride, thiomersal and chlorbutol. EDTA is often present as a synergistic agent. Other agents have also been suggested in the past, e.g. trimethoprim (Editorial, 1985).

Norton *et al.* (1974) tested the antimicrobial efficiencies of contact lens solutions containing a variety of preservatives, including the ones mentioned above. They found a range of activity varying from the adequate to very inadequate. Studies on solutions of preservatives on their own showed benzalkonium chloride to be the most effective against *Staph. aureus* and *Pseud. aeruginosa*.

Soaking solutions for soft lenses contain the same preservatives, with the exception of benzalkonium chloride, because it binds to hydrogel materials and could adversely affect the eye. A controversy exists as to whether benzalkonium chloride can be used with certain gas permeable hard lenses. It has been used for many years in solutions for conventional hard contact lenses, but concern has been expressed about its ability to bind to the surface of some gas permeable materials. Rosenthal *et al.* (1986) found that benzalkonium chloride bound to the surface of silicone/acrylate lenses in a manner different to that of chlorhexidine. Chlorhexidine binding is limited to a monomolecular layer, but benzalkonium chloride builds a self-propagating multi-layer which reduces surface wettability. On the other hand, Richardson, Gee and Meakin (1984) found that the uptake of benzalkonium chloride was less by CAB lenses than it was by PMMA. Wong *et al.* (1986), in a study of both *in vivo* and *in vitro* absorption of benzalkonium chloride, demonstrated that rigid gas permeable lenses do not accumulate significant levels of the preservative. Similarly Walters, Gee and Meakin (1983) found that although benzalkonium chloride bound differently to Boston lenses than it did to PMMA, the actual amount of uptake was significantly different for the two lenses. After 3 months storage in benzalkonium chloride-containing solution, no changes in physical or optical parameters were seen.

Of course it is almost as important that the preservatives do not react with the container in which they are held. Richardson *et al.* (1977) found that some preservatives, particularly thiomersal, reacted markedly with the plastic bottle and as a result the concentration was reduced significantly.

Soaking solutions can be implicated in the development of toxic or allergic reactions, especially in the case of soft lens solutions. Wilson, McNatt and Reitschel (1981) examined 38 patients with ocular signs and symptoms related to soft lens wear. All solutions used by the patients contained thiomersal and 27 patients reponded to thimerosal patch testing.

Wright and Mackie (1982) also examined patients with conjunctival irritation and reduced lens tolerance. In particular, the organic mercurials such as thiomersal were heavily implicated as the cause of the symptoms. Similar results were reported by Mondino and Groden (1980), who reported conjunctival hyperaemia and anterior stromal infiltrates of the cornea in three cosmetic soft contact lens wearers who used chemical disinfection systems containing thiomersal.

Soaking solutions have been traditionally rendered isotonic by the addition of sodium chloride or other electrolytes. One solution on the UK market, however, utilizes a non-electrolyte tonicity agent. It has been assumed that a sodium chloride equivalent of 0.9% would provide the best solution, but Kempster (1984) studied the effect of soaking lenses in solutions of different tonicities and found that solutions between 1.0 and 1.1% w/v produced minimal corneal thickness changes.

Transient disinfecting solutions

Oxidizing agents such as iodine and hydrogen peroxide have antimicrobial effects, especially against anaerobes. Solutions containing iodine have been used in the past. Neutralizing agents reduced the iodine (brown in colour) to the inactive, colourless iodide and the reactions produced a mixture of electrolytes, none of which were foreign to the eyes. Iodine-based solutions failed to find favour.

Solutions of hydrogen peroxide are now used instead. Hydrogen peroxide has been used for many years as a surface disinfectant and for its bleaching effect. Its strength is described in terms of volumes (i.e. 10 volume, 20 volume, etc.). A 10 volume solution produces 10 times its volume of oxygen when it breaks down. In terms of percentage a 10 volume solution is about 3% w/v. Tragakis, Brown and Pearce (1973) found that hydrogen peroxide was very effective against all the organisms used in their tests. Similar results were recorded by Penley *et al.* (1985). Various methods have been used to bring about the breakdown of the peroxide. The original neutralizing process involved soaking the treated lens in sodium bicarbonate (0.5% w/v) and then in two changes of saline, prior to overnight storage in saline. The time-consuming nature of the process prevented the adoption of hydrogen peroxide as a routine disinfecting system until easier neutralizing steps were found. The Septicon system uses a catalyst to break down the peroxide into water and oxygen. This tends to be a little slow and it is possible for the catalyst to become poisoned. Another system uses sodium pyruvate to bring about neutralization. Pyruvic acid is an intermediate in the breakdown of glucose by the glycolytic cycle and is therefore a normal constituent of cells. It can also act as a medium for the growth of bacteria. Sometimes the neutralizing step is forgotten and reactions to unneutralized hydrogen peroxide have been reported (Knopf, 1984).

A chlorine based method involving dichloroisocyanurate, a compound which has been used for water purification, has been introduced. It is naturally unstable and breaks down to hypochlorite, which in turn yields sodium chloride and chlorine. Sodium hypochlorite is the basis of solutions for disinfecting babies' bottles which have been used in the past by some practitioners for disinfection of lenses. Chlorine, like other halogens, acts as a disinfectant and mild cleaning agent.

Although transient agents are neutralized to inactive compounds, the reactions can sometime produce a change in pH. It is thus important that the proper neutralizing solution is used as often this will be buffered. Janoff (1979) noted the acidic shift after the use of peroxide which could overload the buffering capacity of the tears and produce unpleasant symptoms. These could lead to poor compliance by the patient. Whilst these systems were specifically designed for use with soft contact lenses, they could, of course, be used with PMMA or gas permeable hard lenses.

Saline soaking solutions

Heat is a very effective antimicrobial agent (*see* Chapter 3), which has so far only been used for the disinfection of soft lenses. Although the technique involves surrounding the case in steam, the actual contents do not reach boiling point. In fact the maximum temperatures of the contents of the case varied from 78°C to 92°C in a study of nine different heating units (Liubinas, Swenson and Carney, 1987). There were considered to be too high and the authors recommended a temperature of between 70°C and 80°C for 5 minutes. Similarly, Stone *et al.* (1984) recommended that the lens should be subjected to temperatures over 50°C for a minimum time, and 80°C for 10 minutes has been recommended by other authors (Busschaert, Good and Szabocsil, 1978). Even higher temperatures were recorded in a study by Garner (1982). The temperatures achieved are sufficient to kill all vegetative organisms and most spores, providing the biological burden is not too great.

There are several forms of saline for use with boiling systems.

Preserved saline
Solutions of sodium chloride preserved with agents such as thiomersal can be used to store lenses during heating. They have the advantage that simple boiling becomes 'heating with a preservative'—a far more effective antimicrobial method. The presence of the preservative also ensures that the initial level of bacteria is kept to a minimum. However, the presence of the preservative may lead to allergic and toxic reactions.

Shaw (1980) demonstrated the relationship between the preservatives and the incidence of contact lens solution allergy. He used saline solutions containing 0.001% thiomersal and 0.1% EDTA in the lens care regimen of six soft contact lens wearers. Preserved saline solutions containing EDTA as a part of the preservative system have a useful deposit preventing effect compared with an unpreserved saline solution (Moore *et al.* 1980).

Single use sachets
These are ideal as they are produced sterile and remain sterile until they are used. They are more expensive and this may encourage the patient to re-use the saline.

Pressurized containers
These provide a good method of delivering sterile unpreserved saline. They are available both buffered and unbuffered.

Salt tablets
Salt tablets dissolved in the correct amount of purified water can be used to produce normal saline. However, purified water is water that has been purified *chemically*, not *microbiologically*; it can thus be heavily contaminated (Jenkins and Phillips, 1986). Indeed it is this method of producing saline that has been implicated in the outbreak of Acanthamoeba keratitis in contact lens wearers. Three such cases were reported by Moore *et al.* (1986) in which patients were initially diagnosed as suffering from Herpes simplex keratitis or overwear syndrome, but

cultures from the solution bottles revealed the presence of Acanthamoebae. The authors concluded the use of home-made saline should be discouraged.

Saline can also be used as a rinsing solution. Non-sterile nonpreserved saline should be avoided for this purpose, as it can lead to the introduction of potential pathogens (Josse, 1984).

Daily cleaning agents

A daily cleaning regimen is a necessary requirement for all lenses prior to the lens being placed into the disinfecting solution.

As well as micro-organisms, lenses pick up a variety of contaminants including fats and proteins from tears. Other contaminants will occur depending on the patient's lifestyle, e.g. nicotine (Broich, Weiss and Rapp, 1980). Although deposits have been found to occur on hard lenses (Fowler *et al.* 1984) and low and high water content soft lenses (Hosaka *et al.* 1983), the level of deposit formation appears to be proportional to the water content (Fowler, Korb and Allansmith, 1985). Daily cleaning:

(a) Improves the clarity of the lens by removing mucus, lipids and other contaminants. These can become fixed onto the surface of the lens by the disinfecting process.
(b) Prolongs the successful wearing time (Hesse *et al.*, 1982).
(c) Reduces the level of microbiological contamination by physically removing contaminated debris.
(d) Improves the efficacy of the disinfecting agent, whether heat or chemical.
(e) Removes possible nutrients on which organisms can grow.
(f) May reduce toxic effects from the disinfecting solution because contaminants can sometimes bind the preservative to the lens.
(g) Reduces the adherence of organisms to the lens. It has been shown that tear components absorbed onto the lens surface enhance the adherence of micro-organisms to lenses (Butrus and Klotz, 1986), but some may adhere even to clean lenses (Duran *et al.*, 1987)

Daily cleaning is not just a prelude to the disinfection process, it is an integral part of it.

Daily cleaners contain a surface active agent or detergent which reduces the surface tension of fats and other lipophilic substances. As multi-use solutions, they will also contain a preservative, similar to those found in disinfecting and soaking solutions. There is no concern for toxicity, as cleaning solutions should be thoroughly rinsed from the lens before it is inserted. Indeed the lens should be rinsed before it is placed in the soaking solution in order to reduce the contamination of the soaking solution.

Wetting solutions

Wetting solutions are an important part of the care regimen for PMMA and gas permeable hard lenses.

The solutions contain a surface active agent which reduces the contact angle of tears with the contact lens. Properly formulated wetting solutions assist in the insertion, wearing and maintenance of hard lenses.

They provide a coating to the lens, which by being viscous helps to balance the lens on the end of the finger. On insertion the covering provides a mechanical buffer between the lens and the cornea and the lens and the eyelids. This mechanical buffering action continues while the lens is being worn and allows the lids to slide easily over the lens.

Many plastics have a hydrophobic surface and will not be wetted by tears. The unwetted lens will have poor optical properties and retain the foreign body feeling when it is being worn. It will also retain greasy contaminant and be more difficult to clean.

In the past, human saliva has been used as a substitute wetting solution. While being available at no cost and having good wetting and viscoelastic properties, its use involves an unacceptable microbiological hazard.

Wetting solutions contain a wetting agent, a viscosity increasing agent and a preservative. The usual wetting agent found in wetting solutions is polyvinyl alcohol (PVA). It has been extensively employed in artificial tear formulations and to increase the viscosity of eye drops to prolong the contact time in the conjunctival sac and increase penetration.

Thus, as well as acting as the wetting solution PVA also acts as the viscosity increasing agent, but in some formulations other agents such as cellulose derivatives are also added. There is little agreement as to the proper level of viscosity that is required for wetting solutions.

Wetting solutions will be employed after the lens has been removed from the soaking solution, i.e. to a disinfected lens. The function of the antimicrobial preservative is not therefore to disinfect the lens but to only to maintain the initial sterility of the solution in the bottle. The solution in the bottle is expected to be sterile, while that on the lens is not.

It is important that the level of preservative is kept as low as possible while remaining effective in its function.

Benzalkonium chloride is an effective preservative which can be made more effective by the addition of EDTA. It will interfere with tear film integrity if the concentration is too high. A concentration of 0.004% w/v combined with EDTA will give both effectiveness and a reduced effect on the tear film.

Other preservatives may also be incorporated into hard lens wetting solutions. Irrespective of any effect on the tear film, it is imperative that the concentration is kept to a minimum in order to reduce any toxic or allergic effects. Wetting solutions by their very method of use will be in contact with the eye for a prolonged period. They are also used on a daily basis and thus the total exposure time to the eye is quite high.

In use comfort drops

Suitably formulated comfort drops are an optional part of the care regimens for all types of contact lenses.

The eye can tolerate adverse atmospheric conditions. It can also tolerate the wearing of a contact lens but it has difficulty sometimes in dealing with both. In particular dry, smokey atmospheres can produce changes in the lens–tear system which alters an acceptable situation into an intolerable one. Certain drugs such as antihistamines, which have an antimuscarinic effect, can reduce lens tolerance. Hormonal changes in women can also modify the quantity or quality of tears.

In these situations, an in-use comfort drop may be used. These are, in reality, artificial tears with one extra property, i.e. lens compatibility. They will contain a viscosity-increasing substance and (if intended for a hard lens wearer) a wetting agent. If they are in a multi-dose presentation, these drops will contain a suitable preservative. As comfort drops are for 'in use', that is to be applied to the eye while the lens is being worn, the requirement for preservative concentration is the same as for wetting solutions, i.e. they should be kept as low as possible.

Sibley and Lauck (1974) reviewed the usefulness of comfort drops and concluded that their use reduced patient problems and increased comfort.

For hard lenses there are a number of formulations containing polyvinyl alcohol and benzalkonium chloride. The latter should not be of a level greater than 0.004% w/v for the reasons mentioned above under wetting solutions.

For soft lenses, the problem of preservative concentration in the lens reduces the available options. For these lenses, single dose un-preserved saline can be used (but not direct from a pressurized container).

Most artificial tear formulations are isotonic, but Sher and Breslin (1983) found that patients with mild keratoconjunctivitis preferred hypotonic drops.

Protein remover tablets (Figure 12.4)

Protein remover tablets, although originally introduced for use with soft lenses, have found application with gas permeable hard lenses for the removal of the protein film. They may also be used with PMMA lenses (Korb *et al.*, 1983).

A film of protein, mainly lysozyme (Hosaka *et al.*, 1983), but with amounts of albumin and globulin, from the tears can build up on lenses and be difficult to remove with the normal surfactants found in the usual daily cleaning solutions. In order to facilitate the removal of this form of contamination, lenses require periodic treatment with a proteolytic enzyme. Proteins are macromolecules composed of chains of amino acids which are linked by peptide bonds. Proteolytic enzymes hydrolyse these bonds, either at the end of the molecule, stripping off units of amino acids each time, or by breaking the protein into smaller and smaller

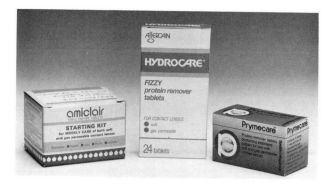

Figure 12.4 Protein remover tablets

multi-amino acid segments. The former are called exopeptidases and the latter endopeptidases. Like all enzymes the proteolytic enzymes have optimum working conditions, i.e. temperature and pH. Tonicity does not seem to be so important, as some tablets can be used in saline while others can be used in purified water. Another property which enzymes share with all proteins is the possibility of producing allergic reactions. Bernstein *et al.* (1984) reported a case of local anaphylaxis resulting from the use of papain; a similar case was reported by Santucci, Cristaudo and Piccardo (1985).

Papain is one of the enzymes routinely used in protein remover tablets. Papain is a thermostable endopeptidase found in the paw-paw fruit. Other enzymes have also been used. For example, Amiclair tablets contains three enzymes, two proteases and a lipase.

It has been suggested that protein remover tablets are unnecessary when hydrogen peroxide solutions are used on soft lenses because this agent causes a swelling followed by a shrinkage upon neutralization and this change in size is thought to dislodge the surface contamination. However, when chemical disinfection and enzymatic cleaning was compared with oxidative disinfection alone (Lasswell *et al.*, 1986), the lenses treated by the former method were significantly better than those treated by the latter.

The use of protein removing tablets is not an alternative to daily cleaners, as the two agents are complementary. Lenses treated with either cleaner were contaminated more than those treated with both (Fowler and Allansmith, 1981).

References

Ahearn, D. G., Penley, C. A. and Wilson, L. A. (1986) Growth and survival of *Serratia marcescens* in hard contact lens wetting solutions. *Contact Lens Association Ophthalmic Journal*, **10/2**, 172–174

Armstrong, J. R., Cohen, K. C. and McCarthy, L. R. (1984) *Haemophilus influenzae* corneal ulcer in a therapeutic contact lens wearer. *Br. J. Ophthalmol.*, **68**, 188–191

Barry, D. J. and Ruben, M. (1978) Contact lens injuries. An analysis of 217 consecutive patients presenting to Moorfields casualty department. *Contact Lens J.*, **9**, 6–10

Bernstein, D. I., Gallagher, J. S., Grad, M. and Bernstein, I. L. (1984) Local ocular anaphylaxis to papain enzyme contained in a contact lens cleaning solution. *J. Allerg. Clin. Immunol.*, **74**, 258–260

Bernstein, H. N. (1973) Fungal growth into a bionite hydrophilic contact lens. *Ann. Ophthalmol.*, March, 317–322

Broich, J. R., Weiss, L., and Rapp, J. (1980) Isolation and identification of biologically active contaminants from soft contact lenses. *Invest. Ophthalmol. Vis. Sci.*, **19/11**, 1328–1335

Brooks, A. M. V., Lazarus, M. G. and Weiner, J. M. (1984) Soft contact lens contamination by *Alternaria alternata*. *Med. J. Aust.*, **2**, 490–491

Busschaert, S. C., Good, R. C. and Szabocsik, A. (1978) Evaluation of thermal disinfection procedures for hydrophilic contact lenses. *Appl. Environ. Microbiol.*, **35/3**, 618–621

Butrus, S. I. and Klotz, S. A. (1986) Blocking Candida adherence to contact lenses. *Curr. Eye Res.*, **5/10**, 745–750

Churner, R. and Cunningham, R. D. (1983) Fungal contaminated soft contact lenses. *Ann. Ophthalmol.*, **15/8**, 724–727

Duran, J. A., Refojo, M. F., Gipson, I. K. and Kenyon, K. R. (1987) Pseudomonas attachment to new hydrogel contact lenses. *Arch. Ophthalmol.*, **105**, 106–108

Editorial (1985) Contact lens solution uses trimethroprim. *Ophthalmol. Times*, **10**, 183

Filippi, J. A., Pfister, R. M., and Hill, R. M. (1973) Penetration of hydrophilic contact lenses by *Aspergillus Fumagatus*. *Am. J. Optom.*, **50/7**, 553–557

Fowler, S. A. and Allansmith, M. R. (1981) The effect of cleaning soft contact lenses. *Arch. Ophthalmol.*, **99**, 1382–1386

Fowler, S. A., Korb, D R., Finnemore, V. M. and Allansmith, M. R. (1985) Deposits on soft contact lenses of various water contents. *The Contact Lens Association Ophthalmic Journal*, **11/2**, 124–127

Sarner, L. F. (1982) A comparison of some heat disinfection methods for soft contact lenses. *Aust. J. Optom.*, **65/1**, 32–34

Hesse, R. J., Kneisser, G., Fukushima, A. and Yamaguchi, T. (1982) Soft contact lens cleaning. A scanning electron microscope study. *Contact and Intraocular Lens Medical Journal*, **8**, 23–28

Hosaka, S. *et al.* (1983) Analysis of deposits on high-content contact lenses. *J. Biomed. Mater. Res.*, **17**, 261–274

Høvding, G. (1981) The conjunctival and contact lens bacterial flora during lens wear. *Acta Ophthalmol.*, **59**, 387–401

Jenkins, C., and Phillips, A. J. (1986) How sterile is preserved saline? *Clin. Exp. Optom.*, **69/4**, 131

Janoff, L. E. (1979) The effective disinfection of soft-contact lenses using hydrogen perioxide. *Optician*, **August 3**, 24–30

Josse, E. (1984) Corneal abscesses from soft contact lenses. *Nursing Times*, **26**, 3–4

Kempster, A. J. (1984) The effect of soft contact lens soaking solutions on corneal thickness. *J. Contact Lens Assoc.*, **7/3**, 137–142

Knopf, H. L. S. (1984) Reaction to hydrogen peroxide in a contact lens wearer. *Arch. Ophthalmol.*, **97/6**, 796

Korb, D. R., Greiner, J. V., Finnemore, M. and Allansmith, M. R. (1983) Treatment of contact lenses with papain. *Arch. Ophthalomol.*, **101**, 48–50

Kreis, F. (1972) La sterilisation des lentilles souples hydrophiles. *Arch. Ophthalmol.*, Paris, **32**, 825–829

Lasswell, L., Tarantino, N., Kono, D., Frank, J. and Nelson, N. E. (1986) Chemical vs oxidative disinfection of high water content extended wear lenses. *Int. Eyecare*, **2/12**, 615–619

Liubinas, J., Swenson, G. and Carney, L. G. (1987) Thermal disinfection of contact lenses. *Clin. Exp. Optom.*, **70**, 8–14

Mondino, B. J. and Groden, L. R. (1980) Conjunctival hyperemia and corneal infiltration with chemically disinfected soft contact lenses. *Arch. Ophthalmol.*, **98**, 1767–1770

Moore, M., McCulley, J., Kaufman, H. and Robin, J. (1980) Radial keratoneuritis as a presenting sign in Ancathomoeba keratitis. *Ophthalmologica*, **93**, 1310

Moore, R. A., Satterberg, L. B., Weiss, S. and Shively, C. D. (1986) Novel temperature dependent model for examining soilant deposition deterrant action. 1 Preserved thermal disinfecting solutions. *Contacto*, **March**, 23–30

Norton, D. A., Davies, D. J. S., Richard, N. E., Meakin, B. J. and Keall, A. (1974) The antimicrobial efficiencies of contact lens solutions. *J. Pharm. Pharmacol.*, **26**, 841–846

Parment, P., Ronnerstam, R. and Walder, M. (1986) Persistance of *Serratia marcescens, S. liquefaciens* and *E. coli* in solutions for contact lenses. *Acta Ophthalmol.*, **64/4**, 456–462

Penley, C. A., Llabres, C., Wilson, L. A. and Ahearn, D. G. (1985) Efficacy of hydrogen peroxide disinfection system for soft contact lenses contaminated with fungi. *Contact Lens Association Ophthalmic Journal*, **11/1**, 65–68

Richardson, N. E., Davies, D. J. G., Meakin, B. J. and Norton, D. A. (1977) Loss of antibacterial preservatives from contact lens solutions during storage. *J. Pharm. Pharmacol.*, **29**, 717–722

Richardson, N. E., Gee, H. J. and Meakin, B. J. (1980) The compatibility of benzalkonium chloride with a CAB lens material. *J. Br. Contact Lens Assoc.*, **3**, 120–124

Rohrer, M. D., Terry, H. A., Bulard, R. A., Graves, D. C. and Taylor, E. M. (1986) Microwave sterilisation of hydrophilic contact lenses. *Am. J. Ophthalmol.*, **101**, 49–51

Rosenthal, P., Chou, M. H., Salamore, J. C. and Israel, S. C. (1986) Quantitative analysis of chlorhexidine gluconate and benzalkonium chloride adsorption on silicone/acrylate polymers. *Contact Lens Association Ophthalmic Journal*, **12**, 43–50

Santucci, B., Cristando, J. and Piccardo, A. (1985) Contact urticaria from papain in a soft lens solution. *Contact Dermatitis*, **12/4**, 233–237

Shaw, E. I. (1980) Allergies induced by contact lens solutions. *Contact Lens Med. J.*, **6**, 273–277

Sher, J. and Breslin, C. W. (1983) Tolerance of wetting agents in contact lens patients with keratitis sicca. *Am. J. Ophthalmol.*, **96/3**, 381–382

Sibley, M. J. and Lauck, D. E. (1974) Contact lens conditioners. New solutions for old problems. *Contact Lens J.*, **8/2**, 10–12

Stone, R. P., Braun, A., Kreutzer, P. and Smith, L. (1984) A new concept in heat disinfection. *Contact Lens J.*, **12**, 5–9

Tragakis, M. P., Brown, S. I. and Pearce, D. B. (1973) Bacteriologic studies of contamination associated with soft contact lenses. *Am. J. Ophthalmol.*, **75/3**, 496–499

Walters, K. A., Gee, H. J. and Meakin, B. J. (1983) The interaction of benzalkonium chloride with Boston contact lens material. Part I Basic interaction studies. *J. Br. Contact Lens Assoc.*, **6**, 42–52

Wardlow, J. C. and Sarver, M. D. (1986) Discolouration of hydrogel contact lenses under standard care regimens. *Am. J. Optom. Physiol. Opt.*, **63/6**, 403–408

Weissman, B. A., Mondino, B. J., Pettit, T. H. and Hofbauer, J. D. (1984) Corneal ulcers associated with extended wear soft contact lenses. *Am. J. Ophthalmol.*, **97**, 476–481

Wilson, L. A., McNatt, J. and Reitschel, R. (1981) Delayed hypersensitivity to thimerosal in soft contact lens wearers. *Transact. Ophthalmol. Soc. UK*, **102**, 3–6

Wong, M. P., Dziabo, A. J. and Kirai, R. M. (1986) Adsorption of benzalkonium chloride by RGP lenses. *Contact Lens Forum*, **May**, 25–32

Wright, P. and Mackie, I. (1982) Preservative-related problems in soft contact lens wearers. *Trans. Ophthal. Soc. UK.*, **102**, 3–6

Chapter 13

Ocular first aid

As a professional involved in health care who is easily accessible to the public, the optometrist will from time to time be confronted by a variety of emergency situations, both ocular and general. The term 'First Aid' is very apt and it is important that procedures should be kept simple and to a minimum.

It is worth stating the underlying principles of first aid which should govern the optometrist's action in an emergency situation.

(1) Separate the patient from the cause of the trauma
If there is an external cause, this should whenever possible be removed from the patient (e.g. a foreign body) or the patient from it. The important words are 'whenever possible' as there are situations in which this aim cannot be achieved or to do so would exacerbate the patient's condition. For example, intraocular and embedded foreign bodies should be left for ophthalmological removal. On the other hand, superficial foreign bodies should be removed if possible and the elimination of chemical splashes on the eye must not be delayed, as in both cases damage will continue to develop while they are in contact with the eye.

(2) Relieve the patient's distress and make him as comfortable as possible
Much of this can be achieved by reassurance from the optometrist. In many simple emergency cases, the patient will believe that he is more injured than he really is, so a confident approach will do much to dispel these fears.

The commendable desire to relieve the patient's symptoms should not, however, lead to indiscriminate use of local anaesthetics.

(3) Seek medical assistance as soon as possible.
The implementation of first aid procedures should not delay the patient's referral for medical assistance.

Of course, the optometrist will be confronted by general emergencies as well as ocular ones. His patients are not immune from such conditions such as epistaxis (nosebleed), syncope (fainting) and heart attacks. A short course in general first aid techniques would thus be useful for the optometrist to attend. In this chapter only ocular emergencies will be covered.

Whatever the emergency, traumatic or medical, serious or trivial, proper records must be kept of each case encountered and should include the following details.

(1) Name and address of patient requesting attention.
(2) Date of treatment.

(3) Brief history and nature of injury, including the time it occurred.

(4) Unaided vision (and visual acuity with spectacles, if worn, of affected eye, taken at earliest suitable opportunity (usually after treatment, before bandaging).

(5) The treatment administered, including any drugs used, and advice given.

(6) In all except minor cases the patient must be referred with a brief note, covering the details listed above, to his own doctor, or a hospital eye department, as appropriate. If the latter, as when specialized ophthalmological treatment is necessitated (for example, in the case of a perforating foreign body or severe chemical burn) a further report must be sent the same day to the patient's own general medical practitioner, with full details of the case, including the procedure followed.

Equipment

A well equipped optometric practice will, as a matter of course, contain most of the instruments and drugs to cope with first aid requirements, such as:

Ophthalmoscope;
Slit-lamp microscope;
Adjustable illumination;
Examination chair.

In addition to the above, the following will be useful:

Glass rods for everting the upper lids;
Cotton wool buds;
Small forceps;
Sterile cotton wool balls.

Careful clinical judgement is necessary in deciding as to whether or not an injured eye should be bandaged. Alternatively, the sterile cotton wool/gauze eyepad may be kept in place with a 2 inch wide (5.1 cm) strip of zinc oxide adhesive plaster extending diagonally from inner forehead to cheek. As Havener (1978) rightly emphasizes, 'patching of an eye promotes the growth of any micro-organisms that may happen to be in this conjunctival sac'. After instillation of an anti-infective preparation only the more seriously injured or painful eyes should be patched, and then only for the shortest period appropriate for that particular case. Sometimes an eyepad is necessitated for superficial corneal abrasions to prevent the pain elicited by movements of the lid across the denuded area. Three hourly instillation of antibacterial eyedrops must be continued until epithelial healing and accompanying absence of discomfort allow discontinuation of drugs and removal of the eyepad.

In addition to the above, certain pharmaceutical agents will be required:

(1) Local anaesthetics, e.g. benoxinate, amethocaine.
(2) Fluorescein in some form, e.g. single use eyedrops or paper strips.
(3) Antibacterial agents, e.g. sulfacetamide, framycetin.
(4) Emollient drops, e.g. castor oil, liquid paraffin.
(5) Normal saline for irrigation.

In most cases where irrigation is required, running water is probably the best medium as it is unlikely that sufficient volume of normal saline will be stocked.

Specific antidotes to cope with chemical injuries to the eye are not worth keeping, as dilution by irrigation is probably the best method.

Common ocular emergencies

The common ocular emergencies are:

Superficial foreign body;
Intraocular foreign body;
Blow with a blunt instrument;
Chemical burns;
Thermal burns;
Exposure keratitis;
Acute closed angle glaucoma.

Superficial foreign body

This is the most common ocular emergency that is likely to be encountered and the stages of dealing with it are as follows:

History;
Local anaesthetic (if necessary);
Location;
Removal;
Staining;
Visual acuity assessment;
Prophylaxis;
Records;
Corneal sensitivity.

History
It is very important to ascertain the circumstances in which the foreign body came in contact with the eye because in every case of superficial foreign body there is always a possibility of an intraocular foreign body and the latter must be positively discounted rather than assumed to be absent. Foreign bodies which result from any kind of explosion, however mild, or are thrown up by moving machinery can sometimes penetrate the eye rather than remaining on the surface.

Local anaesthetic
Foreign bodies cause discomfort and this in turn leads to reflex tearing and blepharospasm. The optometrist is thus confronted by an eye which is closed and difficult to open. Under these circumstances a local anaesthetic can be used to facilitate examination and to alleviate the patient's discomfort. Any of the usual topical anaesthetics are suitable—amethocaine, benoxinate, proxymetacaine or lignocaine.

The use of local anaesthetic is only justified prior to the removal of a foreign body. Problems only arise when local anaesthetics are used to relieve the discomfort which may remain after the foreign body has been removed. Attention has been drawn to the dangers of the over-use of local anaesthetic in the chapter on these agents.

Location
The foreign body should be located if possible. It is not unknown for the reflex tearing to dislodge the object and do the optometrist's job for him. If the foreign body is not immediately visible on inspection it is probably trapped under the upper lid, necessitating eversion of the lid or even double eversion in order to locate it.

Removal
Providing that it is not embedded, the object can be removed, either with a cotton bud or by irrigation with eye lotion or running water. If the particle is embedded, the patient should be immediately referred to the hospital accident and emergency department for medical treatment.

Staining
After removal of the foreign body, staining with fluorescein should be carried out in order to assess the extent of any disturbance to the corneal epithelium. This information will enable the optometrist to decide whether to refer the patient to his general practitioner or whether to ask the patient to return on a subsequent visit for re-examination.

Visual acuity assessment
The patient's visual acuity, both distance and near should be included in the records kept of the incident.

Prophylaxis
In order to supplement the natural antibacterial action of tears, an antimicrobial such as sulfacetamide or framycetin may be instilled. It is debatable how much protection one drop will give, considering the turnover rate of the tear film when the eye is inflamed. It will do no harm providing that it does not lead the practitioner into a false sense of security.

Records
As stated above, full and accurate records are essential and the point is reinforced here because it may be thought that a trivial event such as a foreign body which is easily removed does not warrant the writing up of records. It is just this kind of case which could lead to problems in the future if full details of the history, drugs used, procedures carried out and the results of visual acuity measurement and corneal examination cannot be recalled.

Corneal sensitivity
Finally, if a local anaesthetic has been used, it is important to check that sensitivity has returned to the eye. It would be ironic to say the least if the patient, having had a foreign body removed, were sent out onto the street in a condition in which he would be unaware of the entry of another one.

Intraocular foreign body

Whereas a superficial foreign body may be considered as a relatively trivial problem, an intraocular foreign body is a very serious event which always requires medical attention. Admittedly the eye will tolerate pieces of glass and plastic (for example intraocular lenses) relatively well compared with metals such as copper or iron or organic materials (vegetable or animal), but there is always the threat of infection either from the foreign body itself or by opportunistic organisms gaining access through the entry wound.

There is little an optometrist can do for a patient with an intraocular foreign body other than to refer the patient for medical treatment. His great service to the patient is in the discovery of such an invasion in doubtful cases. The foreign body may be visible by ophthalmoscopic examination or the entry wound may be visible as a rivulet of aqueous. The entry wound may, however, not be visible and the only indication of an intraocular foreign body will be the history. Any suspect case must be referred.

Blow with a blunt instrument

Although the bony orbit provides a good protection against damage, sometimes objects, e.g. squash balls, may penetrate this protection and impact on the eye. Even larger objects can exert such a force to the surrounding tissue as to cause fractures and ocular damage.

The result of a blow can be alarming, with marked swelling and bruising. These will normally resolve spontaneously but there are serious sequelae to blows, e.g.

Detached retina;
Cataract or lens subluxation;
Commotio retinae;
Traumatic macular degeneration;
Blowout fracture;
Iris damage (iridodialysis);
Haemorrhage.

It is important after such an injury that careful ophthalmoscopy is carried out followed by an examination of ocular motility and eye position. If a blowout fracture has occurred one or more extraocular muscles may become trapped, impeding eye movements, and herniation of orbital contents may result in enophthalmos. It is essential that visual acuity is also measured and recorded.

If there is any doubt about the integrity of the eye or other orbital structures, the patient must be referred.

Chemical burns

Both strong acids and strong alkalis can cause damage but the latter are far more harmful to ocular tissues. Chemical splashes can occur in industry but the provision of safety glasses has reduced their occurrence. Potentially harmful substances can also be found in the home and the use of ammonia in 'mugging' constitutes another source of chemical splashes in the eye.

Whether acid or alkali, dilution is the best method of neutralization, preferably using running water. Specific antidotes are necessary and are unlikely to be kept in sufficient quantities to be effective. Irrigation should be maintained for about 20 minutes before referring the patient for medical attention.

Thermal burns

Thermal burns usually involve the face as well as the eye and the patient will probably be in great discomfort. There is no specific treatment and the patient should be referred for medical care as soon as possible.

Exposure keratitis

If the cornea is exposed to short wavelength ultraviolet light for a certain time, it develops a form of keratitis, which normally occurs as snow blindness or arc eye (welder's flash). The patient will complain of a dry, gritty feeling. Arc eye drops, containing adrenaline (a vasoconstrictor) and zinc sulphate (an astringent) have been used in the past, but these are not necessary as the condition is self-resolving.

Acute closed angle glaucoma

This condition can arise spontaneously or as a result of the injudicious use of a mydriatic in an eye with a shallow anterior chamber. Incidence from both causes is very rare but the optometrist must be aware of the signs and symptoms in order to recognize this medical emergency. The patient experiences intense pain which may be severe enough to induce vomiting. The conjunctival blood vessels are dilated, giving the appearance to the inexperienced observer of conjunctivitis. The cornea loses transparency slightly because the high intraocular pressure causes it to imbibe water and swell, which the patient may report as seeing haloes around lights. Through the hazy cornea the pupil can be seen, often mid-dilated (Chandler, 1952) and probably non-circular. The pupil will not constrict to light, accommodation or to the action of miotics. The intraocular pressure, whether measured with a tonometer or assessed digitally, is very high. The situation is an emergency one, but not requiring panic measures. Providing the intraocular pressure is reduced over the ensuing few hours, there should be no long lasting damage.

Although the iris will not react to miotics because of ischaemia, one should still be administered. When the pressure is reduced by systemic methods, it will be present in the aqueous ready to exert its action. A drop of 2% pilocarpine eyedrops should be given to both eyes and repeated at 10 minute intervals (Norden, 1978). There are several first aid methods of trying to reduce the pressure systemically and the decision to use one of these or not will depend on the proximity and availability of expert medical help. The use of glycerol (glycerine) has been recommended as an osmotic agent which can be given orally in orange juice in order to reduce the intraocular pressure sufficiently to allow the miotic to act. About 250 ml of glycerol has been suggested as the amount required for a 70 kg adult (Norden, 1978), but this may not be acceptable to the patient and 100 ml may be more appropriate. If the patient is diabetic, it may be advisable to omit this part of the treatment. In any case, the patient should be referred as soon as possible to an accident and emergency department.

References

Chandler, C (1952) Narrow-angle glaucoma. *Arch. Ophthmol.*, **47**, 695–716
Norden, L. C. (1978) Adverse reactions to topical autonomic agents. *J.A.O.A.*, **48/1**, 75–80

Chapter 14

Legal aspects

The use of drugs by optometrists, in the United Kingdom, is subject to control and regulation by Acts of Parliament in the same manner as the use of drugs by other health professionals or by patients. Much of the sale and supply of drugs is covered by the Medicines Act 1968, which is set out in eight parts and deals not only with sale and supply but also with the licensing of medicinal products, their manufacture or import and other matters such as advertising.

Part I   —Administration of the Act and setting up of Medicines Commission.
Part II   —Licensing
            Manufacture
            Product licenses
            Import and export
            Clinical trial
Part III —Sale and supply (see below)
Part IV —Pharmacies
Part V   —Containers, labelling
Part VI —Promotion and advertising
Part VII —Publications, e.g. *British Pharmacopoeia*
Part VIII—Miscellaneous provisions

A medicinal product is a product intended for one or more of the following purposes:

treating medical conditions;
preventing medical conditions;
diagnosing medical conditions;
contraception;
otherwise modifying the physiological state of the body.

In addition, orders may be made to include products and devices not falling into one of the groups above. For example, an order made in 1976 brought contact lenses and contact lens solutions under some of the provisions of the Medicines Act.

Sale and supply of medicinal products is covered by Part III of the Act which categorizes products into three groups:

General Sale List;
Pharmacy Medicines;
Prescription Only Medicines.

General Sale List (GSL)—section 51

The medicines which are considered to be sufficiently safe that they can be supplied to the general public without supervision of a pharmacist are incorporated into a list of medicines called the General Sale List (S.I. 1980/1922). This list is very detailed and can, for instance, limit the quantity supplied a container. For example, 25 aspirin tablets are a General Sale List medicine but a bottle of 100 such tablets are excluded from the list and become a pharmacy medicine. The list is constantly being updated and amended. Any retailer may sell a GSL medicine providing that he has lockable permanent premises. An optometric practice will certainly satisfy this criterion.

Eye drops and eye ointments are specifically excluded from the General Sale List, whether for human or animal use, irrespective of the drug they contain.

Pharmacy Medicines (P)—section 52

Pharmacy medicines are only available to the general public from a person, lawfully conducting the business of a retail pharmacy, and the sale must be under the supervision of a registered pharmacist. Whereas there are legal lists of GSL and POM medicines, there is no legal list of Pharmacy medicines. Optometrists may supply any pharmacy medicine which is an eye drop or an eye ointment, providing that the supply is (a) in line with his professional practice and is (b) in an emergency. This ability to supply P drugs is due to an amendment order made in 1978 (SI 1978/988).

Prescription Only Medicines (POM)—section 58

As its name suggests, these products are only available to the public on the prescription of a doctor, dentist, or veterinary surgeon. The Prescription Only Medicine List (SI 1983/1212) is very detailed. For many agents there are exemptions from the requirements for a prescription if a maximum dose is specified or if the drug is presented in a particular form. A number of products are exempted, becoming pharmacy medicines if they are intended for external use, providing the external use is not ophthalmic. Eye drops and eye ointments of such compounds remain POM products.

Many of the mydriatics/cycloplegics, miotics, local anaesthetics and antimicrobial agents which the optometrist may wish to use are POM drugs. In order that he may have access to these drugs, specific exemptions are made for registered optometrists. One exemption allows the optometrist to supply the patient directly or via a signed order to the pharmacist, certain medicinal products, e.g. atropine, pilocarpine or sulfacetamide. The direct sale or supply must satisfy the same restrictions as for pharmacy medicines, namely that it must be in the course of the optometrist's professional practice and be in an emergency.

There is another group of drugs which the optometrist may obtain for use in his practice but may not supply to his patients under any circumstances, for example local anaesthetics.

The following is a list of drugs which the optometrist may under the conditions stated above supply to his patient as well as using them in practice.

Atropine sulphate
Bethanecol chloride
Carbachol
Cyclopentolate hydrochloride
Homatropine hydrobromide
Hyoscine hydrobromide
Mafenide
Naphazoline hydrochloride or nitrate
Neostigmine methylsulphate
Physostigmine sulphate or salicylate
Pilocarpine nitrate or hydrochloride
Sulphacetamide sodium
Sulphafurazole
Tropicamide
Any P medicine which is an eye drop or eye ointment

The list of drugs covered by this regulation was initially much longer and included such drugs as ecothiopate, but it was amended in 1978 (SI 1978/987) and is currently incorporated in SI 1983/1212.

The following may only be used by the optometrist in his practice:

Amethocaine hydrochloride
Benoxinate hydrochloride (oxybuprocaine hydrochloride)
Framycetin sulphate
Lignocaine hydrochloride
Oxyphenbutazone
Proxymetacaine hydrochloride
Thymoxamine hydrochloride

This particular list of drugs is not included in the Prescription Only Medicines list, but is the subject of a miscellaneous order provision originally made in 1977 (SI 1977/2132) and subsequently modified in 1978 (SI 1978/989) and currently incorporated in SI 1980/1923. The modifications removed some obscure local anaesthetics and added framycetin.

Sale and supply of contact lens solutions

Contact lens solutions are included in the Medicines Act 1968 by virtue of an order made in 1976. As well as requiring the manufacture and marketing of solutions to be subject to licenses, this legislation can also impose further restrictions as to the sale and supply of solutions.

Unfortunately, contact lens solutions do not fall easily into the normal classification of GSL, P, or POM. Clearly it would be ludicrous for solutions to be subject to the requirements of the Prescription Only Medicines List, but there is a need to restrict sales to outlets at which the patient may receive advice should they request it. Making the product a Pharmacy medicine would only allow the optometrist to supply solutions 'in an emergency'. As can be seen, contact lens solutions do not fit into any of the established categories. They are restricted to sales by registered pharmacists and opticians by mutual agreement between the manufacturers and the regulatory authorities. This restriction only applies to contact lens solutions. Contact lens cases are outside this rule.

Optometrist's formulary

The following is a list of common drugs and preparations that are available for use by the optometrist. The normal volume of a container for eye drops is 10 ml and the weight of a tube of eye ointment is 4 g. Unit dose preparations are usually packed in boxes of 20. When the volumes of branded preparations vary from the above they will be stated.

Mydriatics and cycloplegics

Atropine sulphate available as
    1% w/v drops
    1% w/w ointment
  Branded preparations
    Isopto atropine 1% w/v—5 ml
    (contains a viscolizer)
  Unit dose preparations
    Minims—1% w/v
    Opulets—1% w/v
Cyclopentolate hydrochloride available as
    0.5% w/v drops
    1.0% w/v drops
  Branded preparations
    Mydrilate 0.5% w/v—5 ml
    Mydrilate 1.0% w/v—5 ml
  Unit dose preparations
    Minims—0.5% w/v
    Minims—1.0% w/v
    Opulets—1.0% w/v
Homatropine hydrobromide available as
    1.0% w/v drops
    2.0% w/v drops
  Unit dose preparations
    Minims—2.0% w/v
Hyoscine hydrobromide available as
    0.2% w/v drops
Lachesine chloride available as
    1.0% w/v drops
Phenylephrine hydrochloride available as
    2.5% w/v drops
    10.0% w/v drops
  Unit dose preparations
    Minims—2.5% w/v
    Minims—10.0% w/v

Tropicamide available as
    0.5% w/v drops
    1.0% w/v drops
  Branded preparations
    Mydriacyl—0.5% w/v—5 ml
    Mydriacyl—1.0% w/v—5 ml
  Unit dose preparations
    Minims—0.5% w/v
    Minims—1.0% w/v

Miotics

Carbachol available as
    3% w/v drops
  Branded preparations
    Isopto carbachol 3%
    (contains a viscolizer)
Physostigmine sulphate available as
    0.25% w/v—drops
    0.5% w/v—drops
Pilocarpine hydrochloride (or nitrate) available as
    0.5% w/v drops
    1.0% w/v drops
    2.0% w/v drops
    3.0% w/v drops
    4.0% w/v drops
  Branded preparations
    Isopto carpine 0.5% w/v
    Isopto carpine 1.0% w/v
    Isopto carpine 2.0% w/v
    Isopto carpine 3.0% w/v
    Isopto carpine 4.0% w/v
    (all viscolized preparations)
    Sno pilo 1.0% w/v
    Sno pilo 2.0% w/v
    Sno pilo 4.0% w/v
    (all viscolized preparations)
  Unit dose preparations
    Minims 1.0% w/v
    Minims 2.0% w/v
    Minims 4.0% w/v
    Opulets 1.0% w.v
    Opulets 2.0% w/v
    Opulets 4.0% w/v
Physostigmine and pilocarpine available as
    Physostigmine 0.25% and pilocarpine 2%
    Physostigmine 0.25% and pilocarpine 4%
    Physostigmine 0.50% and pilocarpine 4%

Thymoxamine hydrochloride available as
  0.5% w/v drops
  Unit dose preparations
    Minims 0.5% w/v

Local anaesthetics

Amethocaine hydrochloride available as
  0.5% w/v drops
  1.0% w/v drops
  Unit dose preparations
    Minims 0.5% w/v
    Minims 1.0% w/v
Benoxinate hydrochloride available as
  0.4% w/v drops
  Unit dose preparations
    Minims 0.4% w/v
    Opulets 0.4% w/v
Lignocaine hydrochloride available as
  Unit dose preparation
    Lignocaine hydrochloride 4% w/v with
    Fluorescein sodium 0.25% w/v
Proxymetacaine hydrochloride available as
  0.5% w/v drops
  Branded preparation
    Ophthaine 0.5% w/v—15 ml

Stains

Fluorescein sodium available as
  1% w/v drops
  Unit dose preparations
    Fluorets (paper strips containing 1 mg)
    Minims 1% w/v
    Minims 2% w/v
    Opulets 1% w/v
Rose bengal available as
  1% w/v drops
  Unit dose preparation
    Minims 1% w/v

Antimicrobials

Framycetin sulphate available as
  0.5% w/v drops
  0.5% w/w ointment

Branded preparations
    Framygen 0.5% w/v drops—5 ml
    Framygen 0.5% w/w ointment—3.5 g
    Soframycin 0.5% w/v drops—8 ml
    Soframycin 0.5% w/w ointment—5 g
Propamidine isethionate available as
  Branded preparation
    Brolene—0.1% w/v drops
Sulphacetamide sodium available as
    10% w/v drops
    30% w/v drops
    2.5% w/w ointment
    6.0% w/w ointment
    10.0% w/w ointment
  Branded preparations
    Albucid 10% w/v drops
    Albucid 20% w/v drops
    Albucid 30% w/v drops
    Albucid 2.5% w/w eye ointment
    Albucid 6.0% w/w eye ointment
    Albucid 10.0% w/w eye ointment
    Ocusol 5% w/v drops
    (with 0.1% w/v zinc sulphate)
  Unit dose preparations
    Minims 10% w/v
N.B. There are no preparations of mafenide or sulphafurazole available on the UK
market.

Artificial tears and irrigating solutions

Castor oil available as
  Unit dose preparation
    Minims 100%
Hypromellose available as
    0.3% w/v drops
  Branded preparations
    Isopto alkaline 1% w/v drops
    Isopto plain 0.5% w/v drops
    Tears naturale 0.3% w/v drops
    (with dextran)
Liquid paraffin available as
  Branded preparation
    Lacri-lube ointment—3.5 g
Polyvinyl alcohol available as
  Branded preparations
    Hypotears—1% w/v drops
    (with macrogol)
    Liquifilm tears—1.4% w/v drops—15 ml
    Sno tears—1.4% w/v drops

Sodium chloride available as
   0.9% w/v drops
   Unit dose preparations
      Minims—0.9% w/v
      Opulets—0.9% w/v

Miscellaneous preparations

Antazoline sulphate available as
   Branded preparations
      Otrivine- Antistine 0.5% w/v drops
      (with xylometazoline 0.05% w/v)
      Vasocon- A 0.5% w/v drops
      (with naphazoline 0.05% w/v)
Oxyphenbutazone available as
   Branded product
      Tanderil eye ointment 10% w/w—5 g

Acts of Parliament and statutory instruments

Medicines Act 1968, chapter 67.
The Medicines (General Sale List) Order 1984/769.
The Medicines (Pharmacy and General Sale—Exemptions) Amendment Order 1980/1924.
The Medicines (Products Other than Veterinary Drugs) (Prescription Only Order) 1983/1212.
The Medicines (Sale or Supply) (Miscellaneous Provisions) Amendment Regulations 1978/989.

Chapter 15

Drugs used in ophthalmology—anti-infectives

Products containing antimicrobial substances are the most commonly prescribed medications. Although the title refers to drugs used in ophthalmology, it is the general medical practitioner who sees and treats most of the infections of the anterior eye. Antimicrobial substances are also used for treating more serious infections, and they can be instilled prophylactically before surgery.

Infections can be caused by a variety of micro-organisms, bacteria, fungi or viruses and the appropriate anti-infective must be used in their treatment.

Anti-infective agents are not drugs in the normal sense of the word because their required effect is on the invading organism rather than the host; the title 'Chemotherapeutic Agents' is therefore more appropriate. However, in all other respects such as routes of administration, absorption and excretion, effective dosage and side-effects, the same problems apply to chemotherapeutic agents as those which apply to drugs.

Routes of administration

The route chosen for administration will depend on the site and severity of the infection. As well as the topical application of anti-infectives by the use of eye ointments and eye drops, the medical practitioner may also administer these agents:

(a) orally—in the form of tablets or mixtures;
(b) by injection—intracamerally, intravitreally;
(c) by incorporation into infusion liquids.

Not all anti-infectives will be suitable for all routes. The topical route is only suitable if the agent can be absorbed by the corneal epithelium and so compounds which are very water soluble and poorly fat soluble will not be suitable for this route. This is one of the reasons why penicillin is not favoured as a topical antibiotic.

The success of the oral route will depend on the drug's ability to pass the permeability barriers of the eye, e.g. the blood/aqueous barrier.

Injection of antibiotics carries additional risks either from the physical trauma of the needle or the production of high local concentrations of potentially harmful substances.

Antibacterial agents

The following are the most commonly used antibacterial agents in ophthalmology: chloramphenicol, neomycin, gentamicin, polymixin, tetracyclines, penicillin, bacitracin, erythromycin and tobramycin.

Chloramphenicol

By far the most commonly used topical ophthalmic antibacterial agent, chloramphenicol is effective against a whole range of bacteria and other organisms such as chlamydiae, rickettsiae and spirochaetes. Of the bacteria against which it is effective, there are many ocular pathogens such as *Corynebacterium, E. coli, Haemophilus* and *Streptococci*. It has been recommended for the routine treatment of ophthalmia neonatorum (Pierce, Ward and Seal, 1982). Its effect against chlamydiae has led to its use in trachoma, although its usefulness for this condition is probably in the treatment of secondary infections which are responsible for many of the adverse effects of the infection. It is not effective, however, against most strains of *Pseudomonas aeruginosa*. The bacteriostatic action of chloramphenicol is due to the inhibition of protein synthesis by interaction with the bacterial ribosomes. It penetrates easily into the cell by a process of facilitated diffusion. Resistance to chloramphenicol is brought about by the production of inactivating enzymes.

One of the reasons for the popularity of chloramphenicol as an ophthalmic antibacterial is that it is rarely used systemically and thus there is little chance of cross resistance developing. In a study of 738 patients, only 6% of the organisms cultured were resistant to chloramphenicol. This resistance rate was lower than for any other of the antibiotics tested (Seal, Barrett and McGill, 1982), but much higher resistance rates, e.g. 30.9%, against chloramphenicol have been reported by Mahajan (1983).

The systemic use of chloramphenicol was stopped many years ago because of the incidence of aplastic anaemia producing agranulocytosis. From systemic treatment, the incidence is about 1 in 50 000 patients and from topical use, the incidence is much lower. Trope *et al.* (1979) failed to find systemic absorption after drops were administered every 2 hours for 5–7 days. Topical use can sometimes lead to irritation.

Apart from the potential to cause this rare blood dyscrasia, chloramphenicol is an excellent topical antibiotic. It is available as a 0.5% solution or a 1% eye ointment. Intramuscular injections have been recommended for the treatment of trachoma (Chastain and Newton, 1954). Chloramphenicol has a high lipid solubility and in a study on ovine eyes (Ismail and Morton, 1987) was found to be retained in the cornea at higher levels than the aqueous humour. Ointments gave consistently higher levels in both the cornea and aqueous humour. Solutions of chloramphenicol are not stable at room temperature and must be stored between 2 and 8°C.

Neomycin

Neomycin is one of a group of aminoglycoside antibiotics which include amikacin, streptomycin, tobramycin and gentamicin. All aminoglycosides are rapidly bacteriocidal and inhibit protein synthesis by combining with mRNA but this does not explain their rapidity of action.

Passage into the cells is dependent on electron transport, which in turn can be influenced by transmembrane potential. The transport of the antibacterial into the cell can be reduced by low pH and aerobic conditions. It will also be decreased by Ca^{2+} and Mg^{2+} ions and hyperosmolarity.

As the antibacterial enters the cell it increases the rate at which further amounts can pass in. This leads eventually to disruption of the cell membrane and rapid death of the cell. Resistance can be brought about by the production of enzymes or low affinity of the ribosomes.

Penicillin will aid the passage of aminoglycosides into the cell and thus these two antibacterials should be synergistic. In an experiment study on guinea pigs (Davis, Sarff and Hyndiuk, 1979) no additive or synergistic effect was found when penicillin was injected intramuscularly and an aminoglycoside was applied topically; however, the test organism was *Pseudomonas aeruginosa* and aminoglycosides were found to be the most effective treatment for keratitis produced by this organism.

Neomycin, like chloramphenicol, is favoured as a topical antimicrobial because of the relatively rare systemic use. Neomycin is not absorbed from the gut and is too toxic for parenteral administration. As a result, its use is restricted to either disinfecting the gut prior to surgery or as a topical preparation for skin or mucous membranes.

All aminoglycosides produce nephrotoxicity and ototoxicity but this is not known to occur from topical use. However, keratoconjunctivitis can develop as a result of hypersensitivity to neomycin after ophthalmic use.

Neomycin has a broad spectrum of activity but is not effective against *Pseudomonas aeruginosa*.

Although preparations of neomycin alone (drops or eye ointment) are used, neomycin is most often encountered along with steroids to produce antibiotic cover while treating inflammation.

Gentamicin

Gentamicin is another aminoglycoside antibiotic and has the same toxic effects as neomycin. It is one of the more effective agents in this group and will kill many strains of *Pseudomonas aeruginosa*. It is the treatment of choice for this organism (Seal, Barrett and McGill, 1982), although resistant strains of *Pseudomonas* have been found (Insler, Cavanagh and Wilson, 1985). Gentamicin is given by injection for serious systemic infections when the nature of the invading organism is not known, and therefore it should be kept for serious infections of the eye where other antibacterial agents are ineffective. Unfortunately there is a large number of topical gentamicin preparations and gentamicin-resistant *Pseudomonas* infections have occurred, probably because gentamicin has been used for the treatment of trivial infections such as conjunctivitis.

Absorption across the corneal epithelium is very poor. Hillman *et al.* (1979) found that after application of gentamicin by drops very little appeared in the aqueous humour. Subconjunctival injection produced effective corneal concentrations in 2 hours and these were maintained for 24 hours. If a deep infection of the eye occurs, it is best treated by a slow intravitreal injection. Michelson and Nozik (1979) investigated the use of an implantable osmotic minipump for the administration of gentamicin for the treatment of experimental endophthalmitis in rabbits. Reversible cellular oedema has been reported in the corneal endothelium following anterior chamber injection (Lavine, Binder and Wickham, 1979). Systemic injection will not give rise to sufficient ocular levels because of its poor ability to cross the blood/aqueous barrier. It is usually applied as a 0.3% solution but more concentrated solutions have been recommended for the treatment of bacterial corneal ulcers (Chadhuri and Godfrey, 1987). An intense dosing schedule has been suggested in order to achieve high initial levels (Glasser *et al.* 1985) in the cornea. Loading doses consisting of one drop every minute for 5 minutes produced significant levels in the cornea of rabbits.

Gentamicin is a very toxic compound and like other aminoglycosides can cause damage to the ears and kidneys. Both parts of the ears are affected and so ataxia due to vestibular damage and deafness from cochlear damage are the results of toxic doses.

Polymixin B

Polymixin shares many of the properties of gentamicin. It is effective against many strains of *Pseudomonas aeruginosa* and is recommended by some authors (Mahajan, 1983) as the best drug for the treatment of infections by this organism. It is poorly absorbed from the gut and passage is slow across the blood/aqueous or blood/brain barriers and the intact corneal epithelium. Kidney damage can result from its systemic use. Polymixin is used topically in combination with either bacitracin in ointment form or trimethoprim as drops.

Tetracyclines

Tetracyclines are a group of broad spectrum antibiotics which include chlortetracycline, demethylchlortetracycline, oxytetracycline, tetracycline and minocycline.

There is little to choose between them with the exception of minocycline, which has a broader spectrum and more specific indications. Although the rest of the members of the group are quite similar, cross resistance between them does not necessarily occur.

Tetracyclines are effective against Gram positive and Gram negative bacteria as well as spirochaetes, chlamydiae and other organisms, but *Pseudomonas* and *Proteus* are resistant to these agents.

Tetracyclines taken orally may cause stomach upsets (nausea, vomiting and diarrhoea) but are best known for their effect on bone and teeth in children. They permanently colour teeth yellow and slow bone growth, due to their ability to chelate calcium and magnesium. Adverse effects from topical application are rare due to the low dose of drug that the patient receives in one drop of solution compared with the systemic dose. If a drop of 1% tetracycline solution were to be applied four times a day, it would take 4 months for the equivalent of one oral dose to be administered.

Penetration across the intact cornea is poor and these compounds are best used for surface infections. Topical tetracycline is used in the treatment of trachoma (normally in ointment form) and is becoming the prophylactic of choice for ophthalmia neonatorum. Raucher and Newton (1983) recommend intramuscular penicillin and tetracyclin 1% ointment as a prophylactic agent. If the infecting organism is chlamydial, then tetracycline treatment is to be preferred over other antibiotics (Pierce, Ward and Seal, 1982).

Penicillin

The penicillins are a group of bactericidal agents which interfere with the synthesis of cell walls by binding to certain enzymes in the cell membrane which are responsible for the building of the cell wall, producing morphological changes in the bacteria they affect. Long filamentous cells are produced which fail to divide. Lysis of cells can occur due to the antibacterial action of some autolysins which normally only function during cell division. Benzylpenicillin was the first antibiotic to be introduced into medicine. Newer penicillins have been developed, which are semi-synthetic, but they all share the danger of inducing a possible fatal anaphylaxis in a number of patients. Some of the penicillins are susceptible to breakdown by enzymes (penicillinases) produced by Gram positive bacteria such as Staphylococci. Also, penicillinase-producing Gram negative organisms such as the gonococci have been isolated from cases of ophthalmia neonatorum (Dunlop *et al.* 1950; Pang *et al.* 1979). Newer agents have been produced which are resistant to the action of penicillinase. Resistance to penicillins can also be caused by difficulty of the compound penetrating to the site of action. Penicillins pass across the ocular barriers very poorly and products containing them are rarely used in the treatment of ocular infections.

Bacitracin

This bacteriocidal agent has similar properties to penicillin, especially in its mode of action. It is mainly used externally in combination with other agents, e.g. polymixin. It penetrates the cornea poorly but is effective for surface infections.

Erythromycin

Erythromycin is often used in the treatment of systemic infections but for ophthalmic use is best known for the effect on chlamydiae and other organisms such as Rickettsia, Treponema and mycoplasma. Because of the infrequency of cases in the United Kingdom, preparations of erythromycin are rarely used.

Tobramycin

Tobramycin is an aminoglycoside antibiotic (see gentamicin) and has similar toxic effects to the others in the group (i.e. nephrotoxicity and ototoxicity). It has a better antibacterial efficacy than gentamicin. It is produced in 0.3% solution.

Antifungal agents

Although fungal infections of the eye are much rarer than those caused by bacteria, they are nonetheless very serious when they occur and require prompt and effective treatment if loss of an eye is to be avoided.

Fungal infections occur more frequently in other parts of the body, e.g. athlete's foot and thrush which are infections of the feet and mouth or vagina, respectively. To cope with these a range of antifungal agents has been developed; these include nystatin, amphotericin, natamycin, flucytosine, clotrimazole and miconazole.

Nystatin

Nystatin is probably the oldest and best known antifungal agent. It is produced by a strain of Streptomyces and is fungistatic rather than fungicidal. It is effective against a wide range of fungi but has little effect on other micro-organisms. The compound is poorly absorbed by the cornea, so topical treatment is only effective for surface fungal infection with organisms such as *Candida albicans*. Deep infections require directly injected therapy.

Amphotericin

Amphotericin is also a product of a Streptomyces species and like nystatin is not effective against bacteria and viruses. Its mode of action is to increase permeability of the cell membrane by binding to sterols. This allows other antifungal agents, used in combination to become more effective. Sometimes antifungal agents and antibiotics are combined. Amphotericin was combined with rifampicin (an antibiotic normally associated with the treatment of tuberculosis) in the treatment of experimental *Candida albicans* keratitis and was found to be better than amphotericin alone (Stern, Okumoto and Smolen, 1979). Rifampicin, which is ineffective on its own, passes much more easily through the membrane, which has been made more permeable by amphotericin and inhibits RNA synthesis. Host cells can be similarly affected and this leads to toxicity. Patient's reactions to the drug vary and the dose has to be carefully titrated.

Treatment of fungal infections is much slower than bacterial infections and therapy must often be continued for months. Amphotericin, which is fungistatic, is poorly absorbed and its marked toxicity restricts its use to topical infections.

Natamycin

This fungicidal compound is very effective against a whole range of fungi but not bacteria. Like many other antifungals it penetrates the eye very poorly, but is probably one of the most effective ocular antifungals. It is used as eye drops (5–10%) or eye ointment (1%).

Flucytosine

Flucytosine, which is only active against yeast, is used as eye drops (1.5%). It is a synthetic compound which is well absorbed by the gut and is distributed to all parts of the body after oral administration. Resistance can develop to flucytosine and it is sometimes used in combination with amphotericin, with which it is synergistic.

Clotrimazole

This antifungal agent is most commonly used for fungal infections of the skin, e.g. athlete's foot, and vagina, e.g. thrush. In the eye it is used as a 1% solution.

Miconazole

This broad spectrum antifungal agent produces its effects by acting on the cell wall, by blocking the production of ergosterol. It rivals clotrimazole in its use in skin and genital fungal infections.

Absorption takes place across the intact cornea but if the epithelium is removed much greater absorption takes place.

Antiviral drugs

The number of antiviral drugs is much lower than the number of antibacterial or antifungal agents. Many viral infections still resist treatment and only a few will respond to therapy. Amongst the latter is Herpes simplex, the causative organism of dendritic ulcer. Four agents are in common use as topical treatments for this condition: idoxuridine, vidarabine, trifluorothymidine and acyclovir.

Idoxuridine

This is the oldest antiviral compound and is a derivative of thymidine, one of the organic bases which are incorporated into the nucleic acids. The viral metabolism incorporates the idoxuridine into the nucleic acid and prevents the virus infecting other cells. Idoxuridine competitively inhibits the uptake of thymidine and thus an excess of thymidine will antagonize its action (compare sulphonamides and PABA). It is specifically antiviral and has no effect on bacteria.

It is used as 0.1% eyedrops and 0.5% eye ointment. Penetration into the eye is poor but normally the infection is on the surface of the cornea and clinically effective concentrations can be achieved by topical administration.

Idoxuridine is very selective and does not inhibit epithelial growth (Foster and Pavan-Langston, 1977). The compound is generally non-toxic. It does, however, inhibit stromal healing and causes a reduction of wound strength and cannot be used, therefore, after corneal transplants.

The antiviral agent is only active while it is present and during treatment it must be administered intensively, i.e. every hour. Resistant strains can sometimes develop.

Vidarabine

Vidarabine, otherwise known as adenine arabinoside, is a nucleoside which stops the growth of the nuclear chain. Since its mode of action is different from idoxuridine, it can be used in patients who are allergic to this compound or to treat idoxuridine-resistant cases.

Used in 3% ointment form, it is absorbed to a greater extent than is idoxuridine and can be used topically for herpetic uveitis, but is often given by injection for this condition. Vidarabine drops, of the same concentration, have been tested but they showed up as being significantly poorer than liquid preparations of idoxuridine and trifluorothymidine (Pavan-Langston, Lass and Campbell, 1979) Vidarabine is effective against both strains of H. simplex (I and II), but does not seem to affect the course of infections with adenovirus. Like idoxuridine it does not interfere with the healing of corneal epithelial defects, but will slow the rate of repair of stromal injuries.

The monophosphate derivative of vidarabine—adenine arabinoside monophosphate, otherwise known as AraAMP—has been tested (Falcon and Jones, 1977) as an antiviral in herpetic eye disease. It was found to be better than vidarabine in inhibiting lesions but had similar effects in the treatment of established lesions. It significantly retarded closure of epithelial wounds in rabbits and induced toxic changes in the epithelium (Foster and Pavan-Langston, 1977).

Trifluorothymidine

As the name indicates, trifluorothymidine (TFT F3T) is a thymidine derivative and inhibits the replication of DNA viruses. It is a potent reversible inhibitor of thymidine synthetase and this accounts in part for its mode of action. TFT can also be incorporated into viral DNA to produce defective new virus particles. It has a short half-life when given systemically and is also very toxic when given by this route. Originally designed as an anti-cancer agent, TFT is lipid soluble and crosses the corneal epithelium. It passes into the eye more readily than does vidarabine and idoxuridine and produces levels in the aqueous humour which are effective against deeper viral infections (Pavan-Langston and Nelson, 1979) and therefore it can produce results where idoxuridine (Gilbert and Work, 1980) and vidarabine have had no effect. Like idoxuridine it does not significantly retard the closure of epithelial wounds (Foster and Pavan-Langston, 1977).

Trifluorothymidine was found to be significantly superior to idoxuridine in a study of 78 patients (Wellings *et al.* 1972) on the grounds that the healing time was significantly shorter and the percentage of treatment failures in patients receiving trifluorothymidine was less. Pavan-Langston and Foster (1977) also found a significant difference in the percentage of successfully treated patients. In a coded study 96% of all TFT patients were successfully healed, compared with 75% for idoxuridine.

McKinnon, McGill and Jones (1975) compared trifluorothymidine with vidarabine. Although they found no significant differences, there were trends which suggested that the former drug produced quicker healing, especially in amoeboid ulcers. There were fewer failures and a smaller incidence of further ulceration on this treatment. Slightly different results were found by van Bjisterveld and Post (1980). TFT was found to be slightly slower than vidarabine in producing healing. The healing times was also found to be dependent on the interval between the onset of symptoms and the onset of therapy. Similarly, McNeill and Kaufman (1979) found in an experimental stromal keratitis model that the effectiveness of therapy with trifluorothymidine depended on early treatment.

TFT's superiority in treating amoeboid ulcers was confirmed by Coster, Jones and McGill (1979). Several reasons for this superiority have been put forward. It may be due to superior antiviral activity of the drug in the corneal epithelium or stroma. It may also be due to better absorption across the epithelium or better uptake by the stroma.

Acyclovir

Acyclovir (acycloguanosine) only affects virus infected cells because it utilizes an enzyme thymidine kinase, whose structure and functioning is slightly different in viruses to what it is in cells. Viral thymidine kinase can metabolize acycloguanosine while cellular thymidine kinase cannot. Some viral mutants have modified genes for the production of thymidine kinase but these tend to have low pathogenicity and virulence. Nevertheless, a variant which produces a thymidine kinase with modified specificity has been found (Darby, Field and Salisbury, 1981) which was resistant to acyclovir. The nucleoside is phosphorylated into a tri-phosphate nucleoside which is incorporated into the viral DNA molecule, arresting any further development. It is effective against infections with strains of Herpes simplex I which were resistant to idoxuridine (Trousdale, Newburn and Miller, 1981). Acyclovir was significantly more effective than the other antivirals, even on drug-sensitive strains. Acyclovir-treated eyes showed less corneal epithelial involvement and conjunctivitis and exhibited less iritis and corneal clouding. McGill, Tormey and Walker (1981) compared acyclovir and vidarabine and found that the former had a much better rate of healing and reduction in symptoms, but Coster *et al.* (1980) found no difference between acyclovir and idoxuridine. Because of its very selective action it does not interfere with corneal wound healing, whether epithelial or stromal. Lass, Pavan-Langston and Park (1979) compared the effective on wound healing of acyclovir with that of idoxuridine. Acyclovir had no significant effect on the regenerating epithelium or re-epithelialization of surface wounds or on the collagen content of stromal wounds.

References

Chastain, J. B. and Newton, L. K. (1954) Intramuscular chloramphenicol treatment of trachoma. *Rocky Mountain Medical Journal*, **March**, 191–194

Chaudhuri, P. R. and Godfrey, B. (1982) Treatment of bacterial corneal ulcers with concentrated eye drops. *Transact. Ophthalmol. Soc., UK.*, **102**, 11–14

Coster, D. J., Jones, B. R. and McGill, J. I. (1979) Treatment of amoeboid herpetic ulcers with adenine arabinoside or trifluorothymidine. *Br. J. Ophthalmol.*, **63**, 418–421

Coster, D. J., Wilhelmus, K. R., Michaud, R. and Jones, B. R. (1980) A comparison of acyclovir and idoxuridine as treatment for ulcerative herpetic keratitis. *Br. J. Ophthalmol.*, **64**, 763–765

Darby, G., Field, H. J. and Sailsbury, S. A. (1981) Altered substrate specificity of herpes simplex virus thymidine kinase confers acyclovir-resistance. *Nature*, **289**, 81–83

Davis, S. D., Sarff, L. D. and Hyaduik, R. A. (1979) Experimental *Pseudomas* keratitis in guinea pigs: therapy of moderately severe infections. *Br. J. Ophthalmol.*, **63**, 436–439

Dunlop, E. M., Rodin, P., Seth, A. D. and Kolator, B. (1980) Ophthalmia neonatorum due to β-lactamase producing gonococci. *Br. Med. J.*, **16th August**, 483

Falcon, M. G. and Jones, B. R. (1977) Antivirals for the therapy of herpetic eye disease. *Transact. Ophthalmol. Soc., UK..*, **97**, 330–332

Foster, C. S. and Pavan-Langston, D. (1977) Corneal wound healing and antiviral medication. *Arch. Ophthalmol.*, **95**, 2062–2067

Gilbert, P., and Work, K. (1980) Trifluorothymidine in the treatment of herpes simplex corneal ulcers. *Arch. Ophthalmol.*, **58**, 117–120

Glasser, D. B., Gardner, S., Ellis, J. G. and Pettit, T. H. (1985) Loading doses and extended dosing intervals in topical gentamicin therapy. *Am. J. Ophthalmol.*, **99**, 329–332

Hillman, J. S., Jacobs, S. I., Garrett, A. J. and Kheskani, M. B. (1979) Gentamicin penetration and decay in human aqueous. *Br. J. Ophthalmol.*, **63**, 794–796

Insler, M. S., Cavanagh, H. D. and Wilson, L. A. (1985) Gentamicin-resistant *Pseudomonas* endophthalmitis after penetrating keratoplasty. *Br. J. Ophthalmol.*, **69**, 189–191

Ismail, S. and Morton, D. J. (1987) Ophthalmic uptake of chloramphenicol from proprietary preparations using an in vitro method of evaluation. *Int. J. Pharm.*, **37**, 11–13

Lass, J. H., Pavan-Langston, D. and Park, N. H. (1979) Acyclovir and corneal wound healing. *Am. J. Ophthalmol.*, **88**, 102–108

Lavine, J. B., Binder, P. S. and Wickham, M. G. (1979) Antimicrobials and the corneal endothelium. *Ann. Ophthalmol.*, **11**, 1517–1528

McGill, J., Tormey, P. and Walker, C. B. (1981) Comparative trial of acyclovir and adenine arabinoside in the treatment of herpes simplex corneal ulcers. *Br. J. Ophthalmol.*, **65**, 610–613

McKinnon, J. P., McGill, J. I. and Jones, B. R. (1975) A coded clinical evaluation of adenine arabinoside and trifluorothymidine in the treatment of ulcerative herpetic keratitis. In *Adenine*

Arabinoside: An Antiviral Agent. (ed by Pavan-Langston, D., Buchanan, R. A. and Alford, C. A.), New York: Raven Press

McNeil, J. I. and Kaufman, H. E. (1979) Local antivirals in herpes simplex stromal keratitis model. *Arch. Ophthalmol.*, **97**, 727–729

Mahajan, V. M. (1983) Bacterial infections of the eye: their aetiology and treatment. *Br. J. Ophthalmol.*, **67**, 191–194

Michelson, J. B. and Nozik, R. A. (1979) Experimental endophthalmitis treated with an implantable osmotic minipump. *Arch. Ophthalmol.*, **97**, 1345–1348

Pang, R., Ten, L. B., Rajan, V. S. and Sng, E. H. (1979) Gonococcal ophthalmia neonatorum caused by β-lactamase producing *Neisseria gonorrhoeae*. *Br. Med. J.*, **10th February**, 380

Pavan-Langston, D. and Foster, C. S. (1977) Trifluorothymidine and idoxuridine therapy of ocular herpes. *Am. J. Ophthalmol.*, **84/6**, 818–825

Pavan-Langston, D., Lass, J. H. and Campbell, R. (1979) Antiviral drugs: competitive therapy of experimental herpes simplex keratouveitis.*Arch. Ophthalmol.*, **97**, 1132–1135

Pavan-Langston, D. and Nelson, D. J. (1979) Intraocular penetration of trifluorothymidine. *Am. J. Ophthalmol.*, **87**, 814–818

Pierce, J. M., Ward, M. E. and Seal, D. V. (1982) Ophthalmia neonatorum in the 1980s: incidence, aetiology and treatment. *Br. J. Ophthalmol.*, **66**, 728–731

Raucher, H. S. and Newton, M. J. (1983) New issues in the prevention and treatment of ophthalmia neonatorum. *Ann. Ophthalmol.*, **15**, 1004–1009

Seal, D. V., Barrett, S. P. and McGill, J. T. (1982) Aetiology and treatment of acute bacterial infection of the external eye. *Br. J. Ophthalmol.*, **66**, 357–360

Stern, G. A., Okumoto, M. and Smolin, G. (1979) Combined amphotericin B and rifampicin treatment of experimental *Candida albicans* keratitis. *Arch. Ophthalmol.* **97**, 721–722

Trope, G. E., Lawrence, J. R., Hind, V. M. D. and Bunney, J. (1979) Systemic absorption of topically applied chloramphenicol eyedrops. *Br. J. Ophthalmol.*, **63**, 690–691

Trousdale, M. D., Newburn, A. B. and Miller, C. A. (1981) Assessment of acyclovir on acute ocular infections induced by drug-resistant strains of HSV-I. *Invest. Ophthalmol. Vis. Sci.*, **20/2**, 230–235

van Bjisterveld and Post, H. (1980) Trifluorothymidine versus adenine arabinoside in the treatment of herpes simplex keratitis. *Br. J. Ophthalmol.*, **64**, 33–36

Wellings, P. C., Awdry, P. N., Bors, F. H., Jones, B. R., Brown, D. C. and Kaufman, H. E. (1972) Clinical evaluation of trifluorothymidine in the treatment of herpes simplex corneal ulcers. *Am. J. Ophthalmol.*, **73**, 932–942

Chapter 16

Drugs used in ophthalmology— anti-inflammatory agents

Inflammation is the response of the body to a variety of stimuli, e.g. infection, allergy and trauma.

There are many processes involved in inflammation, but they result in a characteristic reaction which is typified by a reddening of the area (as a result of vasodilation), oedema, loss of function and pain. The process is brought into play to combat and destroy invading organisms, but sometimes the body's own cells are attacked and destroyed and damage to tissues occurs. This is particularly true for the eye, where the delicate, transparent structures are susceptible to damage by scar formation. Permanent loss of vision can be the result of an ocular inflammation and sight can only be preserved if steps are taken to limit the extent of the inflammatory process.

The inflammatory response involves the following processes:

(1) *The increased production of prostaglandins*. Arachidonic acid is produced by the action of phospholipase and this in turn is converted to one of the variety of prostaglandins which have effects on smooth muscle and mediate some of the inflammatory reactions. For example, a mixture of prostaglandins called irin can induce an atropine-resistant miosis which occurs in uveitis.

(2) *The liberation of histamine from mast cells*. This is caused by the allergen–antigen reaction causing an increase in the influx of calcium ions into the mast cells. Histamine, in addition to its ability to stimulate pain and itch nerve fibres, is best known for the production of the 'triple response'. If a small amount of histamine is injected into the skin, a small red area appears at the point of injection, which is due to a direct effect of the histamine on blood vessels, causing vasodilatation. The permeability of the capillaries is increased, causing loss of cells and proteins. The effect of the protein is to raise the osmotic pressure of the fluid, causing increased loss of water into the tissues and consequent oedema. The third component is a diffuse vasodilation, causing a more diffuse red area (flare) around the site of injection.

(3) *Vascular effects*. In addition to the action of histamine, other locally active agents can induce vasodilation and increase capilliary permeability. In the eye, the permeability of the blood/aqueous barrier is increased, leading to a turbid aqueous which contains more protein than normal. Outflow is impaired and an inflammatory form of secondary glaucoma may ensue.

(4) *Fibroblastic activity*. Because of its role in trauma, part of the inflammatory response is to stimulate the mechanism of wound repair, e.g. fibroblast and collagen forming activity, which can sometimes lead to scar formation and, in the cornea, opacity.

(5) *Increased leukocyte activity*. These normally migrate into the site of inflammation in order to attack and kill invading cells. They contain lysosomal vacuoles which can bring about the destruction of cells including the host inflamed cells.

Because the effects of inflammation can be sometimes excessive and in the eye lead to discomfort and loss of vision, it is often desirable to limit the extent by the use of appropriate drugs. Among the drugs which can be used are:

(1) Antihistamines—these combat the action of histamine (Chapter 11).
(2) Non-steroidal anti-inflammatory agents—these interfere with the conversion of arachidonic acid into prostaglandins and reduce leukocyte migration (*see* Chapter 11).
(3) Corticosteroids.
(4) Mast cell stabilizers.

Corticosteroids

The adrenal cortex produces a mixture of steroid hormones which fall into three main groups: glucocorticoids, mineralocorticoids and sex hormones.

Mineralocorticoids are necessary to maintain the electrolyte balance of the body, whilst glucocorticoids affect glucose metabolism and have anti-inflammatory properties. The naturally occurring ones include corticosterone and hydrocortisone, which have sodium retention properties, and in order to separate this latter effect from the anti-inflammatory effects, newer, synthetic and more potent steroids have been developed. Betamethasone and dexamethasone, for example, are 25 times more potent in producing anti-inflammatory effects.

No other group of drugs deserves the title of a 'two-edged sword' as much as the corticosteroids. They are known on the one hand for their useful and sometimes sight-saving effects in the treatment of inflammation, while on the other for the very serious adverse effects which can arise from their use. For example, corticosteroids can assist in the reduction of intraocular pressure when used to treat uveitic secondary glaucoma but can cause a rise in intraocular pressure if used topically in patients who are 'steroid responders'.

Corticosteroids inhibit the inflammatory response to noxious stimuli whether they are radiation, mechanical, chemical, infectious or immunological, affecting the inflammatory process in many ways. They reduce the vasodilatation that is responsible for the redness that accompanies inflammation and stabilize mast cells, thereby reducing the release of histamine. Their use maintains the normal permeability of blood and prevents the development of oedema.

Part of their mechanism of action involves the inhibition of the production of prostaglandins, which mediate some of the effect of inflammation. Prostaglandins are produced by conversion of arachidonic acid by cyclo-oxygenase, and steroids prevent the release of this acid. Corticosteroids not only reduce the early signs of the inflammatory process but also the late manifestations, e.g. proliferation of capillaries and scar formation.

Apart from providing symptomatic relief, corticosteroids are important in ophthalmology in preventing scar formation and loss of transparency of the cornea.

Cortisone and hydrocortisone were the first corticosteroids discovered. Hydrocortisone is so widely used as a topical skin treatment that it is now classed as a pharmacy medicine in this form, providing that the indications are strictly controlled.

The introduction of hydrocortisone was followed by prednisolone, which is five times as potent. This drug has itself been superseded by drugs such as dexamethasone and betamethasone, which are even more effective (50 times the potency of hydrocortisone). They have a better therapeutic ratio than hydrocortisone, being proportionally less sodium and water retentive and causing less potassium loss.

Steroids have many other adverse effects in addition to causing an imbalance in electrolyte levels. When taken systemically they cause weight gain because of increased appetite, exacerbation of peptic ulcers, a deposition of fat leading to the appearance of moon face and cataract (*see* Chapter 18).

Corticosteroids also have marked side-effects when applied topically and their adverse effects must always be balanced against their beneficial ones. For example, they inhibit wound healing and reduce the body's response to infections. If the invading organism is a virus or a non-pyogenic bacteria, then providing the antimicrobial agents are applied at the same time, the steroids will have a beneficial effect by reducing the tissue destruction due to the inflammatory process. If on the other hand, the infecting organism is pyogenic, it will cause tissue damage itself and steroids will delay resolution of the infection.

The effect on wound healing is brought about by changes in the relationship of collagen and cells. Corticosteroids impair fibroblastic and keratocytic activity. They normally inhibit collagenase activity but on some occasions, this can be potentiated, leading to a rapid destruction of the stroma-melting cornea. Wounds have reduced tensile strength as a result of the actions of steroids.

Another adverse reaction to topical therapy is a rise in intraocular pressure in a number of individuals, termed steroid glaucoma. Newer agents such as clobetasone and fluoromethalone are claimed to produce fewer effects on the intraocular pressure, possibly due to differences in absorption.

Sodium cromoglycate (cromolyn sodium)

Sodium cromoglycate was originally indicated for the treatment of asthma and it produces its effect by stabilizing the membranes of mast cells, thus preventing the release of histamine. A topical preparation of this compound has been prepared for the prophylaxis of vernal conjunctivitis and other allergic reactions. It has to be given as a course of treatment and will prevent the symptoms occurring, but will not act as an antihistamine and thus once the histamine is released, produces no effects. It is available as a 0.2% solution or a 4% ointment under the trade mark Opticrom.

Chapter 17

Drugs used in ophthalmology—anti-glaucoma drugs

All glaucoma treatments are aimed at reducing intraocular pressure (IOP), even though it is generally agreed that there is no proven relationship between IOP reduction and visual field preservation. As the level of intraocular pressure is determined by both the rate of production and the rate of outflow, IOP can be reduced by reducing secretion or increasing outflow (Figure 17.1). Most glaucomas are considered to be due to a reduced outflow facility, but it is thought acceptable to approach the problem by modifying the inflow of aqueous humour. The effect of a reduced throughput of aqueous humour has not received a great deal of attention.

Of the primary glaucomas, only open angle glaucoma is amenable to chronic medical treatment. Although acute closed angle glaucoma can be relieved by a combined attack of both topical and systemic treatment, its long term relief will be

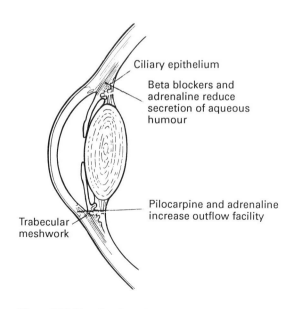

Ciliary epithelium

Beta blockers and adrenaline reduce secretion of aqueous humour

Pilocarpine and adrenaline increase outflow facility

Trabecular meshwork

Figure 17.1 Site of action of anti-glaucoma products

from surgery. Surgical treatment of open angle glaucoma is also an option, especially when medical treatments appear to be losing their effect.

Whatever its form, an anti-glaucoma treatment should satisfy certain criteria.

(1) Reduction of intraocular pressure

The amount by which intraocular pressure must be reduced in order that the glaucoma can be deemed to be 'controlled' varies between different studies. IOPs of below 20 mm Hg are often taken to indicate control, but it is known that different individuals tolerate different tensions, a level of 20 mm Hg not being control for a patient with low tension glaucoma. It is probably more important that the pressure should remain stable and not vary greatly during the day.

(2) Duration of effect

There is little doubt that if the treatment is to be effective then the reduction should last for some hours. As stated above, it is important that the pressure remain stable rather than oscillating.

It is assumed, but not proven, that there is an inverse relationship between the number of doses per day and patient compliance. In other words, twice a day therapy is better than four times a day therapy but not as good as once a day.

(3) Preservation of visual field

With modern diagnostic techniques, most glaucomas today are diagnosed before serious impairment of vision has occurred and the obvious aim of treatment is that no further loss will occur. Since visual field change is a slow insidious effect, it is important that it is monitored

(4) No loss of effect with time

Once a patient has been stabilized on a treatment, it is unfortunate if his therapy has to be modified because the original drug is no longer sufficiently effective.

(5) Compatibility with other treatments

Because drugs can lose their effect with time and because some patients require more vigorous therapy, it is often necessary for more than one drug to be administered. As the possibility exists of modifying pressure by reducing secretion or by increasing outflow, drugs with antagonistic pharmacological actions may have synergistic therapeutic effects.

(6) Lack of topical adverse effects

Often, due to the diligence of the optometrist, glaucoma is detected before the patient is aware of symptoms. The patient does not know that he has a problem which will require a lifetime course of continuing therapy. Having persuaded the patient that it is necessary to apply the drops every day, it is counterproductive if these drops cause problems to him which would lead to lack of patient compliance. Initial stinging is one of the problems that can occur with many eye drops.

Some drops can cause a local anaesthetic effect (e.g. beta-blockers) and this can lead to corneal problems.

Eye drops contain other ingredients as well as the drug and water and these adjuvants may interfere with the anterior surface of the eye. For example, some of the preservatives used to maintain sterility can adversely affect the tear film and can thus exacerbate dry eye problems.

(7) Lack of systemic effects
All topical anti-glaucoma drugs used at the moment produce their action by modifying the effects of the autonomic nervous system. The ANS also innervates many other structures in the body, e.g. the cardiovascular system, the respiratory system and the gastro-intestinal system, and serious systemic effects can result from the topical use of autonomic drugs.

(8) Patient compliance
Treatments must be easy and pleasant to use and this requires attention not only to the active ingredient and its formulation but also to the container in which it is supplied.

   Glaucoma treatments can be administered either systemically or topically.

Systemic treatments

Drugs administered in this manner are given by mouth for chronic treatment or by injection for acute use. Beta-blockers will reduce intraocular pressure when given systemically and have been tested for use in this manner (Tutton and Smith, 1983). Williamson *et al.* (1985) compared topical treatment with timolol and systemic treatment with nadolol. They found that once a day systemic treatment was as efficacious as twice a day topical treatment, and suggested that systemic treatment would be useful for patients who had difficulty in administering drops. However, the only drops used routinely are the carbonic anhydrase inhibitors, acetazolamide and dichlorphenamide. Carbonic anhydrase is present in the ciliary epithelium and is necessary for the secretion of bicarbonate ions. If their secretion is reduced there is a concomitant reduction in the secretion of the accompanying sodium ions. In order to maintain the proper osmotic pressure, the volume of aqueous secreted is less than normal and intraocular pressure falls.

   The carbonic anhydrase inhibitors have some unfortunate side-effects. These include:

   lack of appetite
   paresthesia
   gut disturbances
   fatigue
   kidney stones
   aplastic anaemia

Topical treatments

Topical treatments, with one exception (the Ocusert device), consist of the application of drops to the anterior surface of the eye. There are a number of agents available for use in the treatment of glaucoma, but they fall into three principal groups: miotics, sympathomimetics and beta-blockers.

Miotics

These are the same drugs which can be used to reverse the action of mydriatics. Whereas for the reversal of mydriasis, pupillary constriction is the desired effect, in the treatment of open angle glaucoma, it is an unwanted side-effect. It is the contraction of the ciliary muscle, putting tension on the trabecular meshwork, that is responsible for the increased outflow and reduced intraocular pressure. In addition, direct effects on the trabecular meshwork have been postulated by Barany (1962). Of course, if the filtration angle is narrow, the miosis is an important component of the drug's action but for the majority of patients, it is the cyclospasm which produces the fall in IOP.

By far the most commonly used miotic is pilocarpine, which has been used in ophthalmology for well over 100 years. The concentration employed varies from 0.5% to 8% but the higher strengths are probably 'overkill' as a maximum effect has been reported at 4% (Harris and Galin, 1970). It produces a biphasic, small rise followed by a persistent fall (Korczyn *et al.*, 1982) which lasts for about 6 hours, requiring the drug to be administered four times a day. Its effect is on outflow rather than secretion and thus the drug restores the aqueous flow to a more physiological status.

The miosis and spasm of accommodation are fundamental to the mode of action of these drugs, and there is little that can be done to separate the beneficial effects from the adverse effects. Research into miotics has been aimed at the other disadvantages of pilocarpine, namely:

(1) It is a natural product which means that:
    (a) it tends to be expensive;
    (b) its supplies can be erratic;
    (c) there is a greater possibility of allergic reaction.
(2) Its effects only last for 6 hours and therefore:
    (a) patient compliance is reduced;
    (b) the intraocular pressure goes up and down four times a day.

To avoid these problems, developments have been in two directions, *viz.* new presentations of pilocarpine and new miotics.

New presentations of pilocarpine

These developments have been aimed at increasing the contact time of the drug with the eye, leading to a greater effect and a more prolonged effect. They included:

(a) Viscolized solutions. Viscolizers such as hydroxyethylcellulose or polyvinyl alcohol have been added to make the drop more viscous and thus stay in the eye for longer (Davies *et al.*, 1977). Although a greater and more prolonged fall has been reported following the use of viscolized drops, the duration of effect does not seem to justify a reduction in the number of doses per day.

(b) Gels. Polymers have been developed into which the pilocarpine can be incorporated and from which it is slowly released (Ticho *et al.*, 1979)

(c) Oily solutions. Not only are oils more viscous than water, but the actual alkaloid can be incorporated and thus be better absorbed by the corneal epithelium. Unfortunately oily drops are not as pleasant to use as the aqueous ones.

(d) Soft contact lenses. Hydrophilic lenses can be soaked in pilocarpine solutions and the lens applied to the eye (Marmion *et al.*, 1977), a method of application which does not seem to have been widely accepted.

(e) Ocusert. This consists of viscous solution surrounded by a membrane which allows a slow but constant delivery of pilocarpine into the conjunctival sac (Heilman and Sinz, 1975). The duration of treatment lasts for up to 9 days and because the level of pilocarpine is constant, the side-effects are smaller than from drop application. One of the problems that has been encountered is that sometimes the unit becomes lost and the patient is untreated until the loss is discovered.

New miotics
Many other miotics have been tried in the treatment of glaucoma. These include the following.

(a) Other parasympathomimetics

Aceclidine. This synthetic drug has similar efficacy and duration of action to pilocarpine but does not seem to confer any particular advantage, other than the fact that it can be tolerated when pilocarpine is not (Romano, 1970).

Metachol. A synthetic analogue of acetylcholine.

Carbachol. This drug is similar to metachol but is not broken down by cholinesterase. It is poorly absorbed across the cornea.

(b) Short-acting (reversible) anticholinesterases

Physostigmine. This produces a marked miosis and a reduction of intraocular pressure which last for 12 hours. It is sometimes combined with pilocarpine.

Neostigmine. This is a weaker, synthetic analogue of physostigmine which does seem to have found favour in the treatment of glaucoma.

(c) Long-acting (irreversible) anticholinesterases

Dyflos. DFP was the first organophosphorus compound but this is unstable in water and is administered in arachis oil.

Ecothiopate. This is similarly susceptible to hydrolysis and is supplied dry, being dissolved in a diluent just before use.

Demecarium. This is one of the shorter acting irreversible agents.

Sympathomimetics

The ability of adrenaline to reduce intraocular pressure has been known for a long time, but its application to the treatment of glaucoma was only possible following the development of the gonioscope lens. Because of the ability of adrenaline to cause a dilation of the pupil, it is vital that open angle glaucoma is differentiated from closed angle glaucoma. Sympathomimetics will reduce pressure in the former and increase it in the latter. They produce a triphasic response with a fall, followed by a rise and then a more persistent fall. The effect lasts for at least 12 hours and thus the drops require administration twice a day. The time course of the ocular hypotensive effect is different from the mydriatic effect (Langham *et al.*, 1979). Many different sympathomimetics have been tried but only adrenaline and its derivatives are used routinely.

Adrenaline produces its pharmacological effects by stimulating both alpha- and beta- receptors and by a variety of biochemical effects, e.g. enhanced liver glycogenolysis, leading to a higher blood sugar level and enhanced production of prostaglandins. Its best known biochemical effect is the enhanced production of cyclic adenosine monophosphate from adenosine triphosphate.

Adrenaline produces a beta-mediated increase in secretion by stimulating chloride transport through cAMP production. This increase is, however, more than cancelled out by an alpha-stimulated reduction. It also causes an increase in the facility of outflow by acting beta-receptors.

Adrenaline is not without its adverse effects, producing a red eye in some patients, probably as a result of reactive hyperaemia. It will also cause black deposits in the cornea (Madge *et al.*, 1971), especially if old solutions are used (Krejci and Harrison, 1969). Maculopathy has been reported, especially in aphakic patients (Kolker and Becker, 1968; Mackool *et al.*, 1977).

In order to improve its efficacy, adrenaline has been combined with guanethidine, an adrenergic neurone blocker. It initially causes a release of noradrenaline from the nerve terminals and thus acts as an indirectly acting sympathomimetic. Mydriasis and a fall in intraocular pressure are the result. Since the noradrenaline is not replaced, eventually a chemical denervation syndrome exists. The intraocular pressure returns to normal and the pupil is constricted. The eye is now supersensitive to sympathomimetics and it will respond to a concentration of these agents which would normally have no effect. Crombie (1974) used the combination of guanethidine and adrenaline to control patients who were previously difficult to control. Eltz *et al.* (1978) used a combination of 5% guanethidine and 1% adrenaline and found that the mixture was synergistic.

A recent development has been the production of prodrugs which are modifications of the drug with enhanced lipid solubility. An example is dipivefrin, which is inactive: when it enters the eye, it must be converted to active adrenaline by enzymes before it can produce its hypotensive effect. Kass *et al.* (1979) reported smaller falls with 0.1% dipivefrin than from 2% adrenaline. It was found to be less effective than timolol (Frumar and McGuinness, 1982). In terms of side-effects, the results are disappointing. Reactive hyperaemia (Azuma and Hirano, 1981), endothelial damage (Sasamoto *et al.*, 1981) and follicular conjunctivitis (Theodore and Leibowitz, 1979) have been reported.

Beta-blockers

Beta-blockers were originally developed for the treatment of cardiovascular disorders and this is still the major use for this type of agent. Since it was found that propranolol reduced intraocular pressure, many other beta-blockers have been tried for the treatment of glaucoma. These include atenolol, betaxolol, bupranolol, carteolol, labetalol, levobunolol, metipranolol, metoprolol, nadolol, pindolol, sotalol and timolol.

Beta-blockers reduce intraocular pressure by reducing secretion (Liu *et al.*, 1980). This reduction is probably due to the blocking of the beta-receptors,the stimulation of which causes an increased secretion of chloride ions. Beta-blockers have no effect on outflow resistance (Reiss and Brubaker, 1983).

Not all beta-blockers are the same and they vary in several ways.

(1) Selectivity

Beta-receptors can be divided into two groups—$beta_1$ and $beta_2$. Beta-receptors are found in the heart and kidneys while the bronchi contain $beta_2$. Most beta-blockers are non-selective and have similar potency on both types of beta receptors. However some have a greater affinity for beta-receptors and are called cardio-selective agents. One of the troublesome side-effects of the use of beta-blockers in the treatment of glaucoma is the blocking of the effect of $beta_2$ stimulants, used to dilate bronchi during asthma attacks, leading to aggravation of such attacks (Fraunfelder and Barker, 1984). The use of beta-blockers with reduced activity on $beta_2$-receptors will have less effect on the bronchi and therefore have advantages in patients with obstructive airway disease (Berry *et al.*, 1984). However, they are not completely safe and all beta-blockers must be used with care on asthmatic patients. Harris, Greenstein and Bloom (1986) reported respiratory difficulties in patients receiving topical betaxolol.

(2) Intrinsic sympathomimetic activity (ISA)

These drugs are partial agonists and can stimulate the receptor before blocking it. Many advantages have been claimed for drugs having this property, e.g. less bradycardia, less broncho-constriction but none would appear to have been substantiated by clinical trials. For example, carteolol (a beta-blocker with ISA) causes an inhibition of exercise-induced tachycardia (Brazier and Smith, 1987).

(3) Membrane stabilizing action (MSA)

The membrane referred to here is the membrane of nerve fibres. Membrane stabilizing action is another name for local anaesthetic effect. Propranolol, the first medically used beta-blocker, has marked local anaesthetic effects and because of this all beta-blockers are suspect until proven innocent. Many beta-blockers have small amounts of MSA but for most the effects are not clinically significant.

As well as the embarrassment of respiratory problems, beta-blockers may have effects on other systems, including the cardiovascular system. The effects on the heart are especially noted when increased demands are placed on the system. The heart at rest is often not significantly affected by beta-blockers (Ros and Dake, 1979), but when exercise is taken, the heart has difficulty in speeding up to cope with it. Fraunfelder and Meyer (1987) have reviewed the systemic side-effects of topical timolol and reported effects on the CNS, the skin and the gut as well as the cardiovascular and respiratory systems.

Because it was originally considered possible to separate the ocular hypotensive effects from the systemic effects of beta-blockers by making use of different stereo isomers, Richards and Tattersfield (1987) compared timolol to its D isomer. The isomer is four times less potent in reducing IOP and is four times less potent in causing bronchoconstriction. It does not, therefore, offer any particular advantage for use in asthmatic patients.

Mixtures of agents

Because of their different modes of action, it is possible to mix drugs from different groups in order to achieve an enhanced effect. This is necessary where control is not achieved with a single medication, or the effect of the original therapy wears off with time. It is possible to combine a drug from one group with another from one of the other two groups, e.g.

beta-blockers and miotics;
beta-blockers and sympathomimetics;
miotics and sympathomimetics.

The most common combination is pilocarpine and timolol. One matter of interest is the dose regimen if the drugs are administered in the same drop. Timolol is normally a twice daily therapy while pilocarpine requires administration four times a day. Airaksinen *et al.* (1987) compared timolol and pilocarpine with pilocarpine alone. Not only was a greater effect found with the combination, but the duration of effect was sufficient to allow twice daily administration.

Studies of beta-blockers with adrenaline (Allen and Epstein, 1986) and with dipivefrin (Ober and Scharrer, 1980) have also been undertaken and demonstrated advantages of the combination.

Combining two compounds from the same group, e.g. two miotics or two beta-blockers, is less successful.

It is possible to combine all four forms of medical treatment, i.e. beta-blockers, miotics, sympathomimetics and carbonic anhydrase inhibitors, but usually surgery is employed before this stage is reached.

Future developments

Acetazolamide is ineffective when applied topically but solutions of other diuretics have been tried. Despite encouraging animal tests, none has received widespread clinical use.

Bromocriptine is a dopaminergic receptor stimulant which has been found to be effective in reducing the intraocular pressure in rabbits.

Cannabis, best known as a drug of abuse, contains tetrahydrocannabinol which lowers IOP, but until its effects on the CNS can be separated from the ocular hypotensive effect, there is little future for its clinical use.

Forskolin is a natural product which, like adrenaline, stimulates adenylate cyclase, causing an increase in the intracellular levels of cAMP, but does not involve the reaction with a receptor. It reduces IOP when injected or applied topically (Caprioli, 1985).

References

Airaksinen, P. J. *et al.* (1987) A double masked study of timolol and pilocarpine. *Am. J. Ophthalmol.*, **104**, 587–590

Allen, R. C. and Epstein, D. L. (1986) Additive effect of betaxolol and epinephrine in primary open glaucoma. *Arch. Ophthalmol.*, **104**, 1178–1184

Azuma, I. and Hirumo, T. (1981) Long term topical use of DPE solution in open angle glaucoma. *Acta. Soc. Ophthalmol.*, *Japan*, **85**, 1157–1164

Barany, E. H. (1962) The mode of action of pilocarpine on outflow resistance in the eye of a primate (*Cercopithecus ethiops*) *Invest. Ophthalmol.*, **1**, 712–727

Berry, D. P., van Bushkirk, M. and Shields, M. B. (1984) Betaxolol and timolol. *Arch. Ophthalmol.*, **102**, 42–45

Brazier, D. J. and Smith, S. E. (1987) Ocular and cardiovascular response to topical carteolol 2% and timolol 0.5% in healthy volunteers. *Br. J. Ophthalmol.*, **72**, 101–103

Caprioli, J. (1985) The pathogenesis and medical management of glaucoma. *Drug Dev. Res.*, **6**, 193–215

Crombie, A. L. (1974) Adrenergic hypersensitisation as a therapeutive tool in glaucoma. *Trans. Ophthalmol. Soc. UK.*, **94**, 570–572

Davies, D. J. G., Jones, D. E. P., Meakin, B. J. and Norton, D. A. (1977) The effect of polyvinyl alcohol on the degree of miosis and intraocular pressure induced by pilocarpine. *Ophthal. Dig.*, **39**, 13–26

Ecoffet, H. and Demailly, P. (1987) Middle term double blind study in the treatment of chronic open angle glaucoma: comparison between metipranolol and timolol. *J. Franc. Ophthalmol.*, **10**, 451–454

Eltz, H., Aeschlimann, J. and Gloor, B. (1978) Double blind trial of a guanethidine/adrenaline combination, compared with the two separate components in glaucoma. *Acta Ophthalmol.*, *(Kbh)*, **56**, 191–200

Fraunfelder, F. T. and Barber, A. F. (1984) Respiratory effects of timolol. *New Engl. J. Med.*, **311**, 1441

Fraunfelder, F. T. and Meyer, S. M. (1987) Systemic side effects from ophthalmic timolol and their prevention. *J. Ocular Pharmacol.*, **3**, 177–184

Frumar, K. D. and McGuiness, R. (1982) A study of the intraocular pressure lowering effect of timolol and dipivalylepinephrine. *Aust. J. Ophthalmol.*, **10**, 121–123

Harris, L. S. and Galin, M. A. (1970) Dose response analysis of pilocarpine-induced ocular hypotension. *Arch. Ophthalmol.*, **84**, 605–608

Harris, L. S., Greenstein, S. H. and Bloom, A. F. (1986) Respiratory difficulties with betaxolol. *Am. J. Ophthalmol.*, **102**, 274

Heilman, K. and Sinz, V. (1975) Ocusert—a new drug carrier for the treatment of glaucoma. *Klinische Monatsblatter Augenheilkunde*, **166**, 289–292

Kass, M. A., Mandell, A. I., Goldberg, I., Paine, J. M. and Becker, B. (1979) Dipivedfrin and epinephrine treatment of elevated intraocular pressure. *Arch. Ophthalmol.*, **97**, 1865–1866

Kolker, A. E. and Becker, B. (1968) Epinephrine maculopathy. *Arch Ophthalmol.*, **79**, 552–562

Korczyn, A. D., Nemet, P., Carel, R. S. and Eyal, A. (1982) Effect of pilocarpine on intraocular pressure in normal humans. *Ophthal. Res.*, **14**, 182–187

Krejci, L. and Harrison, R. (1969) Corneal pigment deposits from topically administered epinephrine. *Arch. Ophthalmol.*, **82**, 836–839

Langham, M. E., Simjee, A. and Joseph, S. (1979) The alpha and beta adrenergic responses to epinephrine in the rabbit. *Exp. Eye Res.*, **15**, 75–84

Liu, H. K., Chiou, G. C. Y. and Garg, L. C. (1980) Ocular hypotensive effects of timolol in cats' eyes. *Arch. Ophthalmol.*, **98**, 1467–1469

Mackool, R. J., Muldoon, T., Fortier, A. and Nelson, D. (1977) Epinephrine-induced cystoid macular oedema in aphakic eyes. *Arch. Ophthalmol.*, **95**, 791–793

Madge, G. E., Geeraets, W. J. and Guerry, D. (1971) Black cornea secondary to topical epinephrine. *Am. J. Ophthalmol.*, **71**, 402–405

Marmion, V. J. and Yurdakul, S. (1977) Pilocarpine administration by contact lens. *Transact. Ophthalmol. Soc.*, **97**, 162–163

Ober, M. and Scharrer, A. (1980) The effect of timolol and dipivalyl-epinephrine in the treatment of the elevated intraocular pressure. *Graefes Arch. Ophthalmol.*, **213**, 273–281

Reiss, G. R. and Brubaker, R. F. (1983) The mechanism of betaxolol, a new ocular hypotensive agent. *Ophthalmology*, **90**, 1369–1372

Richards, R. and Tattersfield, A. E. (1987) Comparison of the airway response to eye drops of timolol and its isomer L-714,465 in asthmatic subjects. *Br. J. Clin. Pharmacol.*, **24**, 485–491

Romano, J. H. (1970) Double blind cross-over comparison of aceclidine and pilocarpine in open angle glaucoma. *Br. J. Ophthalmol.*, **54**, 510–521

Ros, F. E. and Dake, C. L. (1979) Timolol eye drops: bradycardia or tachycardia. *Documenta Ophthalmologica*, **48**, 283–289

Sasamoto, K., Akagi, Y., and Itoi, M. (1981) Effects of epinephrine and dipivalyl epinephrine on rabbit corneal endothelium. *Folio Ophthalmol.*, *Japan*, **32**, 1292–1297

Theodore, J. and Leibowitz, H. M. (1979) External ocular toxicity of dipivalyl epinephrine. *Am. J. Ophthalmol.*, **88**, 1013–1016

Ticho, U. *et al.* (1979) A clinical trial with piloplex—a new long acting pilocarpine compound preliminary report. *Ann. Ophthalmol.*, **11**, 535–561

Tutton, M. K. and Smith, R. J. H. (1982) Comparison of ocular hypotensive effects of three dosages of oral atenolol. *Br. J. Ophthalmol.*, **67**, 664–667

Williamson, J., Young, J. D. H., Muir, G. and Kadom, A. (1985) Comparative efficacy of orally and topically administered beta blockers for chronic simple glaucoma. *Br. J. Ophthalmol.*, **69**, 41–45

Chapter 18

Adverse ocular reactions to drug therapy

For a long time it has been realized that some systemic conditions such as diabetes and systemic hypertension may have ophthalmic complications and it has been desirable for the optometrist to take a general medical history before examining the patient. With the realization that the drugs used to treat these systemic conditions can also have effects on the eye, it is now also necessary for him to find out which drugs the patient may be taking. It is important that patients should be questioned on drugs which they purchase for themselves (over-the-counter or o.t.c. drugs) as well as prescription medicines. Kofoed (1986) reported that 40% of patients over 60 use o.t.c. medicines every day. Because they are not considered drugs by patients, they are thought to be safe.

In taking history with regard to medicine, the three 'Ds' are important: namely Drug, Dosage and Duration.

Drug

Patients on long term therapy are very often very knowledgeable about the medicines they are taking, especially if they are being purchased over the counter instead of being prescribed. For any particular drug, the likelihood of a drug causing an undesirable ocular side-effect depends on three factors: prevalence of the condition for which it is prescribed; prescribing habits; and therapeutic index.

Prevalence of the condition

Some pathological conditions are far more common than others, although this may depend on the particular geographical location. In the United Kingdom, patients are far more likely to be suffering from systemic hypertension, rheumatoid arthritis and upper respiratory tract infections than they are from leprosy and malaria.

Prescribing habits

Many drugs have a definite life cycle and go through phases of introduction and growth before becoming standard treatments. Afterwards they go into decline as newer agents are developed and may eventually be discontinued. The amount of drug prescribed during the different phases will vary greatly. Some drugs, however, endure for a long time, notable examples being pilocarpine, aspirin and penicillin.

Therapeutic index

This is a measure of the drug's safety and is the ratio of the lethal dose (LD_{50}) to the effective dose (ED_{50}). The higher the ratio, the safer is the drug. Some agents, such as the antibiotics, have a very high therapeutic index, while drugs used in the treatment of neoplasms have a very low ratio and their use is only justified by the very serious nature of the condition for which they are given. Much pharmaceutical research is aimed at producing drugs with a better therapeutic ratio or formulating existing drugs to maximize the useful effects while reducing as far as possible the unwanted ones.

Dosage

Some drugs have more than one indication and the dosage used for these indications varies greatly. For example, hydroxy chloroquine can be used in three ways: to prevent malaria, to treat malaria and to relieve rheumatoid arthritis.

The dose for malaria prophylaxis is much lower than for its treatment, with the anti-arthritic dose being somewhere in the middle. A patient taking a low dose for a few weeks during and after a trip abroad is most unlikely to exhibit any retinal effects.

Duration

Patients can become tolerant to the side-effects of drugs, especially if they are relatively mild, e.g. small pupil size changes and a loss of accommodation. Such effects are often noted when the treatment is first commenced but as it continues, they become less and less noticeable.

On the other hand, some side-effects are cumulative and only make an appearance when the drug is taken for a long time. For example steroid cataracts are only normally seen after a year's treatment.

Patient variability

Not all patients will exhibit adverse ocular effects. In fact, even when the patient is taking a drug with a well established causal relationship with a particular side-effect, it is by no means certain that the patient will eventually develop that problem.

Factors which influence the occurrence or adverse reactions are:

Age
Sex
Weight
General state of health
Ophthalmic state of health
Concurrent medication
Contact lenses.

Age

Children's metabolism is different to that of adults and they can be subject to certain adverse drug reactions that would not affect adults. For example, aspirin is contra-indicated in children under 12 because it may cause a serious condition called Reye's syndrome, but is safe for patients over that age.

At the other end of the age spectrum, elderly people may not be able to metabolize and detoxify pharmaceutical agents as quickly as younger patients.

Sex

Some drugs interfere with tear production; this is more likely to embarrass middle-aged women who have a greater tendency to become tear deficient than men. Of course, sex hormones may have bizarre effects on the opposite sex.

There is another way in which the sexes differ and that is in the fat/water ratio of the body. For a given weight, women contain a slightly higher level of fat than do men. Drugs which partition between fat and water will behave slightly differently in the two sexes. Sometimes drugs can be taken up by fat stores.

Weight

Weight can influence the incidence of adverse effects in two ways. Overweight people contain proportionally more fat than do thin people and therefore variation in the fat/water ratios will occur. Secondly, the larger the body, the smaller will be the plasma levels resulting from the administration of a given dose of drug. This is especially important in the case of children, who will require proportionally less drug to produce the same effect.

General state of health

Liver and kidney problems will reduce the rate of clearance of drugs and lead to cumulative problems with some drugs.

Ophthalmic state of health

A dilated pupil may be annoying and if the patient has a narrow anterior chamber angle closure is a possibility, although this is not a common occurrence. Similarly, a slightly constricted pupil may only cause a minor problem in normal patients but if he has an early central lens opacity, then the miosis will be a greater problem.

Concurrent medication

Drug interaction is always a possibility when the patient is receiving more than one medicament, even if they are being given by two different routes.

Contact lenses

The successful wearing of contact lenses relies on a normal tear film. If this is reduced in quantity or quality (e.g. a lack of mucin) then the patient may experience problems which a non-wearer would not.

Adverse ocular effects of drugs

These can vary from the mildly irritating, transient effects to the serious cumulative toxic, sight threatening effects. Unfortunately, in much of the general literature on drugs, ocular adverse side-effects are listed merely as 'visual disturbances', 'decreased vision' or 'blurred vision'. There are many underlying causes of such a report. The following are just some of them:

cyclospasm
cycloplegia
corneal oedema
media changes
optic neuritis
retinal changes.

Additionally, a patient may also complain of blurred vision if he fails to wear his proper refractive correction.

The causes vary from the trivial to the very serious and the optometrist is in an ideal situation to be able to differentiate between them.

The most common ocular effects are:

decreased tolerance to contact lenses;
cataract;
decreased accommodation and/or mydriasis;
raised intraocular pressure;
retinal pathologies;
diplopia.

Sources of information

The number and range of products on the market is ever changing and it is difficult to always be aware of the changes in medicinal products. There are many sources of information which are produced mainly with the medical practitioner in mind but which will be a valuable aid to the optometrist if he gains access to them.

Data sheets are produced by the manufacturing company and must be supplied to a doctor if requested. A data sheet carries information such as trade mark, ingredients, indications, dosage and warnings, adverse effects, etc. They are constantly updated where necessary as new information becomes available.

Data Sheet Compendium is a collation of all the data sheets of the products produced by the member companies of the Association of British Pharmaceutical Industry.

MIMS (Monthly Index of Medical Specialities) is a list of all branded medicines (and some unbranded ones) currently on the United Kingdom market. It carries similar information to the data sheet but in a much more concise form.

BNF (British National Formulary) covers all drugs, both branded and generic, and gives a comparison between agents having similar therapeutic effects. The *BNF* carries a supply of yellow cards for the reporting of adverse effects to the Committee on the Safety of Medicines (CSM). If the drug is considered to be a new chemical entity (NCE) then an inverted black triangle will be displayed alongside the approved name of the compound in any product literature or publication. The

CSM requires reporting of all adverse reactions to the drug, irrespective of the nature of severity.

For existing, well-established drugs, only serious side-effects are reported. Well known trivial side-effects need to be notified to the CSM.

Yellow cards have also been issued to optometrists for reporting unwanted side-effects to contact lenses, contact lens solutions and other medicinal products used or sold by optometrists or dispensing opticians. This, of course, will include diagnostic drugs, although the emphasis of the optometrist reporting scheme appears to be on contact lens wear. The form requires the following information:

(i)   Name, sex and age of the patient.
(ii) Type of contact lens and reason for wearing it.
(iii) Contact lens fluid used.
(iv) Other ophthalmic medication.
(v)   Systemic medication.
(vi) Adverse reaction.
(vii) Comments.
(viii) Details of reporting practitioner.

The optometrist yellow card scheme only covers medicinal products which the optometrist uses himself. It does not cover drugs prescribed by the medical practitioner or o.t.c. drugs.

The British College of Optometrists has a reporting scheme of ocular adverse effects of all drugs and this will probably provide a useful source of data in the future.

Both *MIMS* and the *BNF* have a classification in which drugs are broken down into groups according to the anatomical system on which they act. A similar classification will be used in this text to describe some of the more important drugs and their possible ocular effects. The list is not exhaustive and the examples quoted merely give a guide to the more common drugs and their side-effects. Under each heading, the following information will be included.

Indications and usage;
Common examples and trade marks; and
Common ocular adverse reactions.

Drugs acting on the alimentary tract

When drugs are administered orally, the alimentary tract is the first system with which they come in contact. Medicines such as antacids, ulcer healing drugs, laxatives and preparations for the relief of diarrhoea are administered for their action on the gut and often do not require absorption to produce their effect. For this reason, they can be considered as topical agents. Modern drugs are designed or formulated to remain in the gut and to be poorly absorbed. Occasionally absorption does take place from the gut and adverse reactions are possible.

The gut is innervated by the automatic nervous system and stimulation of the parasympathetic division causes increased motility and secretions. Antispasmodics are drugs which have antimuscarinic actions and are used to relieve gastro-intestinal spasms, peptic ulceration and irritable bowel syndrome.

Examples
Dicyclomine (Merbentyl)
Hyoscine (Buscopan)
Propantheline (Probanthine)

Ocular adverse effects
As would be predicted, the ocular adverse effects are mydriasis and cycloplegia, which are mild and transitory. There is a theoretical contra-indication for glaucoma sufferers but there have been few actual cases of closed angle glaucoma resulting from their use.

Drugs acting on the cardiovascular system

These drugs can influence the eye in two ways. Firstly, they can have direct pharmacological effects on the ocular tissues, but they can also cause effects indirectly by producing fluctuations in blood pressure and blood flow. For example, systemic hypertension and glaucoma can co-exist, with the former condition masking the other by maintaining the ocular perfusion. If the blood pressure is reduced by antihypertensives then symptoms of glaucoma may become manifest.

Drugs in this class can be divided into the following groups:

Cardiotonic drugs
Diuretics
Anti-arhythmic drugs
Beta blockers
Anti-hypertensives
Anticoagulants.

Cardiotonic drugs

The best known drugs in this group are the cardiac glycosides which are found in digitalis, in particular digoxin.

Examples
Digoxin (Lanoxin)
Lanatoside C (Cedilanid)
Disopyramide (Rythmodan)

Ocular adverse effects
Digitalis produces toxic effects on the retina which are manifested by a disturbance in colour vision and a glare phenomenon in which objects appear to be surrounded by a white halo. Changes in the ERG and visual field may be recorded. Intraocular pressure is reduced but digitalis produces insufficient effect to be considered as a glaucoma treatment.

A case of mydriasis and cycloplegia equal to that of atropine eye drops was reported after using large doses of disopyramide (Frucht, Freiman and Merin, 1984).

Diuretics

Diuretics promote the flow of urine and are prescribed to reduce oedema in heart failure, essential hypertension, renal dysfunction and other conditions where the water/electrolyte balance of the body is disturbed. There are several different types of diuretic, varying from the very potent loop diuretics, through the moderate diuretics such as the thiazides and carbonic anhydrase inhibitors to the mild potassium- sparing agents.

Examples
Acetazolamide (carbonic anydrase inhibitor) (Diamox)
Bendrofluazide (thiazide) (Aprinox)
Bumetanide (loop diuretic) (Burinex)
Spironolactone (potassium sparing) (Aldactone)
Triamterene (potassium sparing) (Dytac)

Ocular adverse effects
Diuretics are used extensively in modern medicine but produce few ocular adverse reactions. A slight myopia is the most common effect but this usually regresses spontaneously.

Anti-arrhythmic drugs

There are several types of cardiac arrhythmia, e.g.

Atrial fibrillation;
Atrial flutter;
Supraventricular tachycardia; and
Ventricular arrythmias.

Different drugs are used for the different types.

Examples
Amiodarone (Cordarone X)
Disopyramide (Rythmodan)
Verapamil (Cordilox)

Ocular adverse effects
Disopyramide is used in ventricular arrhythmias and has a membrane stabilizing effect. It also has an anticholinergic action whcih can affect the eye, producing blurred vision and mydriasis. If the filtration angle is narrow then glaucoma is a possible problem.

Amiodarone produces yellow-brown deposits in the cornea. This is a fairly common occurrence, and is related to the total dose given. Vortex patterns of deposits are produced in 90% of patients who take the drug for more than a few weeks (Wright, 1978). The deposits will disappear slowly after discontinuation. There have been a few cases of blurred vision.

Beta-blockers

These drugs will be well known to the optometrist for their use in the treatment of glaucoma. Their major use, however, is in the treatment of cardiovascular problems such as hypertension, angina and cardiac arrythmias.

Examples
Atenolol(Tenormin)
Labetalol (Trandate)
Metoprolol (Betaloc)
Oxprenolol (Trasicor)
Propranolol (Inderal)

Ocular adverse reactions
Most beta-blockers are relatively safe and the unwanted ocular side-effects they produce are mild and transient. Practolol (which now has very restricted use) produced an oculomucocutaneous syndrome which was very severe in a number of patients, depending on the duration of treatment. The effect was reversible in the early stages but if the treatment continued then blindness ensued.

Antihypertensives

Essential benign hypertension is one of the most commonly occurring conditions, for which there are a variety of methods of treatment including beta-blockers, diuretics (mentioned above) and centrally acting drugs. Severe hypertension is treated with vasodilator drugs as hydralazine.

Examples
Clonidine (Catapres)
Methyldopa (Aldomet)
Hydralazine (Apresoline)

Ocular adverse reactions
Retinal changes have been reported following the use of clonidine, leading to visual loss. Methyldopa on the other hand affects the anterior eye, being possibly involved with cases of keratoconjunctivitis sicca. Both drugs reduce IOP.

Hydralazine produced a syndrome resembling systemic lupus erythematosus, with accompanying bilateral retinal vasculitis (Doherty, Maddison and Grey, 1985).

Drugs acting on the respiratory system

Respiratory tract infections and bronchospastic conditions figure highly amongst the general practitioner workload. For the latter condition inhalers and insufflators are often the route of administration, and because this form of treatment is more local than systemic, side-effects tend to be limited.

The following drugs are administered systemically for the treatment of respiratory disorders:

corticosteroids (see below);
antihistamines; and
bronchodilators.

Antihistamines

Antihistamines are employed in the treatment of hay fever and are combined with vasoconstrictors for the topical relief of some upper respiratory tract conditions. Many antihistamines have antimuscarinic actions and it is this property which can lead to ocular adverse side-effects.

Examples
Chlorpheniramine (Piriton)
Promethazine (Phenergan)
Terfenadine (Triludan)
Trimeprazine (Vallergan)

Ocular adverse effects
Many drugs in this group have antimuscarinic actions as well as antihistaminic and as would be predicted, a slight mydriasis and cycloplegia are the most common adverse reactions. In addition, the lacrimal gland may be affected, leading to depressed secretion of tears. Contact lens wearers may be particularly affected but sometimes the tears flow is so reduced that the signs and symptoms of keratoconjunctivitis sicca appear.

Bronchodilators

Bronchoconstriction is brought about by the contraction of the smooth muscle which is innervated by the parasympathetic nervous system. This effect can be reversed by antimuscarinic drugs or by sympathomimetic amines. The tendency today is to use sympathomimetic agents because their effects are less. Sympathomimetics are also used in some common cold remedies which are purchased over the counter.

Examples
Ephedrine
Orciprenaline (Alupent)
Pseudoephedrine (Sudafed)
Salbutamol (Ventolin)
Terbutaline (Bricanyl)

Ocular adverse effects
A slight mydriasis is the principal adverse effect arising from their use. Large doses of ephedrine can lead to visual hallucinations (Chaplin, 1984).

Drugs acting on the central nervous system

There are many different types of central nervous system agents and together they represent a large proportion of the prescriptions issued in the United Kingdom. Many of the tissues in the eye, particularly the retina, have neural origins and it is therefore likely that these agents will have effects on the eye. They can also affect the centres in the brain which are responsible for controlling the eye, producing such effects as diplopia.

CNS drugs can be divided into the following groups:

Hypnotics and sedatives
Anti-Parkinsonism agents
Anti-psychotic agents
Anxiolytic agents
Anticonvulsants
Antidepressants.

Hypnotics and sedatives

Hypnotics are drugs prescribed to treat insomnia. In the past, the barbiturates were the major group of drugs used for this purpose. However, because of their addictive properties they have fallen out of favour to a large extent and have been replaced by the benzodiazepines.

Examples
Amylobarbitone (Amytal)
Flurazepam (Dalmane)
Glutethimide (Doriden)
Nitrazepam (Mogadon)
Quinalbarbitone (Tuinal)
Temazepam (Normison)

Ocular adverse effects
Hypnotics are designed to be used short term and when used in this manner will produce few unwanted side-effects. Habitual users of barbiturates may experience problems of the extraocular musculature leading to decreased convergence or nystagmus.

Benzodiazepines have relatively few effects and if they do occur they are normally reversible. Patients sometimes complain of blurred vision caused by either loss of accommodation or abnormal extraocular movements.

Anti-parkinsonism agents

Parkinson's disease has recently received special attention since the advent of the employment of brain cell transplant to produce relief.

Drugs used to treat Parkinson's disease can be divided into antimuscarinic drugs and dopaminergic drugs, which either increase the levels of dopamine in the brain or act directly with the dopamine receptors.

Examples
Amantadine (Symmetrel)
Benzhexol (Artane)
Levodopa (Larodopa)
Orphenadrine (Disipal)

Ocular adverse effects
Amantadine produces few adverse effects apart from visual hallucinations. Antimuscarinic agents include benzhexol and orphenadrine, and their effects include a loss of accommodation and a mydriasis which can be sufficient to cause a closed angle glaucoma in patients whose angle is narrow.

Levodopa produces variable effects. On the pupil, an initial mydriasis is followed by a more persistent miosis. Effects on the lid include ptosis in some patients and intense blepharospasm in others. Involuntary eye movements have also been reported (Davidson and Rennie, 1986).

Antipsychotic agents

This group is sometimes called the major tranquillizers or neuroleptics. The term tranquillizer is confusing as often this effect is secondary to the principal, antipsychotic action. They do not have a hypnotic effect and are used to relieve conditions such as schizophrenia and severe anxiety.

Examples
Chlorpromazine (Largactil)
Haloperidol (Serenace)
Promazine (Sparine)
Thioridazine (Melleril)
Trifluoroperazine (Stelazine)

Ocular adverse effects
Most of the drugs listed above (with the exception of haloperidol) belong to the group known as the phenothiazines, of which the best known is chlorpromazine. The use of these agents is relatively safe in the short term but with longer use, the possibility of adverse effects increases. Like many other classes of drugs, phenothiazines have varying degrees of antimuscarinic effects and these can affect the iris and ciliary muscles, producing mydriasis and cycloplegia.

Chlorpromazine, in chronic therapy, produces pigmentary deposits in the eye which first appear on the lens surface, usually in the pupillary area, then Descemet's membrane becomes affected. The deposits are rarely found in the corneal epithelium. This effect may continue even after the drug is discontinued. Skin pigmentation can also occur and this affects up to 1% of patients who have received large doses for long periods. Corneal deposits occur in 15% of such patients. As the total dosage increases, so does the percentage of patients affected (Bernstein, 1977). The deposits do not appear to interfere with vision and the lens deposits are unlikely to lead to development of cataract (Davidson, 1980). Phenothiazines can, however, cause a retinopathy which is dependent on the total dose administered and results in visual problems (Spiteri and Geraint James, 1983).

Haloperidol (a member of the butyrophenone group) may produce mydriasis.

Anxiolytic agents

In contrast to the foregoing group, anxiolytics are sometimes known as the minor tranquillizers. By far the biggest group of drugs in this class is the benzodiazepines, which are some of the most widely prescribed drugs, and there is a tendency to prescribe them for any stress-related condition. They are really intended for short term use but unfortunately become used chronically, with the development of dependence and withdrawal symptoms on discontinuation.

Examples
Clorazepate (Tranxene)
Diazepam (Valium)
Lorazepam (Ativan)

Ocular adverse effects
There are few ocular adverse reactions to these drugs and those which do occur are reversible. Decreased accommodation and a reduction in corneal reflex may be noted. Some patients can exhibit an allergy to these drugs which can manifest in the eye as allergic conjunctivitis and can cause particular problems to contact lens wearers.

Anticonvulsants

These are drugs used to treat epilepsy by suppressing fits. It is important that the dose of drug be titrated for each patient. The dosage and frequency should be the lowest possible in order to achieve control.

Examples
Ethosuximide (Zarontin)
Phenytoin (Epanutin)
Primidone (Mysoline)
Sodium Valproate (Epilim)

Ocular adverse effects
Nystagmus and diplopia are more commonly the result of overdose than normal side-effects, and will often regress if the dosage is reduced. Phenytoin had a transient effect on the ERG when the drug was perfused through the retinae of rabbits (Honda, Podos and Becker, 1973). A case of Stevens–Johnson syndrome following phenytoin therapy has been reported (Greenberg *et al.*, 1971).

Antidepressants

The more modern tricyclic antidepressants have, to a large extent, superseded the use of monoamine oxidase inhibitors (MAOI) because of the latter's potentially dangerous interactions with some drugs and particular foods (e.g. cheese). Antidepressants are used to treat depressive illnesses, and like the previous group of drugs, it is vital that the dosage is carefully controlled. Some of these drugs have marked sedative properties (e.g. amitriptyline), while in others this effect is much less (e.g. imipramine).

Examples
Amitriptyline (Tryptizol)
Imipramine (Tofranil)
Nortriptyline (Aventyl)
Tranylcypromine (Parnate)
Trimipramine (Surmontil)

Ocular adverse effects
All tricyclic antidepressants have anticholinergic effects to some extent and because they can produce mydriasis and cycloplegia, they are contra-indicated in glaucoma. The effects are reversible and will subside even with continuation of therapy. The lacrimal gland can become affected and the tear flow embarrassed, leading to problems for contact lens wearers.

Monoamine oxidase inhibitors potentiate the effects of sympathomimetics and anticholinergics and care should be taken with the use of mydriatics.

Drugs used in the treatment of infections

There are many different types of organism which can cause infections and a whole range of different compounds must be used to treat them. Although anti-infective drugs are widely prescribed, side-effects are relatively rare. The course of treatment tends to be short and cumulative effects do not have time to develop. Also, anti-infective agents, because of their normally high specificity for the invading micro-organism, have a high therapeutic index.

However, some anti-infectives do require long term therapy and ocular adverse reactions can appear. The following groups will be considered:

Antibiotics
Urinary antiseptics
Antitubercular drugs
Anthelminthics
Antimalarials

Antibiotics

Agents in this class are used for the treatment of bacterial infections and are some of the most widely prescribed compounds in medicine. For most indications (e.g. upper respiratory tract infections), the treatment lasts for a few days but in the treatment of acne, antibiotics are prescribed for months rather than days.

Ideally, the organism should be tested for sensitivity before an antibiotic is prescribed but in practice, therapy is started and modified if necessary.

Examples
These are groups rather than individual drugs:

Penicillins, e.g. penicillin, ampicillin, amoxycillin
Cephalosporins, e.g. cephaloridine, cephalexin, cefuroxime
Tetracyclines, e.g. chlortetracycline, tetracycline, oxytetracycline
Aminoglycosides, e.g. gentamicin, neomycin

Macrolides, e.g. erythromycin
Others, e.g. clindamycin
Sulphonamides

Ocular adverse effects
Of the above, only tetracyclines have been reported to cause ocular adverse reactions. As well as transient myopia and colour vision defects, ocular effects secondary to the penetration of the drug into the cerebrospinal fluid, such as papilloedoma and diplopia, have been reported. Tetracyclines can be secreted in tears and stain soft contact lenses (Aucamp, 1980)

Some antibiotics, e.g. penicillin, can produce allergic responses which may involve ocular tissues.

Sulphonamides have been reported to cause keratoconjunctivitis sicca in dogs (Slatter and Blogg, 1978).

Urinary antiseptics

As their name suggests, these agents are used in the treatment of urinary tract infections.

Examples
Nalidixic acid (Negram)
Nitrofurantoin (Furadantin)

Ocular adverse effects
Ocular irritation and profuse lacrimation leading to problems for contact lens wearers can result from the use of nitrofurantoin, but such problems will regress on drug discontinuation.

Nalidixic acid can affect colour vision and produce symptoms of glare, effects, which are also reversible when the drug is stopped.

Antitubercular agents

The treatment of tuberculosis is a very long term problem because the causative organism, *Mycobacterium tuberculosum*, has a very slow metabolism and grows at a very slow rate. It takes a long time to eradicate the organism and resident strains can occur. Multitherapy is often applied to overcome this latter problem.

Examples
Ethambutol (Myambutol)
Rifampicin (Rifinah)
Isoniazid (used in combination with other drugs)
Streptomycin

Ocular adverse effects
Rifampicin produces a pink coloured by-product which can be excreted in tears and will colour soft contact lenses (Ingram, 1986). It can also cause a conjunctivitis which varies in severity.

Ethambutol is well known for producing optic neuritis, which is slowly reversible in some patients but permanent in others. The optic neuritis takes two forms—an axial and a paraxial form. The axial form affects the central fibres of the optic nerve producing changes in colour vision. Loss of central visual acuity and macular degeneration are often the result. The paraxial form, on the other hand, produces visual field defects, with central acuity and colour vision remaining unaffected.

Toxic effects on the optic nerve can also develop from the use of isoniazid and streptomycin (Spiteri and Geraint James, 1983).

Antimalarials

Probably the majority of use of these compounds is for the prophylaxis of malaria by travellers to malaria-endemic regions, rather than in the treatment of the condition. There are also other uses for some of the antimalarials, e.g. quinine can be used for the relief of night cramps and chloroquine and hydroxychloroquine can be used in the treatment of rheumatoid arthritis.

Examples
Chloroquine (Avlocor, Nivaquine)
Hydroxychloroquine (Plaquenil)
Quinine

Ocular adverse effects
The adverse effects of these drugs are well known. Both retina and cornea can be affected, although the two effects are unrelated and can appear independently of one another.

Effects on the cornea include deposits in the superficial cornea and sub-epithelial layers, which appear greyish white (Sinabulya, 1977), as well as an increased touch threshold and aggravation of existing keratoconjunctivitis sicca. The corneal deposits are often symptomatic (Bernstein, 1977) and do not indicate the discontinuation of therapy.

Pigmentary changes occur in the retina, giving rise to the well-known 'bulls eye maculopathy' (Sinabulya, 1977). Constricted visual fields and scotomata are accompanied by changes in the ERG. The condition is dose related and will continue to develop even if the drug is discontinued. One case of retinopathy, the onset of which was delayed for 7 years after cessation of therapy, has been reported (Ehrenfeld, Necher and Merin, 1986). An early sign of chloroquine retinopathy is blurring of vision.

Quinine amblyopia due to a direct effect on the ganglion cells has been known for a long time and several cases of blindness due to overdosage were reported by Dyson *et al.* (1985). Blindness occurred within hours of ingestion and characteristically the patients had normal fundi when examined. Some of them had dilated unreactive pupils. One case exhibited cholinergic supersensitivity, like Adie's pupil in which the pupil miosed with 0.125% pilocarpine (Canning and Hague, 1988).

As patients recover, paradoxically the fundal appearance changes to show narrowing of the retinal arterioles and optic atrophy. Iris atrophy can occur (Bernstein, 1977).

Anthelminthics

These compounds are used in the treatment of worm infections which, in the UK, tend to be fairly minor and are usually more embarrassing than medically dangerous.

Examples
Piperazine (Antepar, Pripsen)

Ocular adverse effects
Cycloplegia and extraocular muscle paralysis can produce visual problems, but these effects are very rare and only occur in overdosage.

Drugs acting on the endocrine system

These are agents which replace or supplement the natural hormones produced by the endocrine system. Included in this section are:

Drugs used to treat diabetes
Corticosteroids
Oral contraceptives.

Drugs used to treat diabetes

The best known agent for treating diabetes is, of course, insulin but certain forms can be treated with drugs given by mouth rather than injected—the oral hypoglycaemic agents.

Examples
Glibenclamide (Daonil, Euglucon)
Chlorpropamide (Diabinese)
Tolbutamide (Rastinon)
Metformin (Glucophage)

Ocular adverse effects
Diabetes itself, has well known ophthalmic complications and it is important to differentiate any ocular adverse effect of the drug from the problems caused by the condition. Chlorpropamide may produce toxic amblyopia (Davidson, 1971). Overdosage can produce hypoglycaemic attacks, with ocular effects of diplopia and loss of visual acuity.

Corticosteroids

Corticosteroids can be used either physiologically or pharmacologically. In the former manner they are employed for replacement therapy in Addison's disease or after adrenalectomy. For this use, both mineralocorticoid and glucocorticoid activity is required.

   The suppression of disease processes such as inflammation is termed pharmacological use, and corticosteroids are used in this manner in the treatment of rheumatoid arthritis, systemic lupus erythematosus, ulcerative colitis, polyarteritis and chronic active hepatitis.

Examples
Betamethasone (Betnelan)
Cortisone (Cortelan)
Dexamethasone (Decadron)
Prednisolone (Deltacortril)
Fludrocortisone (Florinef)
Triamcinolone (Ledercort)
Methylprednisolone (Medrone)

Ocular adverse effects
Corticosteroids are very notorious for the adverse effects they produce. Systemic use of these agents can result in a cataract which is situated below the posterior capsule and normally occurs after a year's treatment. It affects up to 30% of patients receiving these agents, especially children. Topical use rarely leads to cataract (David and Berkowitz, 1969).

Topical ophthalmic use of steroids can lead to a rise in intraocular pressure in a percentage of patients (steroid responders). This effect can also occur with systemic use, albeit less frequently and after a greater duration of treatment (David and Berkowitz, 1969; McDonnell and Kerr Muir, 1985). Patients who exhibit this reaction are not necessarily in early glaucoma, although like glaucoma there is a familial tendency for the reaction to occur. The increase is due to a reduction in outflow which itself is thought to be due to an accumulation of insoluble, polymerized, acid mucopolysaccharides (Francois, 1984). Newer corticosteroids have been developed which have less tendency to produce a rise in IOP (Morrison and Archer, 1984).

The list of other reported adverse reactions from steroids is long and they would appear to have the ability to produce any and every effect on the eye.

Oral contraceptives

The use of the contraceptive pill in the UK spans over a quarter of a century and it is now the most common method of birth control. There are a large number of pills available today but they can be divided into just two groups—the combined pills and the progestagen only pills. Many of the unwanted side-effects reported following the use of combined pills are from the oestrogen component and the other type is often recommended for individuals who are most at risk from side-effects.

Examples
Combined pills
   Ethinyloestradiol/norethisterone (Brevinor, Gynovlar)
   Ethinyloestradiol/levonorgestrel (Microgynon, Eugynon)
Progestagen only
   Norethisterone (Micronor)
   Levonorgestrel (Microval)

Ocular adverse effects
The contraceptive pill has been taken by millions of women for several years and with all this patient experience, it is surprising that better cause–effect relationships with ocular effects cannot be established. There have been many publications about the possible incompatibility between the pill and the wearing of contact lenses. Goldberg (1970) reviewed the problems of fitting contact lenses to patients taking the pill and suggested that sometimes there is a problem, but his findings are based on 'observation and conjecture'. Chizek and Franceschetti (1969) considered that the signs and symptoms which were reportedly due to the contraceptive pill could be due to overwear, humidity changes and infection. Peturrson, Fraunfelder and Meyer (1981) reviewed the evidence for the relationship between contact lens intolerance and oral contraceptives. A prospective study of 517 patients failed to show any difference in contact lens tolerance between patients taking the pill and those who were not. A similar study by Frankel and Ellis (1978) found no significant difference in tear production or tear break up time between women taking oral contraceptives and women who did not. There is some suggestion that the quality and quantity of tears may be adversely affected, especially during the early stages of their use.

Davidson (1971) reviewed the reported ocular adverse effects of oral contraceptives. The Committee on Safety of Medicines recorded effects secondary to cerebral vascular and neurological events as well as localized vascular problems and visual disturbances. A very small number of patients reported contact lens intolerance. Faust and Tyler (1966) examined 212 patients taking various pills and considered that no pathology existed which would not normally exist in a healthy random sample. Connell and Kelman (1969), in carrying out a similar study, were surprised at the occurrence of abnormalities in the control group but also found no difference between therapy and control groups.

Anti-inflammatory drugs

These are agents which have been developed as alternatives to steroids for the treatment of conditions such as rheumatoid arthritis to avoid the undesirable effects of steroids. They produce their effect in a slightly different manner to steroids and are not as potent. They are referred to as the non-steroidal anti-inflammatory drugs (NSAIDs).

Examples
Ibuprofen (Brufen)
Indomethacin (Indocid)
Ketoprofen (Orudis)
Naproxen (Naprosyn)
Sulindac (Clinoril)

Ocular adverse effects
Reduced colour vision and visual acuity have been reported following the use of ibuprofen and indomethacin. Retinopathy (similar to that produced by chloroquine) has been reported following the use of indomethacin (Bernstein, 1977), involving visual field restrictions, depressed EOGs and a granular appearance of the fundus, effects which are transitory as is the diplopia which can also be

recorded. Fraunfelder (1980) considered most of the ibuprofen-related effects to be unimportant and consistent with 'blurred vision'. Cataract and optic neuritis are serious adverse reactions which have been linked with naproxen, but the actual causal relationship is yet to be established. Benaxaprofen (Opren) has had to be withdrawn because of very serious photoallergic reactions. Optic neuropathy has been reported following the use of this particular compound.

Sulindac is one of the many new agents and any serious adverse effects have yet to be reported.

Drugs acting on the blood

Patients with some conditions require regular blood transfusions. As the donated corpuscles are broken down, the iron is stored and iron overload can develop. To remove this excess iron, a compound which will chelate the iron has to be given regularly. This compound is known as desferrioxamine, and when it reacts with iron it changes to ferrioxamine, which can be excreted in the bile and urine.

Examples
Desferrioxamine (Desferal)

Ocular adverse effects
Arden *et al.* (1984) reported minor alterations in the retinal function as evidenced by alterations in the pattern ERG.

References

Arden, G. B., Wonke, B., Kennedy, C. and Huehns, E. R. (1984) Ocular changes in patients undergoing long-term desferrioxamine treatment. *Br. J. Ophthalmol.*, **68**, 873–877

Aucamp, A. (1980 Drug excretion in human tears and its meaning for contact lens wearers. *Die Suid Afrikaanse Oogkundige*, **39**, 128–136

Bernstein, H. N. (1977) Ocular side effects of drugs in "Drugs and Ocular Tissues". *2nd Meeting of International Society for Eye Research*, 1976

Canning, C. R. and Hague, S. (1988) Ocular quinine toxicity. *Br. J. Ophthalmol.*, **72**, 23–26

Chaplin, S. (1984) Adverse reactions to sympathomimetics in cold remedies. *Adverse Drug Reaction Bulletins*, **No 107**, 369–399

Chizek, D. J. and Franceschetti, A. T. (1969) Oral contraceptives. Their side effects and ophthalmological manifestations. *Surv. Ophthalmol.*, **14/2**, 90/105

Connell, E. B. and Kelman, C. D. (1969) Eye examination in patients taking oral contraceptives. *Fertility and Sterility*, **20**, 67–74

David, D. S. and Berkowitz, J. S. (1969) Ocular effects of topical and systemic corticosteroids. *Lancet*, July 19, 149–151

Davidson, S. I. (1971) Reported adverse effects of oral contraceptives on the eye. *Trans. Ophthalmol. Soc. UK.*, **91**, 561–574

Davidson, S. I. (1980) Drug induced disorders of the eye. *Br. J. Hospital Medicine*, 24–28

Davidson, S. I. and Rennie, I. G. (1986) Ocular toxicity from systemic drug therapy. *Medical Toxicology*, **1**, 217–224

Dodd, M. J., Griffiths, I. D., Howe, J. W. and Mitchell, K. W. (1981) Toxic optic neuropathy caused by benoxaprofen. *Lancet*, 193–194

Doherty, M., Maddison, P. J. and Grey, R. H. B. (1985) Hydrazaline induced lupus syndrome with eye disease. *Br. Med. J.*, **290**, 675

Dyson, E. H., Proudfoot, A. T., Prescott, L. F. and Heyworth, R. (1985) Death and blindness due to overdose of quinine. *Br. Med. J.*, **291**, 31–33

Ehrenfeld, M., Nesher, R. and Merin, S. (1986) Delayed onset chloroquine retinopathy. *Br. J. Ophthalmol*, **70**, 281–283

Faust, J. M. and Tyler, E. T. (1966) Ophthalmic findings in patients using oral contraceptives. *Fertility and Sterility*, **17**, 1–6

Francois, J. (1984) Corticosteroid glaucoma. *Ophthalmologica*, (Basel), **188**, 76–81

Frankel, S. H. and Ellis, P. P. (1978) Effect of oral contraceptives on tear production. *Ann. Ophthalmol.*, **10**, 1585–1588

Fraunfelder, F. T. (1980) Interim reports. National Registry of possible drug-induced ocular side effects. *Ophthalmology*, **87/2**, 87–90

Frucht, J., Freimann, I., and Merin, S. (1984) Ocular side effects of disopyramide. *Br. J. Ophthalmol.*, **68**, 890–891

Goldberg, J. B. (1970) A commentary on oral contraceptive therapy and contact lens wear. *J. Optom. Assc.*, **41**, 237–241

Greenberg, L. M., Mauriello, D. A., Cinattia, A. A. and Buxton, J. N. (1971) Erythema multiforme exudativum (Stevens Johnson syndrome) following sodium diphenylhydantoin therapy. *Ann. Ophthalmol.*, **3/2**, 137–139

Honda, Y., Podos, S. M. and Becker, B. (1973) The effect of diphenylhydantoin on the electro-retinogram of rabbits. *Invest. Ophthalmol.*, **12/8**, 567–572

Ingram, D. V. (1986) Spoiled soft contact lenses. *Br. Med. J.*, **292**, 1619

Kofoed, L. L. (1986) OTC drugs: a third of the elderly are at risk. *Ger. Med.*, **February**, 37–42

McDonnell, P. J. and Kerr Muir, M. G. (1985) Glaucoma associated with systemic corticosteroid therapy. *Lancet*, **2**, 386–387

Morrison, E. and Archer, D. B. (1984) Effect of fluoromethalone (FML) on the intraocular pressure of corticosteroid responders. *Br. J. Ophthalmol.*, **68**, 581–584

Petursson, G. J., Fraunfelder, F. T. and Meyer, B. M. (1981) Oral contraceptives. *Ophthalmology*, **88/4**, 368–371

Sinabulya, P. M. (1977) Chloroquine retinopathy – Case report. *E. African J. Ophthalmol.*, **2/1**, 29/30

Slatter, D. H. and Blogg, J. R. (1978) Keratoconjunctivitis sicca in dogs associated with sulphonamide administration. *Aust. Vet. J.*, **54**, 444–447

Spiteri, M. A. and Geraint James, D. (1983) Adverse ocular reactions to drugs. *Postgrad. Med. J.*, **59**, 343–349

Wright, P. (1978) Effect of drug toxicity on the cornea. *Trans. Ophthalmol. Soc. UK.*, **98**, 377–378

Appendix

UK	USA	Others
Acelidine		
Acetazolamide		
Acetylcholine		Acetazolam
		Choline chloride
		Carbamate
Acyclovir		Acycloguanosine
Adrenaline	Epinephrine	Suparenin, Levorenin
Alcian Blue		
Amethocaine	Tetracaine	
Antazoline		Dicainum
Atenolol		Imidamin
Atropine		
Bacitracin		
Benoxinate		
Benzalkonium		Oxybuprocaine
Betamethasone		
Betaxolol		
Bethanecol		
Bromocriptine		Carbamylmethyl choline
Bupranolol		
Carbachol		
Carteolol		Carbacholine
Castor oil		
Chloramphenicol		
Chlorbutol		Laevomycetinum
Chlorhexidine		
Cocaine		
Cortisone		
Cyclopentolate		
Demecarium		BC48
Dexamethasone		
Dibromo-Propamidine Isethionate		
Dichloro Isocyanurate		
Dichlorphenamide		Diclofenamide
Dyflos	Isofluorophate	DFP, Disopropyl
		fluoro phosphate
Ecothiopate iodine	Echothiophate	Ecostigmine
EDTA	Edetate disodium	Disodium edetate
Ephedrine		
Erythromycin		
Fluorescein sodium		

UK	USA	Others
Forskolin		
Framycetin		Neomycin B
Gentamicin		
Guanethidine		
Homatropine		
Hydrocortisone		Cortisol
Hydrogen peroxide		
Hydroxyamphetamine		Oxamphetamine
Hyoscine		Scopolamine
Hypromellose	Hydroxyl propyl methylcellulose	Hydroxypropyl-methylcellulose
Idoxuridine		
Indomethacin		
Iodine		
Isoprenaline	Isoproterenol	Isopropylarterenol
Labetalol		
Lachesine		
Levobunolol		
Lignocaine	Lidocaine	
Liquid paraffin	Mineral oil	White mineral oil
Mafenide		
Methacholine		Acetyl-β-methyl choline
Metipranolol		Methylpranol Trimepranol
Metoprolol		
Nadolol		
Naphazoline		
Neomycin		
Neostigmine		Synstigmine
Noradrenaline	Levarterenol	
Normal saline		
Oxyphenbutazone		
Papain		
Penicillin		
Phenylephrine		Synephrine Metaoxedrine Mesatonum
Physostigmine		Eserine
Pilocarpine		
Pindolol		Prindolol Prinodolol
Polymixin		
Polyvinyl alchohol		
Propamidine		
Proxymetacaine	Proparacaine	
Rose Bengal		
Sodium cromoglycate	Cromolyn sodium	
Sotalol		
Sulphacetamide Na		
Sulphafurazole	Sulfisoxazole	
Tetracycline		
Tetrahydro Cannabinol		
Tetrahydrozoline		Tetryzoline
Thiomersol		Thiomersalate Mercurothiolate

UK	USA	Others
Thymoxamine		Moxisylyte
Timolol		
Tobramycin		
Trifluorothymidine		F3T
Trimethoprim		
Tropicamide		Bistropamide
Vidarabine		Vira-A adenine
		Arabinoside
Xylometazoline		

Index